CARE P.
for the
OLDER ADULT

Nursing Diagnosis
in Long-Term Care

♦

CARE PLANNING
for the
OLDER ADULT

Nursing Diagnosis in Long-Term Care

◆

Richard S. Ferri, PhD, ANP, RN

Director, Community Outreach
HIV Coordinator
Visiting Nurse Association, Inc.

W.B. SAUNDERS COMPANY
A Division of Harcourt Brace & Company
Philadelphia London Toronto Montreal Sydney Tokyo

W.B. SAUNDERS COMPANY
A Division of Harcourt Brace & Company
The Curtis Center
Independence Square West
Philadelphia, PA 19106

Library of Congress Cataloging-in-Publication Data

Care planning for the older adult : nursing diagnosis in long-term
care / edited by Richard S. Ferri.
  p. cm.
  ISBN 0-7216-2132-5
  1. Geriatric nursing. 2. Nursing care plans. 3. Nursing
diagnosis. 4. Aged—long-term care. I. Ferri, Richard S.
  [DNLM: 1. Long-Term Care—in old age. 2. Nursing Diagnosis.
  3. Patient Care Planning.   WT 30 C2776]
  RC954.C372   1994
  610.73′65—dc20
                                                    92-7916

CARE PLANNING FOR THE OLDER ADULT   ISBN 0-7216-2132-5
Nursing Diagnosis in Long-Term Care

Printed in the United States of America
Last digit is the print number: 9 8 7 6 5 4 3 2 1

For Anna Boerio, my grandmother,
who shared her stories.
For Ken Dawson, former executive director
of Senior Action in a Gay Environment,
for sharing his vision.
And for John E. White for sharing his life.

◆

PREFACE

We are born to age. Older persons comprise more and more of the population throughout the world. They are a highly valuable resource that has been greatly underestimated and overlooked. We, the citizens of this world, need to pay more attention to older people and seek out their advice and knowledge.

The original intent of this book was to look at the special needs and concerns of the elderly that resided in nursing homes either temporarily or permanently. As the book evolved—and all books do—it became clear that a "nursing home clinical reference" was not going to be the sole outcome of this effort. Older people in the nursing home environment are older people in the community. It is important that the whole notion of "nursing homes" be expanded conceptually and literally.

This book has also changed over its creation as the world has changed. The world as we know it today has been greatly impacted by the AIDS epidemic, and older people are not immune to that disease. It is often very easy to dismiss HIV infection in the elderly as nonexistent because of internalized ageism and homophobia. Older people are sexually active; older people can be gay, lesbian, bisexual, or heterosexual.

Cultural diversity is the cornerstone to good nursing practice. Nurses have had the opportunity time and again to demonstate their inclusiveness of all people which is a true hallmark of the profession. The practice of nursing should never be censored or limited. When the elderly are part of a nurse's practice, then that nurse becomes richer for the experience.

Also, it is important to dismiss the notion that nursing practice that is focused on older persons is somehow a lesser practice. No one really wants to say it, but this has been the soft undertone of many professionals. It is simply not true. It also smacks of ageism and health care rationing.

The clinical practice of geriatric nursing is certainly a challenge. It is also a privilege.

The hope and ambition of this book is not to be the definitive text that answers all questions, but it is to be a starting place. It is time to start to look at nursing practice and older persons in a new light.

Richard S. Ferri

CONTRIBUTORS

Elaine Jensen Amella, MA, RNC, CS
Clinical Nurse Specialist—Gerontology
Montefiore Medical Center
Bronx, New York

Self-Perception/Self-Conflict Pattern

Norma Anderson, RN, EdM, MA
Associate Director of Nursing Service
Highbridge Woodycrest Center
Bronx, New York
and
Consultant to LTC facilities
Nursing Management and Educational
    Consultant in Geriatrics

Sleep-Rest Patterns

Jo Anne Bennett, RN, PhD
Consultant
Private Practitioner
New York, New York

*Nursing Diagnosis: The Beginning—The
    Present*

Verna B. Carson, RN, MS
Consultant Director of Psychiatry
Associate Professor
University of Maryland School of
    Nursing
Home Care Service for Bay Area
    Healthcare
Baltimore, Maryland

Value-Belief Pattern

Judith Conway, RN, MS, CS, ET
Adjunct Faculty
Central Connecticut State University
New Britain, Connecticut
and
Patient Care Manager
Transitional Care
Bristol Hospital
Bristol, Connecticut

Elimination Pattern

RoAnne Dahlen-Hartfield, DNSc, RN
Continuing Education Staff Specialist
American Nurses Association
Department of Field Services, Labor
    and Workplace Advocacy
Washington, District of Columbia

Geriatric Update: Research and Action

Jean A. Elmore, MSN, RNC
Assistant Professor
Indiana University, School of Nursing
Indianapolis, Indiana

Cognitive Perceptual Pattern

Richard S. Ferri, PhD, ANP, RN
Director of Community Outreach
HIV Coordinator
Visiting Nurse Association, Inc.
Chatham, Massachusetts

*Health Perception—Health Management
    Pattern*
Sexuality-Reproductive Patterns

James J. Kane, MN, RN, CS
Psychiatric Consultation—Liaison
    Nurse
Mercy Hospital and Medical Center
Behavioral Health Center
San Diego, California
and
Psychiatric Nurse Therapist
Private Practice
San Diego, California

Coping Stress Tolerance Pattern

Sheree Loftus, MSN, RNC
Graduate Nurse Practitioner Program
Pace University
Pleasantville, New York

Sexuality-Reproductive Patterns

Mary Frances Madigan, EdD
Adjunct Instructor—Gerontology
Bloomfield College
Bloomfield, New Jersey
and
Senior Mental Health Clinician
Geropsychiatric Nursing Constultant/
   Therapist
Saint Clares Riverside Medical Center
Denville, New Jersey

Role Relationship Pattern

Kathleen M. Nokes, PhD, RN
Associate Professor
Hunter College, C.U.N.Y.
Hunter-Bellevue School of Nursing
New York, New York
and
HIV Nurse Clinician
Woodhull Medical and Mental Health
   Center
Brooklyn, New York

Activity Exercise Pattern

Moira Shannon, EdD, MSN
Division of Nursing, Bureau of Health
   Professions
Health Resources and Services
   Administration
Public Health Service
U.S. Department of Health and Human
   Services
Rockville, Maryland

Geriatric Update: Research and Action

CONTENTS

13
Coping Stress Tolerance Pattern   316
James J. Kane

14
Value-Belief Pattern   345
Verna B. Carson

Nursing Diagnosis The Beginning—The Present

JoAnne Bennett

◆

Discussions of nursing diagnosis invariably begin with the 1973 American Nurses Association (ANA) *Standards of Medical-Surgical Nursing Practice* (1973), which specified that nursing care must be based on nursing diagnoses; the effort to name and classify diagnoses, which began at a national conference that same year; and the 1980 ANA *A Social Policy Statement* (1980), which defined nursing as the diagnosis and treatment of human responses to actual and potential health problems. These milestone publications, however, are but highlights in our history of independent and collaborative diagnosis. It is easy to lose sight of the long clinical tradition of nursing diagnosis amid the debates about terminology, taxonomy, and turf. To be understood, the course of nurses' diagnoses—whether extensive or limited, well-articulated or unstated, accepted or hotly debated—must be considered along with the course of other aspects of practice and in context with external factors that have impinged on practice. Since others are likely to be unfamiliar with our history, it behooves us to be certain about which directions are new and which paths we have tread for generations.

BARELY A CENTURY OF MODERN NURSING

No historian of health care nor biographer of Nightingale's nurses in England and their successors on this side of the Atlantic could help but notice how nurses' *initiative* in identifying problems and taking *independent* corrective actions reshaped hospital care and improved patient outcomes.

By the 1890s, nurses viewed their work as extending "beyond the care of the sick to the health care of the well through the prevention of illness." They worked in settlement houses, other social agencies, and in the community . . . Prior to 1910 nursing was openly recognized as a branch of applied science that promised to be as important to the patient's health as medicine itself . . . [and] nurses were more certain of their independent functions in the health field than they are today (Ashley 1976). At the turn of the century nursing care was the essential product dispensed by hospitals, considerably more so than today when increasingly high-tech hospitals are also a major source of medical services. The nursing role was that of a versatile generalist, not a specialist; nurses' skills were widely respected and they could insist on a degree of independence. Since the institutional model for running the hospitals was the family, in addition to patient care, nurses "took care of the hospital family" by managing all departments in the hospital, including the kitchen, pharmacy, and supply rooms (Ashley 1976). And in the frequent absence of physicians, nurses assumed full responsibility for decision-making (Ashley 1976, Nahm 1981).

Within three decades, nursing had developed as a separate profession. Scientific developments helped spawn the profession, but hospitals' emergence as businesses shaped nurses' organizational role. "Economic, political and social factors [eventually limited nurses'] contributions and reform" (Ashley 1976). Not surprisingly, many issues in nursing paralleled concerns of other laboring groups and reflected social conceptions of the nature of women and their economic and political place in society.

Nursing's history through the 20th century has been a continuing struggle to wrest control of its education, maintain autonomy in its practice, gain fair remuneration for its services, and set standards to ensure quality. Despite common goals and interests, consistent communication and collaboration between medicine and nursing remains elusive (American Medical Association). However, "the winds of societal change continue to buffet [both] profession[s]" (Ritter et al. 1981). The interdependence of *all* health care providers, rather than prerogatives reserved for any discipline(s), has become more apparent as the health care system has grown more complex, the number of health care disciplines has risen, and consumers have assumed active involvement in planning care and making policy.

Recognition of nurse's independent judgment is reflected in the use of terms such as *nursing assessment* and *nursing orders* in patient records. Some nurses function more independently than others, depending on the setting and individual client's needs. In long-term settings, multidisciplinary care planning is *de rigueur*—legally as well as practically.

◆ What Do We Diagnose—and When?

Until relatively recently the theoretical underpinnings of practice were not extracted and documented (Stevens 1979).

Even a cursory review of our past and current practice reveals its essential core to be an ecologic, holistic approach to health-related problem solving. From the beginning, nurses themselves identified the problems they would tackle and broadly defined health-related problems within a social context. Interventions included personal ministrations to provide relief and comfort, counseling and teaching to promote health, and political advocacy to bring about institutional and community reforms. Until recently, however, we did not try to use specific terms to name the problems identified.

By definition, problem "identification by examination or analysis" is diagnosis (McKechme 1983). The term applies to the process and also to the conclusion reached by the process. Although the connotation of medical assessment is commonly assumed when it is not specifically qualified, the term's use in nursing dates back at least to the 1930s.

The term *nursing diagnosis* appeared with growing frequency in nursing journals and texts through the 1950s and 1960s. Early conceptual discussions of the term suggested what we now refer to as nursing process within which the diagnostic process itself is but a repeated or continuing step—the step of clinical judgment applied to observations and other data collection. The model of nursing practice as a four-step, problem-solving process—assessing, planning, implementing, and evaluating—was elaborated in 1967 (Yura and Walsh 1967). The assessment—i.e., the diagnostic process—combines clinical reasoning with collecting and interpreting information. Planning involves both setting goals and developing strategies to attain them. The evaluation comprises repeated assessment both to confirm the diagnoses that have been made and to measure goal attainment, thus allowing the nurse to determine how appropriate and/or effective implemented interventions have been. A revised plan is often indicated. In fact, many consider revision to be a step in the process.

In the early 1970s, clinicians and educators began to develop specific terms with which to label the problems we identify and treat, i.e., the *phenomena of therapeutic concern to nurses*. The belief that consistent terminology would ensure clear and precise communication underlay this initiative. A parallel concern has been to classify diagnoses in an orderly system—a *taxonomy*. The purposes of a taxonomy are multiple: to further "facilitate communication . . . [and] assist in the development of research hypotheses, point toward future trends, and identify, simplify, and structure hitherto undiscovered characteristics" of these phenomena and thus "provide the necessary conceptual understanding from which the most appropriate intervention choices can be made" (Yura and Walsh 1967).

◆ How We Diagnose

Diagnosis is the process of systematically and logically organizing observations for the purpose of determining what problems exist *and* how to manage them. The label given to the diagnosis has been called just the tip of the diagnostic iceberg. The diagnostic label has four functions:

- ◆ to provide an explanation for the clinical data presented by a particular person
- ◆ to suggest or predict what will follow, including the response to interventions
- ◆ to relate relevant information and theory to an individual situation
- ◆ to link data about a particular individual with the body of general information in order to extend knowledge and confirm relevant theories.

Diagnosing is not a labeling process, however. It is "a complex, sometimes unconscious, integration of critical thinking and data collection . . . the process of inferring the observable state of the client from uncertain, observable data presented. The inference is complex because the relationship between cues and client state is probabilistic—i.e., there is a less-than-perfect relationship between any given cue and a client state" (Tanner 1984). More data help make diagnoses more definite, but also make the diagnostic task more complex because several possible states may be suggested. Thus, diagnosis is a process of differentiating between and among possibilities. *Differential diagnosis* "consists of generating multiple alternatives and systematically testing them against additional information . . . the clinician generates diagnostic hypotheses (possible explanations for the cues) . . . [which are then] informally rank-ordered . . . from most likely to least likely, or most urgent to least urgent and additional data are obtained to assist in ruling in (confirming) or ruling out (disconfirming) the hypothesis" (Tanner 1984).

Four major components of the diagnostic process have been recognized:

◆ cue acquisition or data collection

◆ hypothesis generation—possible conclusions are retrieved from memory. This step includes clustering the data in order to identify significant relationships

◆ cue interpretation—reconsideration of data in relation to how it contributes to each hypotheis.

◆ hypothesis evaluation—weighing and validating data to determine if it confirms an hypothesis. (Bergman and Panetell 1984, Bircher 1975, Carlson et al. 1982).

Some diagnoses may require complex, repetitive assessments for validation. We must avoid premature labeling and facile pigeonholing of patients. When we cannot diagnose a situation definitively, we indicate the tentativeness of our assessment by using the term "possible." If, on the other hand, data suggest a person may be developing a certain problem or is likely to develop it, we indicate this with the term "potential" (Carpenito 1985).

The experienced nurse, or expert, is better able to weigh the relative importance of each piece of data as well as to collate correctly. Experience also teaches the clinician when to pursue more qualitative detail as well as a greater quantity of information. And the experienced nurse can be more efficient at immediately narrowing the range of possible diagnoses (Mitchell 1984). Deduction and induction are adequate for scientific reasoning. Intuition is fundamental (Williams 1980). Benner and others have found that intuitive judgment distinguishes the expert from the novice (and from the computations of a machine) (Benner 1982, Benner and Tanner 1987). Dreyfus has identified six key aspects of intuitive judgment: pattern recognition, similarity recognition, common sense understanding, skilled know-how, sense of salience, and deliberative rationality (Dreyfus and Dreyfus 1985).

Benner and Tanner identified five stages in a nurse's growth to expert practitioner: from novice, to advanced beginner, to competent, to proficient, to expert (Benner and Tanner 1987). Besides experience and intuition, diagnostic competence is affected by a person's theoretical knowledge, intellectual ability, philosophical and conceptual orientation, and data gathering skills (Williams 1980).

FOUR DECADES OF CONFUSION AND DEBATE

The term *nursing diagnosis* did not just slip into common usage. Many nurses have been reluctant to adopt the term, some are adamantly opposed to adopting the term (Levine 1965). Several conceptual debates still continue. First, we had to deal with the confusion of having used various terms more or less interchangeably:

> *patient need*
> *patient assessment*
> *patient problem*
>
> *nursing need*
> *nursing assessment*
> *nursing problem*
> *nursing impression*
>
> *health need*
> *health assessment*
> *health problem*
>
> *defined problem*

These terms emerged from procedure-oriented clinical practice and disease-oriented theoretical content; they were all used to label what was becoming conceptualized as diagnosis (the outcome, not the process). Several authors pointed out the imprecision of the overlapping uses for related terms and the frequent listing of (1) interventions or routine nursing activities under "needs" or (2) diseases or signs and symptoms under "problems" on Kardexes and care plans. It was argued that the confusion existed because the terms themselves were imprecise. Preference for using the term *diagnosis* was posted because *diagnosis connotes a logical and critical analysis and interpretation.*

The concepts *nursing process, nursing diagnosis, taxonomy,* and *diagnostic category* continue to be used imprecisely. Both the diagnostic process and the nursing process are problem-solving processes. As previously discussed, nursing process is a model for the whole nurse-patient interaction. The diagnostic process is part of that process. However, it focuses on only a piece of the puzzle: it seeks to answer two questions: Is there a problem? If so, what is the problem? The nursing process aims not only to find and identify problems, but also to resolve them so that health is restored/promoted: It asks several questions:

1–2 Is there a problem? If so, what is it?

3   How can we eliminate/reduce it most effectively and efficiently?

4–5 How much improvement can be expected? In what time frame?*

6–7 Is the intervention working? How well?

8   Is the patient progressing at the desired pace?

9   Would altering the intervention speed up or improve the outcome?

When the nurse answers the first two questions in a clinical situation, s/he is making a concrete (though sometimes tentative) diagnosis. The diagnosis is the answer to the second question; it identifies and names the client's problem. In the clinical situation, the diagnosis must be as specific as possible—comprehensive yet exclusive. If it is too general or vague or incomplete, its usefulness in pointing to directions for action will be limited.

Most diagnoses that we have recognized and named so far are very broad. In fact, most are really abstract umbrella terms that label *categories* of problems and are rather ill-suited for making specific diagnoses. In other words, they are diagnostic categories. A *diagnostic category* is a cluster or pattern of behaviors that is recognizable as a client state or response to health. Nursing uses the diagnostic category labels clinically as only *part of the problem statement.* A diagnosis is a complete problem statement, which identifies (1) the type of problem (the category), (2) the factors that underlie or have contributed to the origin, continuation, progression, or exacerbation of the problem (the etiology), and (3) the way the individual manifests the problem (signs and symptoms). In other words *the diagnosis is a* concise *summary statement,* which comprises more than just the label for the diagnostic category. One goal of the effort to classify diagnoses is to develop more specific, valid labels that are clinically useful. Perhaps some day we will have more inclusive labels to specify diagnoses without having to use long summary statements.

The format most commonly proposed for diagnostic statements is the P-E-S format, which obviously comprises the three parts just described (some clinicians chart only the P-E portion as the diagnosis in care plans or as the assessment [A] in SOAP notes. This eliminates restating signs and symptoms documented in adjacent notes. The complete statement is nevertheless apparent). Thus, intervention is based on a concrete diagnosis of an individual's situation, not a diagnostic category. Using only diagnostic categories as the basis for planning interventions could result in ineffective, or even unsafe, care.

Between the first National Conference on Classification of Nursing Diagnoses in 1973 and the Eighth Conference in 1988, 103 types of phenomena of therapeutic concern to nurses, mostly diagnostic categories, were identified and *accepted for clinical testing.* Most nurses are familiar with these.

---

*Answers to the fourth and fifth questions indicate prognosis (Ware 1979).

◆ Organizing the Diagnostic Categories into a Coherent Framework

An *alphabetic list* has been a common tool for handy reference. Its obvious limitation is that clinicians do not think alphabetically. That is, we do not make clinical inferences in alphabetic order. So if you do not know whether an accepted label exists for a situation that you have identified, you must search through the entire list. Or, if you are trying to distinguish between two or more types of problems that seem to be clinically related, you may have to jump back and forth on the list because the labels are not next to each other alphabetically (this can be a problem for students too, as they are learning theoretical concepts related to specific diagnoses/clinical phenomena). Another limitation of the alphabetic listing is that broad categories (such as altered thought processes and ineffective breathing patterns) are integrated with more specific categories (such as nutrition more than required and rape trauma syndrome) with no distinction between levels of abstraction. Thus, the alphabetic list simply provides an index of the nomenclature.* Moreover, an alphabetic list is language-specific. Clearly some kind of *taxonomy* using a scheme other than the alphabet to classify the diagnoses would be useful as a cognitive or ideational "search set" in the clinical situation and as a theoretical framework for research (Gordon 1976). A clinically useful system would order diagnostic categories within a conceptual framework that could be used to guide the assessment process itself. Related diagnoses would be near each other so the discontinuity between them could be more readily perceived, aiding differential diagnoses. Also, levels of abstraction would be clear.

There is no single correct way to classify diagnoses. Over the years, several systems of categorization have been proposed. In 1953, Fry suggested five areas of human or self needs on which to base nursing diagnoses:

◆ treatments and medications

◆ personal hygiene

◆ environment

◆ guidance and teaching.

In 1966 Virginia Henderson, who defines nursing as doing for the patient what s/he would do for herself/himself if well,† identified 15 basic functions to be the measure of independence:

---

*The alphabetic list is frequently misused: Nurses transcribe the labels onto charts, Kardexes, care plans, progress notes, and other records in the stilted format of an alphabetic index instead of using them as everyday speech patterns and grammar would suggest. For example, instead of saying, "Mr. Sickman has ineffective airway clearance . . . manifested by coarse rhonchi . . ." some nurses will say, "Mr. Sickman's diagnosis is airway clearance, ineffective," despite the awkwardness of doing so. It is bound to be awkward since we don't think that way. It is also unnecessary.

†Adopted by the International Council of Nurses as its definition of nursing in 1960.

◆ Breathe normally
◆ Eat and drink adequately
◆ Eliminate bodily wastes
◆ Move and maintain desirable postures
◆ Sleep and rest
◆ Select suitable clothing, dress and undress
◆ Maintain body temperature within normal range by adjusting clothing and modifying environment
◆ Keep body clean and well groomed and protect integument
◆ Avoid dangers of environment and avoid injuring others
◆ Communicate with others in expressing emotions, needs, fears, or opinions
◆ Worship according to one's faith
◆ Work in such a way that there is a sense of accomplishment
◆ Play or participate in various forms of recreation
◆ Learn, discover, or satisfy the curiosity that leads to normal development and health
◆ Use the available health facilities.

In 1960 Abdellah et al. examined factors that assisted the therapeutic objectives for nursing care:

◆ to facilitate the maintenance of oxygen to all body cells
◆ to facilitate the maintenance of nutrition to all body cells
◆ to facilitate the maintenance of elimination
◆ to facilitate the maintenance of fluid and electrolyte balance
◆ to promote safety through the prevention of accident, injury, or other trauma and through the prevention of the spread of infection
◆ to facilitate the maintenance of regulatory mechanisms or functions
◆ to facilitate the maintenance of sensory function
◆ to promote optimal activity: exercise, rest, and sleep
◆ to maintain good body mechanics and prevent and correct deformities
◆ to maintain good hygiene and physical comfort
◆ to recognize the physiological responses of the body to disease conditions—pathological and compensatory
◆ to identify and accept positive and negative expressions, feelings, and reactions
◆ to facilitate the maintenance of effective verbal and nonverbal communication

◆ to promote the development of productive interpersonal relationships

◆ to facilitate progress toward achievement of personal spiritual goals

◆ to accept the optimal possible goals in light of limitations, physical and emotional

◆ to use community resources as an aid in resolving problems arising from illness

◆ to create or maintain a therapeutic environment

◆ to understand the role of social problems as influencing factors in the cause of illness

◆ to facilitate awareness of self as an individual with varying physical, emotional, and developmental needs.

Both Henderson and Abdellah stimulated looking beyond what nurses do to why *and* whether we should do what we do. But most nurses continued to describe practice in terms of tasks, not the conditions that necessitated care. In 1974, Gordon began using a typology of 11 functions health patterns, which (depending on one's theoretical orientation) could be conceptualized in areas of self-care agency, adaptation, human need, behavioral systems, or manifestations of the life pattern (Gordon 1976, Gordon 1982).

1. health perception—health management
2. self-perception—self-concept
3. coping—stress tolerance
4. cognition—perception
5. sexuality—reproduction
6. nutrition—metabolism
7. elimination
8. activity—exercise
9. sleep—rest
10. role—relationship
11. value—belief

Gordon correlates her functional health patterns to the 27 (level 2) subcategories of human response patterns* in the taxonomy subsequently developed by the National Conference Group. In 1978 Campbell published a list of 730 nursing diagnoses with definitions, assessment criteria, possible etiologies, and indicated interventions. Although she said she was not

---

*The nine human response patterns are: exchanging, communicating, relating, valuing, choosing, moving, perceiving, knowing, and feeling. Gordon considers growth and development to come under each pattern although in NANDA's Taxonomy I it is a category of the pattern moving.

offering a taxonomy, she defined nursing diagnoses as human responses and resource limitations, presenting 12 categories of the former and two categories of the latter. She also presented seven categories of nursing interventions (assistive, hygienic, rehabilitative, supportive, preventive, observational, and educative) (Campbell 1978).

In 1973, Patricia Lavin and Kristine Gebbie, members of the nursing faculty at St. Louis University, convened a National Conference to address classification of nursing diagnosis. The National Conference Group (NCG) met biannually thereafter. The first five conferences were invitational meetings, which included clinicians, teachers, administrators, researchers, and theorists. They met in working groups and induced diagnoses using empirical data from clinical practice—i.e., observation and experience. Diagnoses proposed in this way were accepted by hand vote of the conference participants. Starting with the Fifth Conference, proposed diagnoses have had to be supported by research or clinical data before being considered.

Constructing the taxonomy, i.e., giving a theoretical order to empirically recognized diagnoses, has been a deductive process. At the Third Conference, Sr. Callista Roy convened the theorists separately to (1) develop a framework for organizing diagnostic categories, (2) make recommendations on levels of abstraction, (3) correlate their theoretical work with the ongoing development of diagnostic categories, and (4) clarify the relevance of the framework for practice. The theorist group analyzed the list of diagnoses that had been induced and identified nine patterns of human responses. This conceptual framework was then refined with input from clinical specialists at the Fourth Conference. Work on developing a taxonomy in 1982 using the theorists' proposed framework began at the Fifth Conference. By consensus, the working Taxonomy Group* began to sort the diagnostic categories that had already been accepted into *nine patterns of unitary persons.* Further sorting into four levels of abstraction was subsequently completed:

◆ patterns of unitary persons/human response pattern
◆ normless assessment categories (alterations in human responses)
◆ categories of phenomena of concern
◆ phenomena of concern.

The hierarchical levels are readily discerned when the taxonomy is outlined or illustrated. This taxonomy, known as NANDA Taxonomy I, was approved in 1986 by mail ballot of the entire membership after the Seventh Conference. Not all branches have been filled; some trees are more complete than others. This reflects the reality that some concepts used in nursing are more developed and better understood than others. Not only do the blanks need to be filled in, but the accepted categories and phenomena have to be validated (through theoretical research and clinical testing). Additional levels, i.e., further subcategorization, may be added. At this point, the taxonomy includes only problems; etiology is not included. Etiologic factors

*This group later became the NANDA Taxonomy Committee.

are inherently part of a problem, however, and thus may eventually be identified as subcategories. This is already possible for some physiologic diagnoses, e.g., urinary incontinence. Theorists have suggested that overriding dysfunctional life patterns can contribute to several specific problems within a problem category and perhaps even to several categories within a pattern and that these should be the focus of nursing intervention.

We take the anatomical-physiological framework of medical diagnoses for granted. It seems so obvious that we rarely are explicit about it. Actually much of the detail of this taxonomy is the result of quite recent knowledge, and it remains far from complete. The systematic description of diseases began in the 18th century as a classification of causes of death. Early medical classifications were based on symptoms. With the rise of pathology in the 19th century, classification in terms of anatomical lesions came to the fore and was then superseded by a system based on physiologic dysfunction. Later, the causes responsible for dysfunctions became the basis for categorizing medical problems (Florence Nightingale was one of the first proponents of accurate statistical record keeping and case classification) (Cohen 1984). By 1893, when the International Classification of diseases (ICD) was first published, 161 diseases had been named (Gordon 1982). Diagnoses continue to be added to this list, which is published every ten years. Some are more vaguely defined than others; some etiologies are better understood than others. And, not driven to a single theoretical umbrella, medicine continues to classify disease in terms of manifestations, lesions, genetics, infective agents, and environmental factors. As particular diseases become better understood in terms of basic biological theories, it is likely that disease classifications will become more uniform, with diseases identified in terms of their causal mechanisms. Some specialty groups, for example psychiatry, have developed other disease classification systems.

Like nursing diagnoses, medical diagnoses are summary statements that indicate the problem, its etiology and its key symptoms (*defining characteristics*). For example, pulmonary disease is classified as restrictive or obstructive, then further delineated: Asthma, bronchitis, and emphysema are obstructive diseases. Chronic asthma is further distinguished from acute status asthmaticus. Both asthma and chronic bronchitis are both more precise and useful for planning medical treatment than the diagnostic category COPD. The broader term is an accurate label, but it is not sufficiently descriptive to be the basis for specific therapy. The therapy aimed at reducing an allergic reaction is quite different from the antibiotic/steroid approaches used to relieve bronchial inflammation. Obviously, the clinician's aim—both in medicine and in nursing—is to maximize diagnostic precision so that the most appropriate intervention can be planned. Of course, sometimes problems are interrelated, and a patient's diagnosis cannot be narrowly defined or labeled. For example, the person with asthma may have some bronchitis too. A person with a left anterolateral myocardial infarction is likely to have impaired circulation to other areas of the myocardium. Neither are nursing diagnoses always cut and dry. A self-care deficit can be related to pain, activity intolerance, anxiety, depression, or perceptual, cognitive, neuromuscular, or musculoskeletal impairments. Or it can contribute to depression, anxiety, ineffective coping, inactivity, and so on. Signs and symptoms are often (more often than not) nonspecific in both nursing and medicine—i.e., the same signs and/or symptoms occur in a lot of problem situations. When signs and symptoms are typically part of a specific problem, we say they are *critical indicators.* These have not yet been clearly established for all nursing diagnoses. How could they be—when we have not yet named or even identified them all? This can be very unsatisfactory, downright frustrating, for the clinician who wants something to use in the here and now. Incompleteness, however, should not make the taxonomy unusable. Clinical discussions do not focus on taxonomic issues. A clinician's purpose is to explain a particular person's state, the behaviors manifested, and to intervene appropriately. The taxonomy will be modified as theoretical and clinical knowledge becomes available. Thus, it is the taxonomy that is limited; it does not limit us. That all the current diagnoses are not based on sound conceptual bases nor precise enough to ensure agreement among nurses viewing the same person or situation is, of course, a serious limitation. But this is a limitation of the state of our art and nursing science, not the taxonomy per se.

Distinguishing nursing diagnosis from medical diagnosis has received considerable, perhaps inordinate, attention over the years and remains a subject of frequent discussion. In fact, some have expressed the view (or hope?) that a nomenclature for nursing diagnosis would "provide the language that is *uniquely* nursing—by which we describe nursing and with which nursing can identify" (Kim 1986). Ironically, much nursing diagnosis discussion has elaborated what nursing is *not* and what nursing diagnoses do *not* describe. Many discussants are adamant that nursing diagnosis must be limited to problems that nurses can treat independently. Gordon has emphasized that what distinguishes nursing diagnoses from medical diagnoses is not diagnostic skill, but who is legally authorized to intervene to correct a problem, who initiates therapy, and who has the major responsibility for related therapeutic decisions. But she asserts that the boundaries of professional domains cannot be totally absolute or rigid (Gordon 1976, Gordon 1987). Physiologic problems are at the center of this controversy. Some people have suggested that labels for physiologic problems are just renaming medical diagnoses making them, as Dracup put it, medical diagnoses in disguise (Dracup 1983, Levine 1965). Stevens observes that "nursing is in a state of flux as to whether it will seek its independence by relating with or differentiating from medicine" (Stevens 1979). Guzzetta and Dossey question whether theoretically dependent or independent roles really exist in practice, pointing out that when nurses fulfill the so-called dependent functions, their actions are not "determined by another [but] reflect the coparticipation of the nurse in assisting the patient and physician in treating illness" (Guzzetta 1983). Kim anticipates that "both nurses and physicians will collaboratively use nursing and medical diagnoses." Her survey of 200 nurses found that all nursing diagnoses involve a considerable degree of interdependent nursing functions; not one was believed to require totally independent nursing functions (Kim 1985).

PATHS TOWARD CONSENSUS

It often may seem as if debate is endless, serving little practical purpose. It is important to appreciate that answers could never be final, once and for all. As knowledge grows, the environment continues to change. New questions arise. Answers that once seemed satisfactory no longer suffice. Theory and practice both evolve, each contributing to the other. Stevens observes, "Theory grows out of nurses' experience in practice and then returns as an intellectual structure [re]organizing that practice . . . with new theory arising from the experiences of nurses functioning under a given intellectual structure (Stevens 1979). The process is circular and ongoing" (Chinn 1983). Thus, the goal is not to achieve an immutable truth or rule. But the continuing refinement of concepts does affect practice. Aydelotte and Peterson remind us, moreover, that we are diverse and serve diverse populations. So we see and describe problems from varying vantage points. As we move to a common perspective (and language), we may adopt more than one major parameter or axis for classifying diagnoses, as medicine has done (Dickhoff and James 1988).

To help nurses acquire and exchange information about diagnostic nomenclature and classification, a Clearinghouse for Nursing Diagnosis was established after the First Conference in 1973 at St. Louis University, initially supported by the School of Nursing. Its first coordinator, Kristine Gebbie, began publication of *NR DX Nursing Diagnosis Newsletter,* which was superseded by "Nursing Diagnosis, The Official Journal of the North American Nursing Diagnosis Association." NANDA was formed at the Fifth Conference, superseding the loose association of National Conference participants and the National Task Force on Classification of Nursing Diagnoses, which had directed conference activities. The ANA, which has sent an official representative to each national conference, established a committee on classification of nursing practice phenomena in 1982. Prior to this committee, several groups had been assigned the task of developing a taxonomy for nursing beyond just diagnoses—including interventions, outcomes, nursing roles and functions and classes of nurses. Proposals were outlined but the only product completed to date is a "working schemata" submitted by ANA in 1986 to WHO to be considered for inclusion in ICD 10. The ANA schemata organized patterns according to nine processes: physiologic, interpersonal, ecologic, decision, cognition, perception, valuation, and activity. The committee which is a committee of the ANA Cabinet on Nursing Practice in collaboration with the Cabinets on Research and Nursing service has maintained a collaborative relationship with NANDA. A more formal model for interorganizational collaboration between ANA and NANDA was adopted just prior to the Eighth Conference. In 1988, the ANA Board of Directors officially "approved recognition of the North American Nursing Diagnosis Association as the body to be utilized by the ANA practice councils for the development, review, and approval of nursing diagnoses [and] . . . the extant NANDA taxonomy as the ANA nursing diagnosis taxonomy".

Nursing specialty organizations have incorporated nursing diagnoses into their practice standards and education programs. NANDA is a member of the Federation of Nursing Organizations (NOLF).

NANDA solicits new diagnosis proposals for review. Diagnoses can be submitted by individual nurses or groups. When a diagnosis is submitted, it is reported in the newsletter. (All proposed diagnoses are in the public domain.) The proposal must include the name or label and definition, (major and minor) defining characteristics, and substantiating materials. Proposed diagnoses are first reviewed by the diagnosis review committee, then by a technical review task force (a panel created to review each diagnosis proposed), then by the Board. The General Assembly reviews and comments on proposals at the biannual meeting, after which the entire membership votes (by mail ballot) on whether to accept the diagnosis for clinical testing and validation.

Many observers note—and applaud—the extensive integration of nursing diagnosis concepts and terminology in practice and education that has taken place over the last two decades. Indeed this so-called implementation has been studied and documented. Some observers, however, argue that implementation has largely been semantic. Can we say that greater precision in terminology has clarified communication? Or even that more precise terminology exists in practice *or* education? Have we developed a vocabulary that remains for many practitioners a language parallel to that which they use in thinking and interacting?

The challenge of diagnostic competency and more precise diagnosing is a challenge to individual practitioners, not just to the profession as a whole. As we practice, we must examine and refine our own diagnostic reasoning. Carnevali suggests two strategies for examining one's own diagnosing: retrospective analysis and concurrent observation or self-monitoring in the clinical situation while actually diagnosing (Carnevali et al. 1984). Aspinall and Tanner identify four potential problem areas in the diagnostic process:

◆ failure to associate initially available data with plausible diagnostic hypotheses

◆ failure to include the accurate diagnoses in the initial set of hypotheses considered

◆ overestimating the probability of one hypothesis because of greater ease recalling defining characteristics or recent experience with other cases of a diagnosis

◆ overestimating the reliability or value of available data (Aspinall 1981).

In 1987 Benner and Tanner studied how novice practitioners acquire expertise and how experienced nurses use intuition in the diagnostic process. Staff development instructors are beginning to address misdiagnosing and inappropriate interventions as well as charting terminology. Attention is also being given to how undergraduate students are taught and learn diagnostic reasoning. And researchers are working to develop methods to enhance the learning of diagnostic skills (Cuddigan et al. 1988, Scheffer et al. 1988).

NANDA's explicit raison d'etre is classification. Considerable taxonomic work still lies ahead. The power of the taxonomy will be its range of application, its usefulness to clinicians, scholars, and theorists, and its degree of relevance to other systems with which nursing must interface. Generating labels is but the first and probably the easiest step (Bergman and Panetell 1984). There is need to validate the existence and definitions of problem categories identified. Some have relatively extensive empirical and theoretical underpinnings, though they may not have been discussed in the literature as nursing diagnoses per se nor with consistent, precise use of terms. More precise distinction between categories and between concrete problems within categories will depend on specifying and clarifying major defining characteristics in observable, measurable ways. Until definitions are thus standardized, we cannot expect consistent use of terms nor can we rely on the labels to reflect accurate diagnosing. Thus, enhanced communication remains elusive. Research is also needed to test the reliability of defining characteristics. As computerized information systems become commonplace and increasingly used to document nursing, concern has been voiced about the potential problems of institutionalizing use of diagnoses that have not been validated.

Taxonomic progress depends not only on validity issues and classificatory questions per se, but also on the state of the art and science of nursing. Phyllis Kritek, who chaired the NANDA Taxonomy Committee through the development of Taxonomy I, points out that "generation and classification of new diagnoses occur in tandem, each enhancing [and challenging] the other" (Kritek 1986). Indeed, at the very time Taxonomy I was first presented to the membership for endorsement, changes were suggested by the General Assembly, thus beginning the work on Taxonomy II. At the next conference, Taxonomy II was *not* discussed. Instead, forums focused on five taxonomic concerns: ideology, clarification of levels of abstraction, sensitivity to cultural diversity, methods of determining probability, and defining "related" in the P-E-S format. In 1988 Dickoff and James raised anew the need for flexible thinking and encouraged receptiveness to theoretical pluralism.

The relative importance—and implications—of identifying etiologies is another area of considerable debate. Though many insist that the focus of nursing intervention is the etiology of problems, numerous authors have said that etiologic relationships do not always reflect cause and effect. Some have said that we deal with possible or probable causes, and causality is never fully established. While pointing out that definitive intervention is not possible without understanding a problem's probable cause, Mundinger and Jauron expressed concern over nurses' assuming the legal burden of proof if we say we are identifying causality. Fitzpatrick has suggested that using the term *influencing factors* might enable us to sidestep some of the debate that the concept of causality engenders and move on to issues she considers to be of more immediate concern. Derdiarian, however, maintains that identifying causal factors is important for diagnoses to guide interventions. She points out that nurses may or may not be able to manipulate influencing factors, i.e., "intervening or extraneous variables that enhance, facilitate, or complicate problem development or exacerbation, but not cause it." Lunney believes etiology comprises the intrapersonal, interpersonal, and nonpersonal factors that nurses can work with to help people restore and maintain healthy, functional behaviors (Levine 1965, Lunney 1986).

Gordon has called for classifications of nursing interventions and outcomes to interface with diagnostic taxonomy (Gordon 1980, Gordon 1987). She points out that nurses have been classified by work setting, education, and the medical diagnoses and ages of their patients, but not according to their diagnostic and therapeutic expertise as nurses. Similarly, work needs to be done on the diagnostic and therapeutic complexity of current diagnostic categories. Entire texts that address specific diagnoses can be envisioned. What level(s) of abstraction will demarcate nursing specialties can now barely be imagined.

DIAGNOSIS IN GERONTOLOGIC PRACTICE

Although the phenomena of concern to nursing cut across all patient groups regardless of medical diagnosis, setting, or age, specific problems are seen more frequently and have higher priority in different clinical areas. Different diagnostic categories predominate as major specialties have different predominant foci. For the experienced nurse, knowing a particular setting or a specific client/patient group leads to specific choices of critical assessment areas, quicker activation of certain diagnostic hypotheses, and facility in identifying which problems most urgently need solution (Mitchell 1984). In long-term care, retrospective nursing epidemiology studies have identified the prevalence of certain diagnoses. Some diagnoses are more or less exclusive to gerontologic practice, e.g. translocation syndrome (Smith 1986).* For other diagnoses, certain defining characteristics or etiologies may be more significant. One might also conclude that nursing diagnoses, more than medical or other diagnoses, predominate among residents of nursing homes and skilled-nursing facilities, where the major goal is not to reverse or correct a biophysical condition, but rather to mediate the impact of the condition(s) on residents' quality of life, activities of daily living, and interpersonal relationships. Although individuals may mainfest different cues, there are commonalities for this population relative to specific diagnoses that are distinct from clients in acute care settings. In recent years, these commonalities have become a frequent focus of discussion in the geriatric nursing literature. And research has underpinned some of this discussion. But more research is needed.

Epidemiologic studies reported for this population show that the prevalence of the most frequent diagnoses are similar in different agencies (Hall GR, Leslie 1981, Rantz and Miller 1987). Continued tracking over a three year period in one agency found a growing prevalence of debilitation—cognitive impairment and physical deterioration—with greater incidence of pain, altered thought processes, potential for violence, and ineffective individual coping (Rantz and Miller 1987). Clearly, there is a place for more such studies to identify trends and changes so that appropriate programs can be planned, with appropriate policies and resource allocation to meet needs as they emerge. Moreover, specific interventions must be explicitly linked to diagnoses and clinically tested for effectiveness.

SUMMARY

Nursing discourse has always addressed nurses' problem-solving from a broad, holistic, ecologic perspective. But most writings in the first half century after Nightingale—reflecting both societal health-care developments and the authors' primary responsibilities—were concerned with education and hospital administration. Although attention to these concerns has not abated in the last 50 years, the explosion in scientific knowledge has brought more extensive literature with a focus on practice itself. With the recognition of patient care as a process rather than as the mere completion of multiple, discrete tasks, individual assessment was seen as basic to the nurse-patient relationship and underlying the rationale for any intervention. How to assess—what to look for in particular situations and how to interpret observations—was emphasized in clinical nursing literature before specific attention was given either to the process of diagnosing or to the use of consistent terms to articulate our assessment findings. Today we are usually referring to the last two decades' attention to developing a nomenclature and taxonomy.

The purpose of the effort to have a consistent nomenclature is to improve practice by facilitating communication among nurses and between nurses and others. The purpose of a taxonomy is to depict the relationships between different diagnoses. Nevertheless, the practitioner may not be as involved (or even interested) in taxonomic development. The clinical priority is making a correct, timely diagnosis in each patient situation and communicating it to all concerned with planning and implementing care. Clinical discussions do not, and need not, focus on taxonomic issues. It is possible to use a framework for categorizing what is wrong or incomplete in significant ways. The clinician *uses* the taxonomy with no intention of modifying it (Albert 1988). (The taxonomist, on the other hand, is not concerned with clinical management, but groups cases in order to promote knowledge.) Several taxonomies may evolve to meet specialized purposes. The priorities of gerontologic practice (and long-term-care of any age group) are essentially nursing concerns, i.e., comfort, self-care, and environment support. Experience enables the clinician to specify what cues are most helpful for making a diagnosis in a particular situation, to determine the exact etiology, to set realistic goals, and to plan the most effective and efficient ways to meet them. Gordon, a pioneer in efforts to develop a nursing diagnosis nomenclature and taxonomy and NANDA's first president, emphasizes that nursing diagnosis is "not an idea that originated in the ivory tower of academe" (Gordon 1982). Practice is the basis for theoretical and clinical research concerning nursing diagnoses. Using theory-based knowledge in practice, tests its accuracy and its relevance, thus forming the basis for subsequent research.

References

Abdellah F, Beland I, Martin, L, Matheney, M. *Patient-centered Approaches to Nursing.* New York: Macmillan; 1960.

Albert DH, Munson R, Resnik MD. *Reasoning in Medicine: An Introduction to Clinical Inference.* Baltimore: The Johns Hopkins University Press; 1988.

Alfano G: Healing or caretaking—which will it be? *Nurs Clinics No Am.* 1970; 6:273–280.

American Nurses' Association. *Nursing: A Social Policy Statement.* Kansas City, MO: The Association; 1980.

American Nurses' Association: *Standards of Medical-Surgical Nursing Practice.* Kansas City, MO: The Association; 1973.

Ashley J. *Hospitals, Paternalism, and the Role of the Nurse.* New York: Teachers College Press; 1976.

Aspinall MJ. Use of a decision tree to improve accuracy of diagnosis. *Nurs Research.* 1979; 28:128–185.

Aspinall MJ, Tanner CA. *Decision Making for Patient Care.* New York: Appleton-Century-Crofts; 1981.

Aydelotte M, Peterson KH. Keynote address: nursing taxonomies: State of the art. In McLane A. *Proceedings of the Seventh Conference on the Classification of Nursing Diagnoses.* St. Louis: C.V. Mosby; 1987.

Baretich DM, Anderson LB. Should we diagnose strengths? No: stick to the problems. *Am J Nurs.* 1987; 87:1211–1212.

Benner P: From novice to expert. *Am J Nurs.* 1982; 82:402–407.

Benner P, Tanner C. Clinical judgment: How expert nurses use intuition. *Am J Nurs.* 1987; 87:23–31.

Bergman DA, Panetell RH. The art and science of medical decision making. *Journal Pediatrics.* 1984; 104:649–656.

Bircher AU. On the development and classification of diagnoses. *Nurs Forum.* 1975; 14:10.

Brady PF. Labeling confusion in the elderly. *J Gerontolog Nurs.* 1987; 13:29.

Brown M. Epidemiologic approach to the study of clinical nursing diagnoses. *Nurs Forum.* 1974; 13:346–359.

Campbell C. *Nursing Diagnoses and Interventions in Nursing Practice.* 1st ed. New York: John Wiley and Sons; 1978.

Carlson JH, Craft CA, McGuire AD. *Nursing Diagnosis.* Philadelphia: W.B. Saunders; 1982.

Carnevali DL. Strategies for self-monitoring of diagnostic-reasoning behaviors: Pathway to professional growth. In Carnevalli DL, Mitchell PH, Woods NF, Tanner CA. *Diagnostic Reasoning in Nursing.* Philadelphia: J.B. Lippincott; 1984: 225–228.

Carnevali DL, Mitchell PH, Woods NF, Tanner CA. *Diagnostic Reasoning in Nursing.* Philadelphia: J.B. Lippincott; 1984.

Carpenito LJC. Actual, potential, or possible. *Am J Nurs.* 1985; 85:458.

Chinn PL, Jacobs MK. *Theory and Nursing: A Systematic Approach.* St. Louis: C.V. Mosby; 1983.

Cohen IB. Florence Nightingale. *Scientific American* 1984; 128–137.

Cuddigan J, Norris J, Nilson P, Mockelstrom N, Wellman C, Dixon E, Graves J. Clinical evaluation of an artificial intelligence. Presented at the Eighth Conference, 1988.

Derderian A. Etiology: Practical relevance. In McLane A. *Proceedings of the Seventh Conference on Classification of Nursing Diagnoses.* St. Louis: C.V. Mosby Co.; 1987: 65–77.

Dickhoff J, James P. Theoretical pluralism for nursing diagnosis. Presented at Eighth Conference on Classification of Nursing Diagnosis; March 14, 1988; St. Louis.

Douglas DJ, Murphy EK. Nursing process, nursing diagnosis and emerging taxonomies. In McCloskey JC, Grace HK (ed). *Current Issues in Nursing.* 1st ed. London: Blackwell Scientific Publications; 1981; 50–57.

Dracup K. Nursing diagnosis: A rose by any other name. *Heart and Lung.* 1983; 12:211.

Dreyfus H, Dreyfus S. *Mind Over Machine: The Poser of Human Intuition and Expertise in the Era of the Computer.* New York: Free Press; 1985.

Durand M, Prince R. Nursing diagnosis: process and decision-making. *Nursing Forum.* 1966; 5:50.

Ellis B. Winds of change sweep nursing profession. *Hospitals.* 1980; 54:95.

Elstein AS, Schulman CS, Sprafka SA. *Medical Problem-solving: An Analysis of Clinical Reasoning.* Cambridge MA: Harvard University Press; 1978; 64–121.

Fitzpatrick JJ. Etiology: conceptual concerns. In McLane A (ed). *Proceedings of the Seventh Conference on the Classification of Nursing Diagnoses.* St. Louis: C.V. Mosby; 1987; 1–64.

Fox EGN. New sources of nursing power. *Public Health Nursing.* 1942; 34:246–280.

Fry VS. The creative approach to nursing. *Am J Nurs.* 1953; 53:301.

Gebbie K, Lavin MA. Classifying nursing diagnoses. *Am J Nurs.* 1974; 74:250.

Gordon M. Nursing diagnosis and the diagnostic process. *Am J Nurs.* 1976; 76:1298–1300.

Gordon M. Determining study topics. *Nurs Research.* 1980; 29:83–87.

Gordon M. *Nursing Diagnosis: Process and Application.* 1st ed. New York: McGraw-Hill; 1982.

Gordon M. Structure of diagnostic categories. In Hurley ME (ed). *Proceedings of the Sixth Conference on Classification of Nursing Diagnoses.* St. Louis: C.V. Mosby; 1986.

Gordon M. *Nursing Diagnosis: Process and Application.* 2nd ed. New York: McGraw-Hill; 1987.

Gordon M. *Report of the President.* St. Louis, NANDA, 1988.

Guzzetta CD. Nursing diagnosis: framework, process, and problems. *Heart and Lung.* 1983; 12:281–291.

Hardy MA, Maas M. Nursing diagnosis of long-term-care residents: A descriptive comparison. Presented at Eighth Conference, 1988.

Henderson V. *The Nature of Nursing: A Definition and Its Implications for Practice, Research, and Education.* New York: Macmillan; 1966.

Jacoby MK. Eliminate the double standard. *Am J Nurs.* 1985; 85:281–285.

Kim MJ. Nursing diagnosis: a Janus view. In *Proceedings of the Sixth Conference on the Classification of Nursing Diagnoses.* St. Louis: C.V. Mosby; 1986.

Kim MJ. Without collaboration, what's left? *Am J Nurs.* 1985; 85:281–284.

Kritek PB. Development of a taxonomic structure for nursing diagnoses: A review and an update. In Hurley M (ed): *Classification of Nursing Diagnoses: Proceedings of the Sixth Conference.* St. Louis: C.V. Mosby; 1986, 23–38.

Kritek PB. The struggle to classify our diagnoses. *Am J Nurs.* 1986; 86:722–723.

Lash AA. Nursing diagnosis: Some comments about the gap between theory and practice. In McCloskey JC, Grace HK (ed). *Current Issues in Nursing.* 1st ed. London: Blackwell Scientific Publications; 1981; 44–50.

Leslie FM. Nursing diagnoses: Use in long term care. *Am J Nurs.* 1981; 81:1012–1014.

Levine ME. Trophicognosis: An alternative to nursing diagnosis. In ANA Regional Clinical Conference. 1965; 55–70.

Lunney M. Nursing diagnosis: refining the system. *Am J Nurs.* 1981; 81:1012–1014.

Lunney M. The PES system: A time for change. In Hurley M (ed). *Proceedings of the Sixth Conference on the Classification of Nursing Diagnoses.* St. Louis: C.V. Mosby; 1986; 215–225.

Maas M, Hardy M. A challenge for the future. *J Gerontol Nurs.* 1988; 14:8–13.

McCloskey JC, Grace HK. Nursing definitional issues. In McCloskey JC, Grace HK (ed). *Current Issues in Nursing.* 1st ed. London: Blackwell Scientific Publications; 1981; 3–5.

McCormick JS. Diagnosis: the need for demystification.

McKechnie JL (supv. ed). *Webster's New Universal Unabridged Dictionary.* 2nd ed. New York: Dorset & Baber; 1983; 1434.

McShane CM. In a letter to *Image.* 1987; 19:158–159.

Mitchell PH. Diagnostic reasoning in clinical practice. In Carnevali DL, Mitchell PH, Woods, NF, Tanner CA. *Diagnostic reasoning in nursing.* Philadelphia: J.B. Lippincott; 1984; 105–106.

Mundinger M, Jauron GD. Developing a nursing diagnosis. *Nursing Outlook.* 1975; 23:94–98.

Nahm HE. History of nursing—a century of change. In McCloskey JC, Grace HK (ed). *Current Issues in Nursing.* 1st ed. London: Blackwell Scientific Publications; 1981; 14–26.

Nightingale F. *Notes on Matters Affecting the Health, Efficiency, and Hospital Administration of the British Army Founded Chiefly on the Experience of the Late War and Subsidiary Notes as to the Introduction of Female Nursing into Military Hospitals in Peace and War.* London: Harrison; 1858.

Palmer IS. Origins of education of nurses. *Nursing Forum.* 1985; 22:102–110.

Popkess-Vawter S, Pinnell N. Should we diagnose strengths? Yes: Accentuate the positive. *Am J Nurs.* 1987; 87:23–31.

Rantz M et al. Nursing diagnosis in long-term care. *Am J Nurs.* 1985; 85:916–917.

Rantz M, Miller TV. How diagnoses are changing in long-term care. *Am J Nurs.* 1987; 87:360–361.

Ritter T, Crulich M, Mcentegart A. Nursing practice: An amalgam of dependence, independence and interdependence. In McCloskey JC, Grace HK (ed). *Current Issues in Nursing.* 1st ed. London: Blackwell Scientific Publications; 1981; 5–14.

Roy C. A diagnostic classification system for nursing. *Nurs Outlook.* 1975; 23:90–94.

Scheffer B, Rabenfeld G, Watson K. The LEAD model: Learning efficient and accurate diagnosing. Presented at the Eighth Conference, 1988.

Smith BA. When is "confusion" translocation syndrome? *Am J Nurs.* 1986; 86:1280.

Stevens BJ. *Nursing Theory Analysis, Application, Evaluation.* Boston: Little Brown; 1979.

Tanner CA. Factors influencing the diagnostic process. Pp 61–82. In Carnevali DL, Mitchell PH, Woods PH, Tanner CA. Philadelphia: J.B. Lippincott 1984. Diagnostic Reasoning in Clinical Practice. Pp 105–106.

Ware AM. Using nursing prognosis to set priorities. *Am J Nurs.* 1979; 79:921.

Williams AB. Rethinking nursing diagnosis. *Nurs Forum.* 1980; 19:357–363.

Yura H, Walsh MB. *The Nursing Process: Assessing, Planning, Implementing, and Evaluating.* 1st ed. Washington DC: CUA Press; 1967.

2

The Older Adult—What Are the Differences?

◆

People are living longer. Longevity has affected the individual and society. Where, how, and with whom a person lives are topics that are frequently discussed and that have resulted in the ongoing search for meaning and the quality of life. Advanced technology, legislative regulations, changing family roles, and ethical and moral issues are a few of the areas that have created the need for health care professionals who can adequately assess the physical, mental, emotional, and spiritual needs of this population and, in addition, develop, implement, and evaluate subsequent plans of care.

In order to relate to this specialized group, it is necessary for health care professionals to be able to communicate effectively. This means that nurses must be able to listen with a "third ear" in order to understand the verbal and non-verbal interactions occurring between them and their clients. They must be able to recognize their own thoughts, feelings, expectations, and perceptions as well as those of their clients. They must also be able to assess their own attitudes and behavior toward the older adult in order to understand those of their clients. Nurses must be aware that their attitudes toward aging are reflected in their behavior, and many frustrations will be alleviated if they understand the specific characteristics associated with the aged.

In addition to understanding the communication process, nurses must also be aware of how they and their clients have learned to satisfy their individual needs, and how they have learned to cope with the frustrations that occur when these needs are not satisfied. Being able to recognize various defenses or coping mechanisms can reduce the conflicts that frequently occur when nurses and their clients interrelate. This recognition will also facilitate the development of the individualized care plans and the acquisition and utilization of interdisciplinary personnel.

It is important for nurses to recognize and accept the fact that their role will be greatly expanded when dealing with the older client and, depending upon the client's diagnosis, that they will be expected to provide nursing care related not only to the client's physical problems but also to their psychosocial and environmental problems. Thus, nurses caring for the older adult must possess effective observational, listening, and clinical skills.

In order for nurses to adequately care for the older adult who is living in the community, a skilled nursing facility, or a health-related facility, they must understand the aging process. Since people age chronologically, biologically, and psychologically, it is erroneous to generalize and use the label "old." No two people age the same way. We frequently meet people who are old chronologically but quite young psychologically, and we meet people who are old psychologically but young chronologically. Why is this? What causes this difference among people? The following questions and answers can be used to facilitate an understanding of the aging process and its implication for nursing.

WHAT IS AGING?

To understand the aging process, it might be helpful to define aging as the journey through life during which we have many experiences. These experiences assist our growth and development.

◆ What Occurs During the Years from Birth Through Early Adulthood?

We refer to the following designated paths on our aging journey as periods: infancy, childhood, adolescence, and adulthood. Although each path is different and there are various challenges encountered on each, people proceed through all of them. As we follow an individual through life or as we reflect on our own journey, we should be able to understand the factors that have influenced us and taught us to think, feel, and behave the way we do.

During infancy we are completely dependent on someone else (usually our mother) for the satisfaction of our needs, and as we develop we become increasingly more independent. We want to be in control of what happens to us, and we learn to communicate accordingly. Since our language skills are not yet developed, we must rely on nonverbal behavior; thus, crying assumes an important function. Facial expressions and tactile contact from the provider also teach the infant how his or her needs may be gratified.

During childhood, words are added to the crying and other body language formerly used; our world expands to include peers and significant others rather than being limited to mother; our conscience develops as we become aware of right and wrong; various academic and social skills crystallize due to our entrance into school; sexual curiosity and sex role identification emerge; and we learn various defensive behavior or coping mechanisms to protect ourselves from anxiety-provoking experiences. These are the crucial years in the formation of our personality. These are the years that ultimately produce the "older" adult, and these are the years during which the needs that have been identified by Abraham Maslow become more visible. These needs include security, socialization, recognition, and self-fulfillment.

When we reach adolescence, we experience a period of transition because many unexpected changes occur. Although our physical appearance has changed during the years, we now discover the development of secondary sex characteristics, unexplained emotional feelings, a desire for independence with a co-existing need for dependence, and the emergence of the question: "Who am I?" Our positive or negative self-image emerges, and this accompanies us along the next path of our journey—adulthood.

Adulthood is divided into three phases: early, middle, and later adulthood, and each phase has its specific characteristics. During the early adulthood phase, the individual usually leaves home to establish his or her sense of complete independence; interests center on preparing for and acquiring a career; deciding to remain single or marry; and deciding what kind of family life to have. Many decisions and adjustments have to be made during this period, and it is during this time of life that an individual's level of maturity will be tested and observed.

◆ Why Is Middle Adulthood Considered a Critical Aging Period?

Middle adulthood is a phase of development that is being studied relatively recently. It is the time when life styles change and individuals go through transitional periods described by Gail Sheehy in her book *Passages.*

Middle adulthood is that period when women and men experience the climacteric phase of their lives due to alterations in their hormonal levels. For women, it is the culmination of their fertility and reproductive ability. It begins around the age of 40 years when a decrease and irregularity of the menstrual flow is noticed, and it ends around the age of 50 or 60 years when menses ultimately ceases. In addition changes also occur in the ovaries, Fallopian tubes, uterus, and vagina, and some women may experience the discomfort of hot flushes.

As opposed to women, men do not lose their fertility and reproductive ability. During middle adulthood, it is their psychological and emotional outlook which is primarily affected. During this time, both sexes will begin to notice subtle changes which include: the appearance of gray hair or the loss of hair in some men, "laugh lines" around the mouth, increased weight and a change in shape, increased fatigue and breathlessness following certain activities, and change in vision and hearing. This is also the time when illnesses such as heart attack, stroke, and other chronic conditions may strike causing permanent disabilities or even sudden death.

Middle adulthood is the time when children leave home to establish their own independence and identities, and this creates the "empty nest syndrome" for many parents; a midlife pregnancy may occur; grandchildren are born causing the middle-aged adult to assume the role of grandparent; people may decide to change careers or accept early retirement. Both men and women may experience a mid-life crisis—that is, the time when they ask themselves "Is this all there is?" even though they may have what appears to be everything—good marriage, good home, good family, good job, and so on. Unexplained feelings of discontent arise and cause them to experience inner turmoil, because they often feel that their lives are no longer fulfilling. Insecurity is aroused by the expectations imposed by the family and society which conflict with those of the individual. This is often due to the dichotomy existing between the need to fulfill the functions associated with a stereotype role/image compared to that portrayed by new and changing concepts. Men and women often try to discover how to satisfactorily meet their own needs while satisfying and conforming to those of others. Family relationships and life styles may be affected and this may culminate in marital separations and divorce. Sons or daughters may acquire the responsibility of caring for their parent(s) and/or parent(s)-in-law, and this may force them to alter or abandon their personal goals and assume the role of caretaker. These and other situations may result in the middle-aged adult assuming roles and responsibilities for which they are not prepared. Such challenges often create feelings of anger, fear, resentment, restlessness, and depression which, if not recognized and treated, lead to deeper problems. The individual may choose to use various means to escape from the feelings he or she can't understand or the changes he or she can't accept, rather than admitting that the feelings exist and seeking help to alleviate or solve the problem. The middle-aged adult must recognize that this is another time of growing up. The crises encountered during this period are vital to entering and adjusting to those crises that will occur during the next phase of life.

◆ What Inter-Generational Problems Can Arise Within a Family Caring for an Older Adult?

At some point in middle adulthood, a son and/or daughter may assume the role of caretaker of their parent(s). Usually some kind of confused behavior is displayed, which alarms the adult child. This behavior may be manifested as periods of forgetfulness taking the form of wandering or memory lapses, outbursts of anger at inappropriate times, episodes of sadness, inappropriate sexual behavior, and so on. When children see this disturbing behavior, they may decide that their parent is becoming senile and that action must be taken to insure the parent's safety and well-being. Without consulting the older adult, decisions are made concerning who will assume the ultimate responsibility for making alternate living arrangements for the older adult and who will oversee his/her affairs. If there is more than one child in a family, problems may arise among the siblings.

Since inter-generational problems can arise within a family when a son/daughter assumes the role of caretaker for an aged parent, it is very important to consider family interactions. Attention should be paid on how the various members of the family relate to each other. Dysfunctional relationships within the family can be magnified by caring for an older adult. Living arrangements, finances, relationships, responsibilities, and life styles are affected.

Inter-generational conflicts are complex issues usually occurring due to the need for power and/or control, and they result in behavior which is either overt or covert in form. Families, including both elders and adolescents, usually experience problems associated with power, and when an older adult's need for power, control, or independence is threatened or removed, they may display behavior which reflects their feelings. For example, it is not unusual for an older adult to use illness and dependency to gain attention or for family members to use overindulgence or withdrawal to cope with their guilt or frustration. Other feelings which will evoke various behaviors include love, tenderness, respect, compassion, fear, sadness, contempt, anger, shame, and hostility. Although these feelings may be repressed and/or denied, they do not disappear. They will manifest themselves in some manner. They will also be intensified if the caregiver is burdened with other problems and is being reminded of his or her own aging.

When dealing with inter-generational problems, health-care professionals must be able to recognize family interactions and behaviors that not only create dysfunctional situations but are also used to maintain family harmony.

CHANGES OF LATER ADULTHOOD

◆ What Additional Physical Changes Occur During Later Adulthood?

As individuals advance in age, additional physical changes will be noted. The skin texture and pigmentation change causing additional wrinkling and sagging, "bags" to appear under the eyes, and brown pigments (sometimes referred to as "age spots") to appear. The skin also loses some of its softness. Sensitivity to temperature and touch decreases making the person less adaptable to the cold and less aware of painful stimuli.

Older adults notice that their sense of smell and taste changes and this, together with changes in the structure of their gums and teeth may greatly affect their desire and enjoyment of food, as well as their subsequent nutritional status. The change in taste occurs because the number of taste buds decrease, and taste buds are not as sharp as they were prior to late adulthood.

Movement in the older person may become more difficult. Susceptibility to fractures increases due to changes in the musculo-skeletal system. Bones become porous and fragile, joints stiffen, and muscles loose their elasticity. Because spinal discs may degenerate, a change occurs in the vertebral structure causing the individual to acquire a curvature as well as to decrease in height.

Digestion slows down with age because the process of peristalsis is impeded by the decrease in muscle tone and activity increasing the time needed for food to be digested and eliminated.

With advancing age, several changes occur within the heart and blood vessels that can impede the flow of blood. The heart muscle may become damaged, valves may lose their elasticity, and arteries may become constricted or clogged with fatty deposits. These changes result in decreased circulation which, in turn, may cause arrythmias, increased blood pressure, and a decreased blood supply to the other systems.

Respiration is affected by a change in the respiratory organs. The lungs, rib cage, and chest muscles undergo alterations resulting in a change in lung and breathing capacity as well as in the exchange and utilization of oxygen and other gases.

Changes continue to occur in the reproductive system. In women, the hair on the external genitalia becomes thinner, and the labia loses its firmness. The size of the cervix, uterus, and ovaries decreases. The vaginal lining becomes thinner; there is decreased elasticity; and vaginal secretions decrease. The muscle tone of the pelvic floor weakens, and there is a possibility that the uterus may prolapse. The breasts become smaller and lose their firmness. With age, men may be troubled by an enlargement of the prostate gland causing urinary frequency and/or incontinence. Men will also note that their scrotum hangs lower and that it will take longer to reach and recover from orgasm. Despite these changes in the reproductive organs, the need for love and affection does not change for either sex. Although sex may be less frequent and less intense, it is still meaningful and important, and it continues among many older adults.

As people age, they may notice that they have to urinate more frequently. Men, especially, may notice this since the amount of urine their bladder can normally hold will greatly decrease.

Changes in the nervous system and brain also occur as a person ages. Although the brain may change in size, weight, and wetness, no drastic changes occur in its cognitive functioning. It is most important to remember than an individual can learn no matter what his or her age *unless* there is some interfering pathology. In the past it was common to label older adults as "senile," because society applied a stereotyped image to the "aged" or "old" person.

If an older adult has memory lapses or begins to wander, has inappropriate outbursts of anger, displays inappropriate sexual behavior, or manifests signs of depression or confusion, it is extremely important to determine if the cause is physical, psychological, or interactional. Memory can be affected at any age by stress, emotional upsets, poor health, medications, vitamin deficiencies, or poor nutrition. For this reason, it is vital that a correct diagnosis be made. In view of this, professionals must understand the condition known as organic brain syndrome (OBS).

Organic brain syndrome (OBS) is the technical term to denote that the cause of memory lapse is due to physiological change. It consists of two types: acute brain syndrome (ABS), which is brief and reversible, and chronic brain syndrome (CBS), which is irreversible and of long-term duration. Both young and old can be affected by ABS, which can be caused by physical illness or drug interactions. Elders are more affected by CBS, caused by strokes or some destructive disease of the nervous system. The results of CBS are wasting away of areas of the brain and behavior changes. Because OBS is a term that includes both ABS and CBS, it is extremely important that a differentiation be made. Misdiagnosis may allow reversible conditions to progress to the irreversible state.

Another change in the older adult occurs in the immune system. Susceptibility to infections is not uncommon within this age group.

It is also very important to remember that, as a result of physical changes, the older adult is susceptible to many diseases that can ultimately lead to death. These illnesses include heart disease, accidents, chronic obstructive pulmonary disease, malignancies, diabetes, influenza, pneumonia, chronic liver disease, cirrhosis, and atherosclerosis. Suicide is also a cause of death for many older people. It may be linked to depression or may not be due to any specific pathology.

◆ What Emotional and/or Psychological Problems May Affect the Older Adult?

The various losses that ultimately result in changes in the life style of older adults may produce various emotional and/or psychological problems. Depending upon the personalities they developed early in life to fit their temperament and meet their needs, some individuals will adapt to changes and others will rebel.

When older people experience changes in their lives, lose loved ones, or become concerned about their health, finances, or living arrangements, it is normal for them to become sad, to express feelings of anger, resentment, envy, jealousy, loneliness, and deprivation, and to display behaviors that express these feelings. This is their way of expressing grief—a necessary step toward feeling better. After a reasonable length of time, they will usually return to the active, productive, stimulating, and satisfying life which they previously enjoyed. It is important to remember that the length of time it takes to recover depends upon the gravity, suddenness, and duration of the incident, the individual's personality, and the proximity of any additional losses.

Individuals who find it difficult to accept losses and changes in their lives, as well as those who have a predisposition to problems, will develop emotional and psychological problems; these will vary in severity. These problems include the following: anxiety, depression, alcohol abuse, drug abuse, hypochondriasis, confusion, senility, paranoia, and suicide. Noting the similarities manifested by several of these conditions and emphasizing the necessity of acquiring an accurate diagnosis prior to treatment are very important.

Anxiety is a symptom aroused when an individual feels afraid of things to come but is unable to state the reason for this fear. Various physical and psychological reactions occur which, if not recognized and treated, may cause the individual to become depressed.

Depression is an illness often mistakenly diagnosed because its symptoms appear to resemble those of other psychological problems. Although the individual's behavior and complaints usually follow some significant loss, depression may also be due to heredity or some biological disturbance. People may be mistakenly labeled "senile" because they exhibit forgetfulness and confusion, express feelings of sadness, cry easily, sometimes appear hyperactive, derive no enjoyment from former interests, complain of feeling fatigued and energyless, and display many other behaviors. If the depression becomes severe, they may become paranoid and display more psychotic behavior. If their depression has existed for a long time, it may be difficult to diagnose because its longevity facilitates its eventual incorporation into the individual's total personality. Depression can usually be treated with psychotherapy and medication, if necessary. It is important, however, to acquire an in-depth history and to do an extensive physical assessment prior to initiating any form of treatment. It is also important to be aware of the fact that people may mask their problem by denying its existence or by abusing alcohol and/or drugs. If people resort to such behavior, the problem will increase.

Although the older adult may, like other individuals, resort to *alcohol abuse* as a means of alleviating the problems, he or she will soon learn that the feelings of depression increase rather than disappear. Even though large amounts of alcohol may not be consumed, the older adult's tolerance decreases and this results in an inability to function. It may also produce and/or increase the severity of physical changes.

Drug abuse, another problem found among older adults, differs from that found in the younger population. Older adults typically misuse over-the-counter and prescription drugs. Poor vision predisposes them to reading labels erroneously. Having several physicians provides older adults with an abundant supply of varying medications which, taken incorrectly, may be hazardous and lethal. Being prone to confusion makes older adults susceptible to overdose. In addition, various physical and mental problems predispose them to using too many pain medications, laxatives, tranquilizers, and sleeping pills.

Many older adults develop *hypochondriasis.* This is the emotional disturbance in which the individual is convinced that they have a physical ailment despite negative findings on examination. The person goes from doctor to doctor insisting that they are ill. Although the specific cause of hypochondriasis is unknown, it is believed that there are several predisposing psychological factors and that it usually follows a major stressful event. Persons afflicted with this problem have real symptoms and need treatment. Although they may not receive medication or other palliative measures, they do receive attention and an expression of concern from others.

The most difficult psychological problem that may appear in an older adult is *confusion.* Like anxiety, confusion is a symptom rather than an illness. It can be caused by pathological as well as non-pathological factors. Any stressful event, adverse reactions to medications, change in diet or familiar surroundings can trigger the confusion. Because confusion is reversible and will disappear when the underlying cause is removed, the older adult should be thoroughly examined and never receive drugs or be hospitalized without a complete evaluation of possible causes of confusion. It is imperative that a careful physical and mental assessment be done.

What is seen as *senility* may or may not be reversible. It is a term frequently and incorrectly applied to older adults who become forgetful, whose ability to comprehend decreases, and whose behavior becomes abnormal. It is, unfortunately, assumed by many that these individuals will continue to deteriorate and, in view of this, they are often ignored. Their independence is frequently taken away by caregivers who, due to fear for the person's safety and well being, remove them from familiar surroundings and assume the responsibility for their finances. The individual often loses the freedom to make their own decisions and must become submissive to those of others. It is sad to note that when these older adults are taken for a medical/psychological assessment, they are often misdiagnosed and subsequently receive incorrect treatment. As a result, a condition which was reversible becomes irreversible.

Dementia, termed by the layperson *senility,* develops slowly and results in the complete destruction of the intellect and memory. Severe depression is frequently confused with dementia but can be distinguished from it because the symptoms of depression are reversible if treated correctly. Although there are several forms of dementia, Alzheimer's disease and multi-infarct-dementia are common. Alzheimer's disease is a form of dementia which occurs more frequently in women. Its cause in unknown at present despite extensive research. Deterioration of memory, personality, intelligence, and physical health are slow, but death usually occurs within five to ten years after the symptoms begin. Multi-infarct-dementia usually occurs in persons afflicted with atherosclerosis and heart disease. It takes several months or years to develop, with the individual experiencing periods of mental clearness during this time. Death occurs early due to heart disease, stroke, or pneumonia rather than to mental deterioration.

Another psychological problem that affects many older people is *paranoia.* People experience unreasonable suspiciousness and anxiety, which alienates them from others. They interpret everything (both good and bad) personally, and they often accuse others of insulting them.

The final psychological problem, probably a culmination of all the other problems, is *suicide.* Older adults kill themselves more frequently than any other age group. Seventy and eighty year old white males have the highest incidence of suicide. Individuals who have serious physical illness; have continuous pain; are deeply depressed; abuse alcohol; suffer with hypchondriasis, confusion, or dementia; have attempted suicide before; have a poor self-image; or are grieving over the loss of someone close may also commit suicide. Older adults usually give no pre-warning. They make a decision and act. Their actions are, sadly to say, usually successful.

HOW DO OLDER ADULTS VIEW DEATH AND DYING?

Death is a part of life that becomes more prominent in the thoughts of older people. Although older people do not develop a morbid curiosity, most become concerned about when and how they will die. In today's society, the use of modern technology to prolong life or to restore its sudden cessation creates a fear in many older adults that they will merely exist rather than be allowed to leave this world with dignity. The stereotyped image of the dependent, nonresponsive individual produces an additional fear of being aborted from society by the hands of others. Just as they want to control the activities of their daily living, most older adults want to have control over the way they die. It is unfortunate that although people may have a "living will," this document is not universally accepted throughout the states. Older adults, however, are able to accomplish this same objective if they have children or others with whom they can discuss their wishes and be assured that they will be implemented.

Older adults become more aware of death with each passing year, especially when they see the deaths of relatives and close friends. Although these deaths produce grief in the older adult, many of them have already experienced grief. It is not unusual to note older adults' interest in the obituary column of the daily newspaper, their concern about setting their affairs in order, and their increased spiritual awareness. If older adults are unable to physically attend spiritual services, they may listen to spiritual programs on the radio or television; they will read their Bible or other materials devoted to spiritual topics; and they will avail themselves of visits from clergy. They may be comforted by the thought that there is an afterlife where they will be united with loved ones and will finally see God. For the older adult, discussing death may be a great consolation. Although they may be afraid of how they will die, older adults are usually not afraid of death itself.

Some older adults, however, reject death and continuously deny its approach. Although they may pass through the stages of anger, bargaining, and depression that have been described by Elisabeth Kubler-Ross, they never reach the final stage of acceptance. These individuals usually do not derive solace from having a spiritual awareness because they do not believe in an afterlife. They believe that there is nothing after death. They feel their existence ceases completely. These individuals are usually afraid, not only about how they will die, but also about death itself.

It is important to note that most older adults do not usually fear death, even though there are exceptions. Some older adults welcome death as a means of ending their suffering, loneliness, and boredom. The fact that older adults do not talk about death does not mean that they are not thinking about it.

WHAT ARE THE NURSING IMPLICATIONS FOR THE OLDER ADULT LIVING IN A LONG-TERM FACILITY?

Nursing care of the older adult is similar to nursing care of any other age group in so far as it requires the utilization of the nursing process. This means that the nurse must be able to assess, plan, implement, and evaluate the needs of the client and make revisions accordingly. This process is required whether the client is in the hospital, at home, at a short or long-term care facility.

Nursing care in a long-term facility warrants special consideration because the resident will need either skilled or health-related nursing care, and regardless of why he or she is in the facility, the resident will require nursing staff who can provide for his or her physical and psychological needs. Depending upon how long he resides there, a special relationship will usually develop because for many, this will probably become their home. They will, therefore, suffer, not only the loss of their physical health—the main reason they are there, but they will also suffer the loss of familiar surroundings, possessions, family, and social contacts. They may also lose much of their independence, because they will be dependent on others to provide for their various needs. These changes will require the client to make several major adjustments that will evoke many feelings. The client, in turn, will manifest behavior that will either be accepted or rejected.

In order to adequately assess the needs of the client or family member(s), nursing staff must be able to listen, observe, and ask pertinent questions. Although the resident's history will provide valuable identifying data (age, religion, occupation, marital status, financial resources, etc.), as well as information regarding his or her physical and social status, nothing can substitute for the personal interaction between resident and staff member. Seeing a tense body or tearful eyes, hearing a changed tone or loudness of voice, or receiving silence in place of a verbal response to an inquiry are messages that no written document can communicate. In view of this, nursing staff must be aware of the normal physiological, mental, and emotional changes that occur in the older adult, so that they can adequately assess the possibility of pathology and provide appropriate intervention.

Because different stimuli can cause mental confusion in the older adult, which can result in physical or verbal behavioral outbursts, nursing staff must be knowledgeable in psychological behaviors and able to distinguish between normal and abnormal conduct. They should also be aware of the implications for using restraints and p.r.n. medications, as well as the results of incorrectly labeling behavior.

In addition to assessing the needs of the resident, nursing staff should be available to assist family members by listening to them and observing their interactions with the resident. Family members who have assumed the caretaker role also need reassurance and support, because they may frequently feel very guilty about placing their loved one in the facility. They may also be the recipients of the resident's feelings of anger and resentment. Counseling may be necessary and should be provided by qualified, professional nursing staff.

Following the assessment of the resident's needs and determining a nursing diagnosis, the plan of care can be developed. It should be written in behavioral or measurable terms in order to facilitate easy evaluation, and it should be developed by all professional and non-professional staff responsible for the client's care in order to provide continuity of care. Staff from all shifts and, if possible, the resident should be consulted for input.

Nursing staff who implement the plan and care for the resident must consider all his or her needs on a daily basis, even though evaluations are mandated to be done at other specific times. Although other disciplines may supplement the care (e.g., physical therapist, occupational therapist, speech therapist, etc.), total nursing care must include activities that will stimulate and maintain the adequate functioning of all the body systems. In addition, social activities must be provided not only to facilitate interaction but also to satisfy individual preferences. For this reason, long-term care facilities should have a means by which residents can participate in recommended activities.

Opportunities should be provided to allow residents to express and share their feelings and views. Nursing staff should be aware that the clients' behavior may be indications of their anxiety or sadness over their losses and changed life-style.

THE OLDER ADULT—WHAT'S THE DIFFERENCE?

The older adult is an individual who has passed through five phases of growth and development—infancy, childhood, adolescence, early adulthood, and middle adulthood—and is now in the final phase of later adulthood. During each of these phases, physical and psychological changes have occurred. Specific needs that have been identified by Abraham Maslow—physiological needs, the need for security, the need for self-fulfillment—had to be met either by the individual or by someone else. The manner in which the individual adjusted to these various changes and stresses depended on the coping mechanisms that had been developed according to his or her individual personality. Inability to cope resulted in various physiological and psychological problems that may or may not have needed intervention.

The older adult is a living paradox. A total human being has been formed over the years and is a still-evolving individual facing life. Providing expert care to these individuals is one of nursing's major opportunities.

References

Kubler-Ross, E. *On Death and Dying.* New York: Macmillan; 1969.

Maslow, A. *Toward a Psychology of Being.* Princeton, NJ: D. Van Nostrand; 1962.

Matteson, MA, McConnell, ES. *Gerontological Nursing: Concepts and Practice.* Philadelphia: W. B. Saunders; 1988.

Yurick, AG et al. *The Aged Person and the Nursing Process.* Norwalk, Connecticut: Appleton and Lange; 1989.

3

Geriatric Update: Research and Action

RoAnne Dahlen-Hartfield
Moira Shannon

♦

PURPOSES OF NURSING RESEARCH

One of the ways in which gerontological nursing will gain further recognition as a distinct and separate specialty within the broader discipline of nursing is through nursing research. Nursing research assists in developing the scientific base to all phases of the nursing process in the care of the older adult.

♦ Assessment

Nursing research has helped in the development and validation of assessment instruments that assist the nurse in the planning of individualized care for the older adult. These instruments have been geared toward the older adult by inclusion of the normal changes related to aging, as well as those changes related to specific disease processes. With the use of these validated instruments, the nurse is able to do a more complete and thorough assessment to ensure identification of the correct nursing diagnosis within a related functional pattern.

♦ Planning and Intervention

Nursing research has helped to determine, through experimental studies, those interventions that appear to be most effective in caring for the older adult. Relationships useful in predicting and controlling the effects of nursing interventions have been identified.

♦ Evaluation

Nursing research has developed evaluation techniques, forms, and protocols to assist nurses in program evaluation and subsequent program planning and development.

◆ Other Purposes—Achievement of Accountability and Professional Recognition

Nursing research serves to assist gerontological nurses in achieving accountability, which has been a longstanding problem. Researchers stated that the knowledge level of nurses in the practice setting was vague. Specific nursing interventions lacked a grounding in a theoretical base. Once nurses in long-term care settings are able to validate their practice through nursing research, they should be able to experience increased accountability and subsequent recognition.

◆ Review of Past Gerontological Nursing Research

A review of past gerontological nursing research completed during the period of 1955 through 1992 reveals that much progress has been made. There are a number of excellent reviews of gerontological nursing and research (Bassen 1967, Gunter and Miller 1977, Brimmer 1979, Kayser-Jones 1981, Dye 1983, Thompson and Steffl 1984, Burnside 1985, Adams 1986, Haight 1989, Peters 1989, O'Leary et al. 1990, and Engle and Graney 1990).

These reviews help demonstrate the increase in the number and type of studies done in gerontological nursing research, as well as indicating a broadening of focus and areas of interest. The reviews vary, as do the references reviewed by the author: nursing journals, other gerontological research journals, unpublished theses and dissertations, and textbooks in gerontological nursing.

Bassen's review (1967) reported for the period of 1955 to 1965. Of the total of 515 papers, only 12 percent of the articles were research-based.

Gunter and Miller (1977) characterized gerontological nursing research as emphasizing the psychosocial realm and included psychosocial needs and characteristics of the elderly, the caretaker's attitudes and interventions, and interventions to meet the psychosocial needs of the elderly.

Brimmer (1979) further substantiated the steady increase in the literature of articles about gerontological nursing. Of the papers reviewed, only 7 percent focused on the chronically ill and rehabilitative needs of the elderly.

Kayser-Jones (1981) found nurse researchers continuing to focus on the psychosocial needs of the elderly in institutional settings. There was a continuing interest in attitudes (especially those of nurses, and student nurses) toward the elderly, aging, and institutional settings such as nursing homes. She noted an increase in the number of studies that focused on clinical problems.

Dye (1983) cited only 13 percent of the studies reviewed as having a clinical focus. There continued to be a lack of replication of previous studies.

Burnside (1985), in her review of studies by gerontological nurse researchers from 1975 to 1984, identified 39 percent of 113 studies that examined nursing activities and attitudes. Drugs (8 studies) and accidents and falls (6 studies) were the most prevalent clinical problems studied. She noted the following trends: inclusion of a variety of theoretical frameworks as a base for the research; increased collaborative research efforts; more sophisticated design; statistical and computer analysis; and innovative clinical demonstration projects.

Haight (1989) in her review of nursing research in long-term care facilities from 1984 to 1988 noted that nurse researchers had changed direction from the studying of attitudes and nursing students to examining physical problems such as incontinence, pressure sores, falls, sleep, drug interaction and fluid intake, and psychological problems related to communication, interaction, behavior, and confusion. Research studies related to these problems are summarized according to author, journal, purpose, sample size, design, and results.

Peters (1989) reviewed the current research which examined quality of care in long-term settings from the perspective of patient outcomes. This type of research generally considers: (1) the scope of health care in long-term care; (2) the criteria which need to be measured, and (3) a framework for measurement. The impetus for this examination of quality was driven by the Omnibus Reconciliation Act (OBRA) of 1987 which mandates the development of a resident assessment process including patient outcome measures suitable for national use by all nursing home facilities participating in Medicare and Medicaid funding.

O'Leary (1990) evaluated the potential usefulness of the research which was generated in 1986 to 1988 within nursing, medicine, the behavioral sciences, and through multidisciplinary efforts to gerontological nursing practice.

Engle and Graney (1990) explored the value of meta-analysis for literature integration and research which will strengthen the validated body of knowledge of this practice.

In summary, these reviews recognize that the historical development of gerontological nursing, gerontological nursing research, and its recognition as a specialty within the profession of nursing have been directly linked.

◆ Research in Nursing Diagnosis and Functional Patterns

Research in nursing diagnosis is at an even earlier stage than gerontological nursing research. The nursing diagnosis research efforts have been directed toward identifying new nursing diagnoses and clinically validating those nursing diagnoses found on the current list of nursing diagnoses approved by the North American Nursing Diagnosis Association.

The process for identifying new nursing diagnoses is not an easy one. The nurse researcher queries a national sample of nurse clinical specialists about the characteristics, signs, and symptoms most commonly found in 100 patients demonstrating the proposed nursing-diagnosed problem. Groups of patients may also be used to assist in the identification of general, defining, and critical characteristics, as well as the associated etiological factors.

Once this descriptive process is completed, the Nursing Diagnosis with its accompanying characteristics and proposed etiological factors is subjected to clinical validation by clinical nurse specialists. These nurse specialists independently interview and assess the same patients. Their written assessments are compared to determine the percent of agreement on the specific nursing diagnosis, presence of defining and critical characteristics, and identified etiologies.

The studies described in this chapter will be organized according to the functional patterns for nursing diagnosis which were proposed by Gordon. These functional patterns include the following: Health Perception-Health Management Pattern; Nutritional-Metabolic Pattern; Elimination Pattern; Activity-Exercise Pattern; Sleep-Rest Pattern; Cognitive-perceptual Pattern; Self-Perception–Self-Concept Pattern; Role-Relationship Pattern; Sexuality-Reproductive Pattern; Coping-Stress Tolerance Pattern; and the Value-Belief pattern.

Each pattern will be defined and subsequent research detailed.

◆ Health Perception-Health Management Pattern and the Value-Belief Pattern

The Health Perception-Health Management Pattern describes the older adult's perception of health status; general health care behavior, such as adherence to preventative health practices, nursing and medical prescriptions, and follow-up care; and their efforts for future planning.

The Value-Belief Pattern describes the values, goals, or beliefs that guide older adults in making choices and decisions in their lives and about their personal health.

Crucial variables regarding the individual's genetic, behavioral, and attitudinal characteristics exist in relation to health. The nurse or the individual cannot change the genetic characteristics, but there is evidence that changes in health-related behaviors and attitudes can have significant impact on health outcomes. Some of these are described in the research studies presented.

McGlove and Kick (1978) conducted a study on the effects of good health habits. In a study of 52 patients over the age of 30, health habits included keeping active physically and mentally, eating properly, staying thin, moderation in use of alcohol, and absence of smoking.

Kee (1984) examined some of the "facts" about old age that inaccurately portray this as a time of dread. Health promotion to minimize the deficits of old age was seen as a needed intervention to change the perception of the elderly (and others) in relation to this inaccurate portrayal.

Melillo (1985) described a project that provided health examinations to elderly women focusing on preventive medicine practices. Medicare reimbursement practices as of the writing do not support this type of preventive care. Helping the elderly person to perceive the value of preventive health care in light of such reimbursement practices is a challenge.

Parent and Whall (1984) described the relationship between physical activities and self-esteem and found physical activity to be supportive to self-esteem. They also examined the correlation between self-esteem and depression and found they were negatively and strongly correlated. This means that as the person's self-esteem increased, the level of depression decreased. These findings support the encouragement of physical activity in older persons.

Kolanowski and Gunter (1985) studied the health practices of retired career women. Behaviors that were seen to influence well-being in this group included social connectedness, activity, flexibility, integrity, and transcendence.

Gunter (1985) described a project for training peer counselors to capitalize on elder strengths as a resource for their peers. This experiment benefited the counselors, as well as those who were counseled.

Several of the studies appropriate to this section also relate to environmental concerns (Wolanin 1978, Louis 1981, and Lester and Baltes 1978). Gioiella (1987) described the preferred personal space aspect of the environment of the elderly and further cofirmed earlier findings that the nurse must assess the preference of the individual before assuming personal space preference.

Bahr and Gress (1985) described the importance of healthy sleep in their study group. Sleep is seen as a vital component of health care, especially in elderly persons, and will be discussed more extensively under the Sleep-Rest Pattern.

In an institutional setting, the nurse has maximum control over the residents' environment, especially for factors that involve activities of daily living and treatments. This influence can be used to impact positively on the health of the residents and to maximize potential for physical and psychosocial functioning.

A major nursing and medical treatment area controlled by the nurse is drug therapy with its assessment, administration, and teaching aspects. Brown, Boosinger, et al. (1977) described a pilot study that examined the potential for clinically significant drug to drug interactions and adverse drug side effects in residents in a rural nursing home and an urban nursing home. The preventive measures of periodically reviewing the resident's drug profile and evaluating the drug effectiveness were seen as essential to prevention of drug interactions. PRN drugs involving tranquilizers, hypnotics, and sedatives created a potential hazard. Laxatives produced significant abnormalities in the older adult so as to warrant limitation in use. Aspirin, as a commonly prescribed drug, produced gastric irritation and bleeding and should only be given with food or large quantities of fluid. The most common drug interaction occurred when cardiac glycosides were used in conjunction with potassium depleting diuretics.

Kim and Grier (1981) examined the effects of varying the pace of medication instruction on the older adult's learning and retention as measured by pre- and post-test scores. Findings showed that older adults who are taught at a slower paced speech rate will have a greater gain in pre-post drug information test scores than those taught at a normal pace or those who received no instruction. The slowed speech allowed the older adult to more adequately integrate the information. Use of printed information in conjunction with this teaching program was also emphasized.

Naylor and Shaid (1991) analyzed patient information needs of hospitalized elderly persons and identified the need for information not only about their current problem, but also about health promotion, disease prevention, and the availability of resources.

KEY POINTS

◆ Good health habits include physical and mental activity, proper eating, weight control, moderate alcohol consumption, absence of smoking, and healthy sleep.

◆ Physical activity increases self-esteem and decreases depression.

◆ Health promotion, as an intervention, decreases dread of old age.

◆ Use of peers as counselors for support is effective.

◆ The individual's preference of personal space should be addressed.

◆ Drug interactions can be decreased by careful monitoring of the resident's medications by the nurse, the physician, and the pharmacist.

◆ Slow-paced drug instruction programs with written materials lead to greater learning retention and self-care capabilities. Nurses who are aware of self-care behaviors that enhance health can reinforce such behaviors when they exist and try to encourage the person to develop them through education and motivational interventions.

◆ Nutritional-Metabolic Pattern

The Nutritional-Metabolic Pattern describes the older adult's patterns of food and fluid consumption time—type and quantity of food and drink preferred and consumed and use of nutrient and vitamin supplements. The effects of this pattern on skin, skin lesions, healing ability, hair, nails, mucous membranes, body temperature, height, and weight are also noted.

The taste abilities of institutionalized elderly, noninstitutionalized elderly, and young adults were compared by Spitzer (1988). The bitter detection threshold increases with age. There is also a significant increase in the sour detection threshold for institutionalized elderly on medication. The sweet taste ability is unrelated to age.

Longman and Dewalt (1986) recognized the influence of oral health on the life style, appetite, food consumption, and quality of life of residents in nursing homes. Many of these residents require daily assistance by nursing assistants with their oral care. The nurse researchers developed and tested *An Oral Assessment Guide for Nursing Assistants* to determine the effectiveness of this oral hygiene program on oral health. Improvement in the oral health of the residents was noted. A teaching and training program for the nursing assistants was developed and implemented with positive results.

In an experimental study, using 48 institutionalized older adults, Dewalt (1977) identified and compared the effects produced on oral mucosa and teeth by applying oral hygiene at two-, three-, and four-hour intervals, eight hours a day, 5 days a week, for a two week period with either a tooth brush or soft glycerin swab. An assessment rating instrument was developed and scored 9 variables that reflected oral health: salivation, tongue moisture, tongue color, moisture of palates, condition of gingival tissue, color of membranes, lip texture and moisture, and soft tooth debris. The findings substantiated that nursing intervention can produce significant and observable changes in the oral tissues of the geriatric patient. These responses do not appear to be cumulative over time, which speaks to the need for continued daily oral hygiene.

Food and fluid intake of organic brain syndrome patients was examined by Eaton (1986). Touch, as a symbol of caring, was used by care givers during meal time which had become a caring social event rather than a task. Both staff and patients seemed to benefit from the improved meal atmosphere.

Pritchard (1988) compared the use of the small-bore feeding tube to the larger-bore Levine type of naso-gastric tube in relation to infections and safety. The small-bore tube was associated with fewer pneumonias, tube displacements, and incidents of aspiration in the residents.

Volicer (1989) reported finding little difference in mortality rates of terminal stage dementia patients who are tube fed or who were encouraged to eat by mouth. These findings were inconsistent with Michaelsson (1987), who reported that most end-stage patients were able to be spoon fed and did not require a feeding tube.

Skin and its integrity is viewed as an important component of this functional pattern. Nurse researchers have examined this area from the perspective of assessment, intervention, and evaluation. In the area of assessment, Jones and Millman (1986) devised a three-part system to combat pressure sores. This enabled the nurse to identify those patients who were at the highest risk of developing pressure sores. Protocols were instituted to ensure consistent interventions. The incidence of pressure sores that originated in the institution decreased by almost half. The severity of the pressure sores and the mortality of the patients with pressure sores also decreased.

Development of the Standards of Care (patient outcomes) and Standards of Nursing Practice in the prevention and treatment of pressure sores in the resident was described by West (1991). These Standards incorporated an assessment tool adapted from the Norton and Waterlow Scales, a wound grading scale, and recommended treatment protocols.

Boykin and Winland-Brown (1986) compared the effectiveness of hydro-colloid occlusive dressing to the providone-iodine therapy in the treatment of pressure sores in 21 elderly residents. The pressure sores treated with the hydro-colloid occlusive dressing showed a decrease in size twice that of the providone-iodine treated pressure sores.

Accidental hypothermia, which is defined as a core (rectal) body temperature of below 95 degrees F, was addressed by Kolanowski and Gunter (1981) in their descriptive study of 101 subjects age 65 and over, who resided in a nursing home, high rise apartment, or their own home. Data were collected during the month of February when the mean temperature was 24.7 degrees F. Implications for nursing practice included the need to use low-reading thermometers which should be shaken down to their lowest point before using them. If a very low oral temperature is recorded, the older adult's temperature should be measured again using a rectal thermometer. Loss of sub-cutaneous fat, orthostatic hypotension, and falls were contributing factors to the problem of hypothermia.

KEY POINTS

◆ Taste abilities change as a result of aging or in some cases by the use of medications. Bitter and sour detection increases. Sweet tasting is unrelated to age.

◆ An accurate and complete assessment and use of systematic intervention protocols are needed in order to maintain and improve oral health and subsequent improvement in appetite and nutritional status of the resident.

◆ Mealtime should become a social event rather than a task. Touch enhances the element of caring.

◆ Use of small-bore feeding tubes result in fewer instances of pneumonias, tube displacement, and aspiration.

◆ Results of comparing different treatment interventions for pressure sores are available in the nursing research literature.

◆ Incidents of accidental hypothermia in the resident is prevented by accurate temperature readings and teaching programs.

◆ Elimination Pattern

The Elimination Pattern describes the patterns of excretory function of bowel, bladder, and skin, including the use of laxatives or devices to influence the pattern.

Wichita addressed the concern of bowel incontinence, which was occurring in half of the 200 residents within a skilled facility. A clinical demonstration project was developed using a group of residents who were self-fed and a group of residents who were fed by staff. A month of baseline data as to the number of incontinent accidents, anal dilitations, suppositories, and enemas for each subject was obtained. The uses of increased fiber diet and use of bran on cereals was instituted for one month. Comparisons of baseline to post-diet indicated significant reductions in percent of incontinent accidents, use of suppositories, and enemas. The finding had implications for cost savings, staff time, and most important for the older adult's feelings of dignity and self-worth.

Davis, et al. (1986) also recognized the potential importance of upgrading bowel management programs in hope of improving the self-esteem and dignity of older clients. This nursing research study evaluated the use of a quality assurance program with implementation of bowel management standards, audit and updated ongoing general education in service programs on the incidence of bowel incontinence. Positive effects were noted.

Urinary incontinence has been viewed not as a disease, but rather as a non-specific symptom of an underlying medical, psychological, or environmental problem. Urinary incontinence is the second most common cause for institutionalization of the elderly. The range of urinary incontinence in the institutionalized elderly is 13 to 89.3 percent (Brocklehurst 1985). Burgio (1988) examined 154 residents who were continent and incontinent. Fifty-four percent of the patients displayed impairments in cognition and mobility. It is not only a major social problem for the elderly, but a major financial burden for society. Recently nurse researchers have been addressing the use of various experimental interventions such as education programs that focus on biofeedback and kegel exercises as a means of reducing the incidence of urinary incontinence (Wells and Jiovec 1985, Burns, et al. 1985).

Ouslander (1987) determined in 50 continent and 50 incontinent residents that there was no significant differences in participation in social or recreational activities. The difference was more related to their level of agility.

Taylor and Henderson (1986) reported on their pilot study in which they also examined the effects of biofeedback on pubococcygeal muscle strength and simple urinary stress incontinence in a small sample of 12 post-menopausal women. Effective use of kegel exercises appears to be related to teaching the exercises correctly, assisting the older adult in identifying the correct muscle to contract, allowing enough time for the exercise sessions, and using the visual personal perionometer. As part of a larger study which was designed to test the efficacy of a noninvasive behavioral treatment approach called Pattern Urge Response Toileting (PURT) for urinary incontinence (UI) in nursing home residents, Campbell (1991) examined 166 staff members in four nursing homes. In the treatment group, there was a slight increase in the staff's knowledge about UI and its treatment; maintenance of positive outlook over 9 months; 72% compliance with the toileting protocol by residents with staff assistance; and evidence of reduced UI in the residents. Currently this area of nursing research is receiving federal and private funding and holds much promise for replication and additional experimental research efforts.

KEY POINTS

◆ Increased fiber and bran cereals help to maintain the bulk of the diet and improve the consistency of the bowel movement.

◆ Implementation of bowel management programs for the residents and upgrading the in-service education programs for staff are successful in helping to alleviate the problem of bowel incontinence.

◆ Accurate assessment of the underlying causes of UI is important to be able to identify those residents whose problem of UI would be amenable to an education-Kegel exercise program.

◆ There is validity in the use of Kegel exercises, education, biofeedback, toileting programs, and selected equipment for UI.

◆ Activity-Exercise Pattern

The Activity-Exercise Pattern describes patterns of exercise, activity, leisure, and recreation. Included are activities of daily living, hygiene, and cooking. Neuromuscular deficits, cardiac-pulmonary dysfunctions, and other factors that interfere with this pattern are also included.

Body movement (exercise, activity) has been the focus for several of the research studies. Fitzpatrick and Donovan (1978) examined the differences in body movement and an individual's temporal experience of the past, present, and future in an institutionalized group and a non-institutionalized group of older adults. Those elderly found within institutions were more past oriented, less concerned with present and future, and displayed more body movement. This latter finding appeared to be related to the fact that they were interviewed within their own familiar surroundings. Non-institutionalized elderly appeared to be more concerned with their present life and activities. Knowledge of the older adult's orientation to past, present, and future will be useful in the planning, designing, and delivering of health care services.

In an experimental nursing research study: *Movement Therapy and the Aged,* Goldberg and Fitzpatrick (1980) examined the effects of participation in a movement therapy group on morale and self-esteem in a sample of 30 institutionalized older adults. Participants in the experimental group demonstrated significant improvement in total morale and attitudes toward their own aging as compared to the control group. Movement Therapy is viewed as a nursing intervention, since nurses are oriented to the wholeness of the individual.

Nursing has long recognized the importance of foot care in the routine daily care of the older adult. Foot health is vital to mobility and helps to determine the quality of one's existence. In a descriptive study, Schank (1987) surveyed 125 members of a large urban senior center. Among those indicating foot problems, women outnumbered the men 89% to 61%. The five most frequently cited foot complaints were corns (41 percent), callouses (30 percent), toenail problems (24 percent), bunions (22 percent), and edema (19 percent). Only one-third of the subjects sought medical advice for foot problems. Self-care practices included foot soaks, medicated corn pads, self-filing, and cutting of own corns and toenails.

Once the finding of this descriptive nursing research study were reviewed, the need for a well-developed foot care education program became evident. Conrad described the development of this program, which was implemented in five senior centers. Nurses and podiatrists worked closely in the planning and implementation of the program. In the reported program evaluation study, response and attendance of the elderly were most positive. Of the 377 persons examined, 102 were contacted for follow-up. Follow-up revealed the need for further clarification of podiatrist's recommendations, counseling regarding specific foot care practices, and general health teaching.

Inherent in mobility and activity is the potential problem of older persons falling and injuring themselves. According to the National Center of Health Statistics, more than one third of the deaths from unintentional injury in people 65 and over are attributable to falls.

Patient falls have always been a major area of concern for nurses in all health care settings. It is viewed by other health disciplines as a "nursing problem." In their descriptive study, Morse, et al. (1985) examined those patients who had fallen twice in one month or three times in one year. Comparisons were made of two groups of 20 subjects each that were matched according to diagnosis, age, and sex. No differences were noted between the two groups for weight, temperature, vital signs, hemoglobin, drug risk, sensory impairment, or mental status. Of importance was the significant difference in the patients' gait and mobility capabilities. The multiple faller group were more apt to exhibit impaired gait secondary to old age, spastic hemiparesis, or Parkinsonian tremors than the control group.

Hernandez and Miller (1986) conducted a two-year nursing project on a 21 bed geropsychiatric unit in order to identify precipitants and predictors of falls, develop and test levels of fall precautions, and decrease the incidence of falls. The goals of this project were met. Recommendations for nurse administrators and staff were identified and included identification of risk factors, *Fall Assessment Instrument,* and the Fall Precautions Program.

Craven and Burns (1986) identified the predictors for falls in a convenience sample of 99 non-institutionalized ambulatory elderly living in an inner city area. The risk factors identified were in agreement with the previous nursing research findings. The factor set of age, living alone, visual deficits, balance problems, and neurologic problems had 66 percent ability to predict falls. This set of predictors may be used to identify those older adults who may be in need of learning preventive behaviors and measures.

Evans and Strumpf (1989) reported that in the course of a year, more than 500,000 older persons are tied to their beds and chairs in hospitals and nursing homes. The Health Care Financing Administration (1988) identified that from 1976 to 1988, the use of restraints has increased from 25% to 41% in nursing home settings. The Omnibus Budget Reconciliation Act (OBRA) of 1987 legislates a mechanism for decreasing the use of restraints by protecting patients from being restrained for discipline or convenience purposes. Janelli et al. (1991) examined the knowledge level of nursing home staff regarding the proper use and application of physical restraints. This was part of a larger study which also examined nursing practice and staff attitudes about restraints. Of the 118 nursing staff, there were 63 aides, 38 LPNs, and 17 RNs who worked all three shifts in a county nursing home. Knowledge was measured by 18 true or false questions and examined the different types of restraints, procedures for applying these restraints, and circumstances or legality of application of restraints. Significant differences were found related to level of knowledge in RNs versus LPNs and NAs. There was no relationship between the level of knowledge and age of staff, shift they worked, and years in gerontological nursing. Implications for role playing, demonstration and discussion for staff and family members were described.

A fractured hip is often the sequelae to a fall. Post-operative nursing care greatly contributes to the ease and speed of the older adult's recuperation and rehabilitation. Correct positioning has been stressed as being of utmost importance to this process. Lamb (1979) determined there was no significant relationship to comfort in turning patients following open reduction and internal fixation with pins/plate of fractured hip to either the operated or unoperated side. There was also no relationship between the subject's preferred side to sleep on and their subsequent comfort level. Body weight made no significant difference in comfort level.

The Activity-Exercise Pattern also includes cardiac-pulmonary dysfunctions, such as chronic bronchitis and emphysema. Perry (1981) evaluated the effectiveness of the educational component of a rehabilitation program for 20 patients ages 51 to 70 with chronic bronchitis and emphysema. This study indicated maximizing the subjects' involvement in the rehabilitation program fostered their ability to make decisions and take actions required in order to cope with their illness.

In summary, the finding of the above nursing research studies should be viewed only as preliminary due to small sample sizes. However, these articles are in sufficient detail to permit and encourage replication.

KEY POINTS

◆ The positive effects of body movement and exercise on the older adult's total morale and perceptions of their own aging has been documented.

◆ Nursing assessment and education programs to address the problems of foot care, prevention of falls, and rehabilitation of the older adult with chronic bronchitis and emphysema is useful.

◆ Following implementation of OBRA in 1987, there exists legal means to protect the residents from being restrained for discipline or convenience purposes.

◆ Sleep-Rest Pattern

The Sleep-Rest Pattern describes the patterns of sleep and rest—relaxation periods during a twenty-four hour day. It includes the type of night-time medications and routines an individual may use. Perceptions of quality and quantity of sleep and resulting energy levels are also addressed.

Nurse researchers in addressing the Sleep-Rest Pattern have been interested in identifying, describing, and comparing sleep patterns of the older adult in a variety of settings. Pacini and Fitzpatrick (1982) examined the sleep patterns of 38 individuals between the ages of 60 and 82: Half were hospitalized in the acute care facility and the other half resided in their own homes or with relatives. The variables of nocturnal sleep time (sleep at night), other sleep time, bedtime, and time for awakening were examined. Findings indicated the hospital environment has some influence in terms of alternating measured patterns of sleep, other sleep time, nocturnal sleep time, and bedtime. Apparently, health status, state of mind, and state of fatigue also contribute to the alteration in sleep patterns of the hospitalized older adult. In the event of the older adult needing to be hospitalized, it would be important for the nurse in the long-term care setting to convey in the transfer note, information about the resident's sleep patterns and routines in order to ensure as smooth a transition as possible.

Patterns of sleep were also examined by Hayter (1983). She identified the primary changes in sleep associated with aging which include increased time spent sleeping including nap time; increased night-time awakenings; and changes in the stages of sleep. After the age of 85, there is a change to an earlier bedtime, a longer time required to get to sleep, and the total time sleeping.

The interventions of giving sleep medication at an earlier time was examined by Dittmar & Dulski (1977). Outcomes of this intervention indicated an improvement in activities of daily living and a high incidence of negative social behavior with family, staff, and other patients. The authors suggested this negative social behavior when linked with improved activities of daily living, may be viewed as positive. The older adult is seen as mobilizing energy and becoming reactive to the environment and their present situation.

Jean Hayter Muncy (1986), in a later study, reviewed the existing nursing and other research on sleep. She described ten measures with extensive scientific rationale that nurses should use in order to enhance sleep in the older adult.

Bowe (1989) reviewed the various research studies that examined the self-regulation techniques of progressive muscle relaxation (PMR), Benson's Relaxation Response, biofeedback, yoga, and imagery. Progressive Muscle Relaxation was developed by Bernstein and Borkovec to produce skeletal muscle relaxation and reduce stimulation of other bodily systems. The resident learns to sense the presence of tension and consciously produce a state of relaxation. This relaxation is accompanied by a reduction in mental processing such as worrying, negative mental images and an increase in an experience of peace. PMR was used successfully in improving insomnia for 22 older adults over a 4-week time period. However, improvement was not retained (Engle-Friedman, 1986). The Relaxation Response, which focuses on breathing and meditation, helps to produce a state of relaxation. Biofeedback focuses on achieving physiological reactions through voluntary control of internal body responses. Yoga, a meditation and breathing technique, is used to produce a serenity of the mind which is essential for a healthy body. Imagery employs the imagination of the resident in focusing on settings filled with happiness and relaxation rather than stressful situations. Validity of many of these studies must be questioned because of the weaknesses of the research design. Sample sizes are not clearly identified.

KEY POINTS

◆ Nurses need to include information about the resident's sleep patterns and routines in the transfer note from the nursing home to the hospital.

◆ Sleep medications are to be given at an earlier time in the evening.

◆ Use of self-regulation techniques of progressive muscle relaxation such as Benson's Relaxation Response, biofeedback, yoga, and imagery are encouraged.

◆ Self-Perception–Self-Concept Pattern and the Role-Relationship Pattern

There are common problems of the older adult which are able to be addressed under the combined patterns of Self-Perception–Self-Concept Pattern and the Role-Relationship Pattern. The Self-Perception–Self-Concept Pattern includes the individual's attitudes about self; perception of their own cognitive, affective, and physical abilities; body image; identity; self-worth; and general emotional pattern. Body posture, movement, eye contact, voice, and speech patterns are also included. In the Role-Relationship Pattern, the individuals' perceptions of their current major roles and responsibilities in life and their level of satisfaction in relationships with family, work, and others are included.

One of the prevailing problems of elderly persons seems to be the various types of losses they experience. Loss of persons who have been important in their lives, places, roles, cognitive functions, as well as physical functions and loss of independence frequently surface. Disengagement and depression are often observed. It is important for those caring for the elderly person to understand these variables in order to effectively intervene and assist the individual in coping with such losses.

Wolanin (1978), in her review of research on relocation of the elderly, noted that relocation can be life-threatening if not accompanied by needed planning and preparation of the individual. The principles that contributed to successful relocation in her study included the patient's right to information and participation in the move; the right to make choices, whenever possible; inclusion of families and staff in any move; maintaining familiar features in the new environment; and orienting the person to the new environment.

Old age, with its general slowing down, impacts on health. Differences and commonalities on how this impact is experienced by men and women has been identified. Cowling and Campbell (1986) researched the literature and concluded that health, retirement, dependency, and sexuality are the major concerns of older men.

McElmurry and LiBrizzi (1986) developed an instrument to evaluate the self-reported health concerns of older women, using field research or research conducted in actual clinical settings. Findings from their study indicated that the profile of older women suggest health and independence with a capacity for self-care. This profile contradicts the common stereotype of the older woman as ill and dependent. Since psychological well-being is a predictor of health, it can be inferred that a positive image of old age in women will contribute to their well-being. Nurses can project that positive image to their patients in their everyday interactions by stressing the patients' assets and strengths.

One way to strengthen feelings of independence and self-esteem in the resident is by teaching a program of self-medication (Webb, 1990).

Another common change that occurs in old age and represents a major role change, as well as a loss, is the death of a mate. Richter (1984) researched the literature about this phenomenon and described a conceptual model for the crisis of mate loss that emphasizes the nurses' role in facilitating rsources to a spouse during the dying process of the mate. The major resources identified were the interpersonal support provided by other people, their own religious spiritual beliefs, and their interpersonal coping skills in dealing positively with their own difficulties.

Loss of independence with resulting dependency behaviors can be devastating to the individual. Miller (1984) reviewed studies and found that the dependency is more often the result of the patient's interaction with the institutional environment than the effect of medical or physical factors. She proposes that nurses often inadvertently reinforce dependent behaviors, when a medical approach or treatment of disease is the focus of action rather than the focus being a behavioral approach and treating the person as a whole being. Lester and Baltes (1978) also described the relationship between social environment in institutions and the behavior of the elderly. They concluded that dependent behaviors are given more positive verbal reinforcement by nursing personnel than are independent behaviors. They suggested the importance of the nurse as the change agent in fostering independent and dependent behaviors.

Depression is a frequent occurrence in older adults. Newman and Gaudiano (1984) examined depression and its relationship to decreased perception of time by the older adult. Their findings suggest that depression may be a contributing factor to this diminished sense of time. Increased sense of time adds to the quality of life of the older person and the value of focusing on intra versus inter activity is seen. This includes reminiscing about past events that are meaningful to the person.

According to Zerhusen et al. (1991), group cognitive therapy is also effective for depressed elderly persons. In this study, nursing home residents made substantial positive gains using cognitive therapy techniques.

Whether disengagement or gradual withdrawing from social involvement is a normal function of aging is questioned in a study by Henthorn (1979). Results of this study, which compared nursing home residents and community registered voters, suggested that situational factors add to the disengagement process. This process is also viewed as being reversible. Social learning principles used by personnel to reinforce active behavior rather than extinguishing or punishing such behavior can influence the disengagement process and foster more positive actions and attitudes.

KEY POINTS

◆ Older adults need orientation to new situations and environments.

◆ Familiar features should be included when relocating.

◆ Nurses need to encourage independent behaviors and not reinforce inappropriate dependent behaviors in residents.

◆ Techniques such as reminiscence and cognitive therapy may help promote positive self-perceptions and prevent depression.

SIDEBAR

The importance of an assessment that allows an accurate nursing diagnosis cannot be overemphasized.

With an accurate nursing diagnosis, the nurse can then look for available research finding to support nursing interventions.

An inability to find the necessary researched scientific support may provide the necessary motivation and impetus for the staff nurses to institute a small clinical research study in their own setting.

◆ Sexuality-Reproductive Pattern

A review of the literature reveals no current nursing research that has addressed the Sexuality-Reproductive Pattern area. This pattern describes the reproductive pattern and the individual's perceived satisfaction or disturbances in their own sexuality. Also included are post-menopause and other perceived problem areas.

In the past, nurse researchers have studied this pattern area from the perspective of attitudes of others toward sexuality in the older adult. There are many myths and misconceptions. The lack in this area of formalized nursing research does not negate its importance. Rather, it highlights the need for nurse researchers to address this area. Literature from other health disciplines identifies that sexuality need not diminish with age. This is also confirmed by the older adult population.

KEY POINTS

◆ Changes due to aging may affect sexual behaviors but these changes do not negate sexuality in older persons.

◆ There is a need for research in sexuality in old age.

◆ Cognitive-Perceptual Pattern and the Coping-Stress Tolerance Pattern

For several years, nurse researchers have examined interventions to enhance cognitive and behavioral functioning of the older adult. These studies encompass both the Cognitive-Perceptual Pattern and the Coping-Stress Tolerance Pattern. The Cognitive-Perceptual Pattern includes the sensory modes of vision, hearing, taste, touch, and smell, as well as the cognitive functional abilities of language, memory, and decision-making. The Coping-Stress Tolerance Pattern includes the older adult's capacity to resist challenges and stress to self-integrity, modes of handling stress, types of family and other support systems, and the perceived ability to control and manage life's situations.

Armstrong-Esther and Browne (1986) investigated nurse patient interaction on a geriatric ward in relation to cognitive and behavioral functioning. Results showed generally low levels of staff-patient communication with even lower rates of interaction with confused patients. Although patients were observed to spend most of their time doing nothing, nursing staff perceived their main function as providing physical care rather than psychosocial interaction or types of restorative activities. These findings raise questions about common perceptions of nursing staff regarding their ability and responsibility to provide non-physical types of care to patients, especially those who are mentally impaired.

Interactions between nursing staff and institutionalized cognitively impaired Alzheimer's Dementia (AD) residents also have been described by Burgener and Barton (1991). Approaches which improve the management of these situations were identified. Staff's relaxed behavior and flexibility were related to the residents' flexibility, ability to relax, remain calm, and be cooperative. Use of the personal approach rather than an authoritarian or task-oriented manner was also found effective. The amount of staff's verbal output was more important than the actual content in stimulating the resident's interest or cooperation. Use of distraction and redirection by the staff was effective in avoiding an uncooperative, tense, or agitated incident with a resident. The presence of a second caregiver was also important in AD persons prone to paranoia or swift changes in affect.

Baily, et al. (1986) described a 24-hour reality orientation program, which included organizing reality orientation support groups, providing encouragement, and bringing in outside groups to participate in the program and provide additional resources and support. This was done in a long-stay geriatric ward. Their findings indicated that such a program maintained functional levels in the subjects and, in some cases, slightly improved the level of function. This was done primarily through environmental interventions and demonstrated the effectiveness of interdisciplinary efforts by all staff concerned with the care of these patients.

Hughes (1979) studied the future orientation of older adults living in an institution and found that residents were not future-oriented. Their orientation also became less recent the longer they stayed in the institution. The findings of this study suggest that many nurse patient interactions focus on the person's limitations and tend to discourage the patients from positive planning and participation in activities. It is suggested that persons caring for patients in an institution be educated about the impact of their messages to individuals, especially as these messages may convey deterrents to trying new and interesting activities, based on excessive fear of injury or illness.

Jones and van Amelsvort Jones (1986) studied verbal communication between nursing staff and elderly residents in a long-term care facility and compared these patterns based on different ethnic backgrounds of the residents. Although this study had a model sample size (N = 41), the findings showed that residents who were not Canadian-born or born in the United Kingdom were communicated to with significantly less frequency than those who were of similar ethnic background as the staff. This study raises an issue that is an ongoing challenge to nursing staff as they work to overcome language barriers and cultural differences that interfere with care and communication with older persons who have relocated from other cultures.

Louis (1981) described an empirical study of the personal space boundary needs of older persons. Her findings supported the concept of individual differences in preference for personal space. Subjects needed less space when approached frontally than when they were approached from the side or the back.

Krause (1986) studied the effect of social support in lessening the impact of stressful life events on depressive symptoms in a community sample of older adults. Findings showed that these supports did not help when the stressful event was global.

Specific types of social support were found to assist individuals in specific types of stressful situations. One of these was in bereavement, where there is often an accompanying life transition.

Sheehan (1986) studied informal support among tenants in public senior housing projects by using self-administered questionnaires and interviews. Results showed the existence of this type of support, but noted that frail and impaired tenants received less support than tenants in stronger health. Frail tenants sought less involvement with others. These findings have implications for nurses who work in community settings and are in a position to identify frail, elderly persons and assist them in participating in needed informal support activities.

Hollinger (1986) studied the relationship between nurses, touch, and the verbal responses of the hospitalized elderly during nurse-patient interactions. Findings support the importance of initial introduction of nurses to elderly persons and the importance of assessing the individual patient's comfort level with touch. Touch was seen as a communication technique within a holistic view of elderly persons and their environment.

Palmateer and McCartney (1985) compared use of a standardized screening tool to nursing assessment techniques in order to identify cognitively impaired elderly patients. Nursing assessment techniques failed to identify a significant number of these patients on admission. Although the researchers noted the limitations of the findings, study results raise a question which has been addressed by others in relation to improvement of assessment techniques used to evaluate cognitive deficits.

Clites described a group project designed to assist elderly survivors in coping with loss of close friends and relatives. This was seen as a successful experiment and a useful form of mental health intervention.

Schwab, et al. (1985) described a program called SERVE which is an acronym for Self-Esteem, Relaxation, Vitality, and Exercise. This program was initiated to deal with nursing problems and improve functioning in patients with dementia. It was part of a Teaching Nursing Home program. Results to date indicate that this is an effective intervention.

KEY POINTS

◆ Staff interactions in a relaxed, flexible, and personal manner are important to being able to work effectively with all patients, most particularly with those who are cognitively impaired or confused.

◆ Use of reality orientation support groups can help patients who are cognitively impaired.

◆ Staff needs to find ways to overcome barriers to patient communication due to language and cultural differences.

◆ Touch may be used therapeutically as a communication technique when it is acceptable to the resident.

SUMMARY

This chapter has reviewed selected gerontological nursing research studies conducted within the period of 1955 through 1992 by nurse researchers and described in selected nursing journals. There is inconsistency as to the use of theoretical frameworks, rigor of the research design, sampling method, appropriateness of sample size, and methods of data analysis. The instruments used have either been created by the researcher or taken from other research studies. Despite these limitations, gerontological nursing research has begun to move beyond the descriptive phase to examination of the effectiveness of various nursing interventions in helping the older adult to maintain a high quality of life. Choice of intervention will depend on the individual resident, nursing diagnosis, and available resources. Research findings may also provide the necessary support and rationale needed to substantiate nursing's request for additional resources and personnel.

Future directions have been identified for several well-known gerontological nurse experts and researchers. Clinical nursing must now become the major focus for gerontological nurse researchers. Haight and Bahr (1991) identified the Nursing Research agenda in long term care for the 1990s. The top 10 items included: patient outcomes, functional status-assessment and intervention; effects of institutionalization; safety/environmental features; post-discharge care; falls; depression; quality assurance, restraints and sensory deprivation or overload.

Hall (1991) further advocated the need to do clinical research on residents in the end stage of dementia in order to be able to answer the question of, "What can we do when we can't do any more?" These are but a few of the day-to-day problems in long-term care and chronic illness that need to be evaluated. The staff nurse in the long-term care setting is in an excellent position to have a major role in gerontological nursing research.

By keeping their knowledge base current, either by reading the nursing and nursing research journals and/or by attending workshops and continuing education classes, the gerontological nurse is able to incorporate those research findings applicable to their given work setting into their own nursing practice. This incorporation of additional scientific rationale will serve to strengthen and expand their practice. It will also assist in helping them to gain additional professional recognition and accountability.

◆ The Role of the Staff Nurse in a Long-term Care Setting in Gerontological Nursing Research

The staff nurse is one of the most critical elements in nursing research. Without his or her expertise and knowledge in nursing, research could not provide the realistic enhancements to an older adult's life that it does. Some roles for the staff nurse in research are to identify problem areas suitable for research; to assist in helping to make the research design realistic and workable in the given setting; to introduce the principal nurse researcher to the residents and staff member of nursing and other health disciplines; to assure the ethical principles required are adhered to for the protection of the resident subject; to assist in the collection of data; to serve as a co-presenter of the study's findings at a local, regional, or national nursing/research conference; to be a co-author on an article reporting on the research study and submit it for publication.

However, the most important outcome of involvement of the staff nurse in gerontological nursing research will be the enhancement and improvement of the quality of care they are able to provide for the older adults who are trying to maintain their individuality, independence, and quality of life.

References

Adams, M. Aging: Gerontological nursing research. In *Annual Review of Nursing Research.* 4th ed. New York: Springer Publishing Company; 1986; IV: 77–103.

Armstrong-Esther, CA, Browne, KD. The influence of elderly patients' mental impairment on nurse-patient interaction. *J. of Advanced Nursing.* July 1986; 11:379–387.

Bahr, Sr. RT, Gress, L. The 24-hour cycle: Rhythms of healthy sleep. *J. of Gerontological Nursing.* April 1985; 11:14–17.

Bailey, EA, Brown, S, Goble, REA, Holden UP. Twenty-four hour reality orientation: Changes for staff and patients. *J. Advanced Nursing.* March 1986; 11:145–151.

Bassen, PH. The gerontological nursing literature. *Nursing Research.* 1967; 16:267–272.

Bower, M. Self regulation techniques in the elderly. *J. of Gerontological Nursing.* January 1989; 15:15–20.

Boykin, A, Winland-Brown, J. Pressure sores: Nursing management. *J. of Gerontological Nursing.* May 1986; 12:17–21.

Brimmer, PF. Past present and future in gerontological nursing research. *J. of Gerontological Nursing.* 1979; 5:27–34.

Brocklehurst, JC. *Textbook of Geriatric Medicine and Gerontology.* Edinburgh: Churchill Livingston; 1985.

Brower, T, Crist, MA. Research priorities in gerontologic nursing in long-term care. *Image: The Journal of Nursing Scholarship.* Winter 1985; XVII:22–27.

Brown, M, Boosinger, J, Henderson, M, Rife, S, Rustia, J, Taylor, D, Young, W. Drug-drug interactions among residents in homes for the elderly: A pilot study. *Nursing Research.* January–February 1977; 26:47–52.

Burgener, S, Barton, D. Nursing care of cognitively impaired, institutionalized elderly. *J. of Gerontological Nursing.* November 1991; 17:37–43.

Burgio, LD, Jones, LT, Engle, BT. Studying incontinence in an urban nursing home. *J. of Gerontological Nursing.* May 1988; 14:40–45.

Burns, P, Mareki, M, Dittmar, S, Bullough, B. Kegel's exercises with biofeedback therapy for treatment of stress incontinence. *Nurse Practitioner.* February 1985; 28–35.

Burnside, I. Gerontological nursing research: 1975 to 1984. In NLN (Eds). *Overcoming the bias of ageism in long-term care.* NLN Publication #20-1975. New York: NLN Publication Company; 1985:121–140.

Campbell, E, Knight, M, Benson, M, Colling, J. Effect of an incontinence training program on nursing home staff's knowledge, attitudes and behavior. *Gerontologist.* December, 1991; 31:788–794.

Clites, J. Maximizing the memory retention in the aged. *J. of Gerontological Nursing.* August 1984; 10:34–39.

Conrad, C. Foot education and screening programs for the elderly. *J. of Gerontological Nursing.* November–December 1977; 3:11–15.

Cowling, WR, Campbell, V. Health concerns of aging men. *Nursing Clinics of North America.* March 1986; 21:75–83.

Craven, R, Burns, P. Teach the elderly to prevent falls. *J. of Gerontological Nursing.* August 1986; 12:27–33.

Davis, A, Nagelhout, M, Hoban, M, Barnard, B. Bowel management a quality assurance approach to upgrading programs. *J. of Gerontological Nursing.* May 1986; 12:13–17.

Dewalt, EM. Effect of timed hygienic measures on oral mucosa in a group of elderly subjects. *Nursing Research.* March–April 1977; 13:104–108.

Dittmar, SS, Dulski, T. Early evening administration of sleep medication to the hospitalized aged: A consideration in rehabilitation. *Nursing Research.* July–August 1977; 26:299–303.

Dye, C. The aging society and nursing research. In *The Aging Society: A challenge for nursing education.* Atlanta, Georgia: Southern Regional Educational Board; 1983.

Eaton, M, Bitchell-Bonair, I, Friedmann, E. The effect of touch on nutritional intake of chronic organic brain syndrome patients. *J. of Gerontology.* September 1986; 41:611–616.

Engle, VF, Graney, MJ. Meta-analysis for the refinement of gerontological nursing research and theory. *J. of Gerontological Nursing.* September 1990; 16:12–15.

Engle-Friedman, M. An evaluation of behavioral treatments for insomnia in the older adult. Dissertation Abstracts International. 1986; 46:2803B.

Evans, LK, Strumpf, NE. Tying down the elderly: A review of the literature on physical restraints. *J. of the American Geriatrics Society.* January 1989; 37:65–74.

Fitzpatrick, J, Donovan, MJ. Temporal experience and motor behavior among the aging. *Research in Nursing and Health.* 1978; 1:60–68.

Gallagher, E. Capitalize on elder strengths. *J. of Gerontological Nursing.* June 1985; 11:13–17.

Gioiella, E. The relationships between slowness of response, state anxiety, social isolation, and self-esteem, and preferred personal space in the elderly. *J. of Gerontological Nursing.* January 1987; 4:40–43.

Goldberg, W, Fitzpatrick, J. Movement therapy with the aged. *Nursing Research.* November–December 1980; 29:339–346.

Gorden, M. *Nursing diagnosis: Process and application.* New York: McGraw-Hill; 1982:84–97.

Gunter, LM, Miller, JC. Toward a nursing gerontology. *Nursing Research.* 1977; 26:208–221.

Haight, B. Update on research in long-term care: 1984–1988. NLN Pub. 1989; #20-2292:7–51.

Haight, B, Bahr, Sister RT. A report: Long-term care nursing research agenda for the 1990's. NLN Publ. 1991; #41-2382:77–102.

Hall, G. Editorial: Examining the end stage: What can we do when we can't do any more? *J. of Gerontological Nursing.* September 1991; 17:3–4.

Hallal, J. Nursing diagnosis: An essential step to quality care. *J. of Gerontological Nursing.* September 1985; 11:35–38.

Hayter, J. Sleep behaviors of older adults. *Nursing Research.* 1983; 32:242–246.

Health Care Financing Administration. Medicare/Medicaid nursing homes information: 1987–1988. ISSN 0364 6750. Washington, D.C.: U.S. Government Printing Office. 1988.

Henthorn, B. Disengagement and reinforcement in the elderly. *Research in Nursing and Health.* 1979; 2:1–8.

Hernandez, M, Miller, J. How to reduce falls. *Geriatric Nursing.* March–April 1986; 7:97–102.

Hollinger, L. Communicating with the elderly. *J. of Gerontological Nursing.* March 1986; 12:8–13.

Hughes, E. Institutionalized older adults and their future orientation. *J. of the American Geriatrics Society.* March 1979; XXVII:130–134.

Janelli, L, Scherer, Y, Kanski, G, Neary, M. What nursing staff members really know about physical restraints. *Rehabilitation Nursing.* November–December 1991; 16:345–348.

Jones, P, Millman, A. A three-part system to combat pressure sores. *Geriatric Nursing.* March–April 1986; 7:78–82.

Jones, P, van Amelsvort Jones, G. Communication patterns between nursing staff and the ethnic elderly in a long-term care facility. *J. of Advanced Nursing.* May 1986; 11:265–272.

Kayser-Jones, J. Gerontological nursing research revisited. *J. of Gerontological Nursing.* 1981; 217–223.

Kee, C. A case for health promotion with the elderly. *Nursing Clinics of No. America.* June 1984; 19:251–262.

Kim, K, Grier, M. Pacing effects of medication instruction for the elderly. *J. of Gerontological Nursing.* August 1981; 7:464–468.

Kolanowski, A, Gunter, L. Hypothermia in the elderly. In *Geriatric Nursing.* September–October 1981; 2:362–365.

Kolanowski, A, Gunter, L. What are the health practices of retired career women? *J. of Gerontological Nursing.* December 1985; 11:22–30.

Krause, N. Social support, stress, and well-being among older adults. *J. of Gerontology,* July 1986; 41:512–519.

Lamb, K. Effect of positioning of post-operative fractured hip patients as related to comfort. *Nursing Research.* September–October 1979; 28:291–294.

Lester, P, Baltes, M. Functional interdependence of the social environment and the behavior of the institutional aged. *J. of Gerontological Nursing.* March–April 1978; 4:23–27.

Longman, A, Dewalt, ZM. A guide for oral assessment. *Geriatric Nursing.* September–October 1986; 7:252–253.

Louis, M. Personal space boundary needs of elderly persons an empirical study. *J. of Gerontological Nursing.* July 1981; 7:395–400.

McElmurry, B, LiBrizzi, S. The health of older women. *Nursing Clinics of No. America.* March 1986; 21:161–171.

McGlove, F, Kick, E. Health habits in relation to aging. *J. of the American Geriatrics Soc.* November 1978; XXVI:481–488.

Melillo, K. Who needs health maintenance? *J. of Gerontological Nursing.* February 1985; 11:18–21.

Michaelsson, E, Norberg, A, Norberg, B. A quality of life issue: Feeding methods for demented patients in the end stage of life. *Geriatric Nursing.* September 1987; 8:69–73.

Miller, A. Nurse/patient dependency—a review of different approaches with particular reference to studies of the dependency of elderly patients. *J. of Advanced Nursing.* December 1984; 9:479–486.

Morse, JM, Tylko, SJ, Dixon, HA. The patient who falls and falls again. *J. of Gerontological Nursing.* November 1985; 11:15–18.

Muncy-Hayter, J. Measures to rid sleeplessness. *J. of Gerontological Nursing.* August 1986; 12:6–11.

National Safety Council, Home Department. Older Americans accidents facts age 65 and over. Chicago: The Council; 1980.

Naylor, M, Shaid, E. Content analysis of pre and post discharge topics taught to hospitalized elderly by gerontological nurse specialists. *Clinical Nurse Specialist.* Summer 1991; 5:111–116.

Newman, M, Guadiano, J. Depression as an explanation for decreased subjective time in the elderly. *Nursing Research.* May–June 1984; 33:137–139.

Nichols, B. *Nursing shortage and nursing within the long term setting.* Unpublished testimony before the House Select Committee on Aging; 1980.

O'Leary, P, McGill, J, Jones, K, Paul, P. Gerontological research: Is it useful for nursing practice. *J. of Gerontological Nursing.* May 1990; 16:28–32.

Ouslander, JG, Morishita, L, Blaustein, J, Orzeck, S, Dunn, S, Sayre, J. Clinical, functional, and psychosocial characteristics in an incontinent nursing home population. *J. of Gerontology.* November 1987; 42:631–637.

Pacini, CM, Fitzpatrick, JJ. Sleep patterns of hospitalized and nonhospitalized aged individuals. *J. of Gerontological Nursing.* June 1982; 8:327–332.

Palmateer, L, McCartney, JR. Do nurses know when patients have cognitive defects? *J. of Gerontological Nursing.* February 1985; 11:6–16.

Parent, C, Whall, A. Are physical activity, self-esteem, and depression related? *J. of Gerontological Nursing.* September 1984; 10:8–11.

Pease, R. Praise elders to help them learn. *J. of Gerontological Nursing.* March 1985; 11:16–20.

Perry, J. Effectiveness of teaching in the rehabilitation of patients with chronic bronchitis and emphsyema. *Nursing Research.* July–August 1981; 30:219–222.

Peters, D. An overview of current research relating to outcomes of care. NLN Publ. 1989; #20-2292:61–79.

Pritchard, V. Tube feeding related pneumonias. *J. of Gerontological Nursing.* July 1988; 14:32–36.

Richter, J. Crisis of mate loss in the elderly. *Advances in Nursing Science.* July 1984; 45–54.

Schank, MJ. A survey of the well elderly: Their foot problems, practices, and needs. *J. of Gerontological Nursing.* November–December 1987; 3:11–151.

Schwab, M, Rader, J, Doan, J. Relieving the anxiety and fear in dementia. *J. of Gerontological Nursing.* May 1985; 11:8–15.

Sheehan, N. Informal support among the elderly in public senior housing. *The Gerontologist.* April 1986; 26:171–175.

Spitzer, M. Taste acuity in institutionalized and non-institutionalized elderly men. *J. of Gerontology.* May 1988; 43:71–74.

Taylor, K, Henderson, J. Effects of biofeedback and urinary stress incontinence in older women. *J. of Gerontological Nursing.* September 1986; 12:25–30.

Thompson, LF, Steffl, BM. Research in gerontological nursing. In B. Steffl (ed.). *Handbook of Gerontological Nursing.* New York: Van Nostrand Reinhold; 1984:513–528.

Utley, Q, Rasie, S. Coping with loss. *J. of Gerontological Nursing.* August 1984; 10:8–14.

Volicer, L, Seltzer, B, Rheaume Y, Karner, J, Glennon, M, Riley, M. Eating difficulties in patients with probable dementia of the Alzheimer type. *J. of Geriatric Psychology Neurol.* June 1989; 2:188–195.

Webb, C, Addison, C, Holman, H, Saklaki, B, Wagner, A. Self medication for elderly patients. *Nursing Times.* April 18, 1990; 16:46–49.

Wells, TJ. *Problems in geriatric nursing care.* New York: Churchill Livingston; 1980.

Wells TJ, Jiovec, MM. *Factors associated with urine control in elderly with degenerative brain disease.* Paper presented at annual meeting of the Gerontological Society of America; November 1985; New Orleans, LA.

West, J, Brockman, S, Scott, A. Action research and standards of care. The prevention and treatment of pressure sores in elderly patients. *Health Bulletin.* November 1991; 49:356–361.

Wichita, C. Treating and preventing constipation in nursing home residents. *J. of Gerontological Nursing.* November–December 1977; 2:35–39.

Wolanin, M. Relocation of the elderly. *J. of Gerontological Nursing.* May–June 1978; 4:47–50.

Zerhusen, J, Boyle, K, Wilson, W. Out of the darkness: Group cognitive therapy for the depressed elderly. *J. of Psychosocial Nursing and Mental Health Services.* 1991; 29:16–21.

4

Health Perception— Health Management Pattern

Richard S. Ferri

◆

HEALTH MAINTENANCE ALTERATION

◆ Nursing Diagnosis

The inability to identify, manage, and/or seek out help to maintain health. This phenomenon occurs in all age groups. In the very young, health may not be independently maintained due to developmental immaturity and primary inability to self-manage. In the elderly, physical and/or psychosocial deterioration may affect the ability to identify and/or seek health maintenance assistance. In all other age groups, illness may affect the individual's ability to self-manage; lack of available resources, both financial and community-based, may involuntarily restrict the individual from meeting identified health needs.

ASSESSMENT

A practitioner can identify an individual as having the nursing diagnosis of Health Maintenance Alteration as part of the overall nursing history and general assessment. The resident will demonstrate a lack of knowledge of basic health practices, may or may not realize that knowledge deficit, and may or may not express an interest in obtaining a fuller awareness. The individual may be directly observed as having the inability to adapt behaviors to meet basic health requirements. This may be the case in the lone elderly. Conversely, a significant other may report observations of impairment or a lack of necessary resources.

AGE-RELATED PHENOMENON

As individuals age, physical changes occur in the ability to identify, manage, and/or seek out help to maintain health. A major occurrence, arteriosclerosis, affects this segment to varying extents. This is a disorder of the large arteries that can be described as a thickening or hardening of the arterial wall. Risk factors associated with arteriosclerosis include aging in itself, sex, and genetic traits; these are factors that the individual cannot control. On the other hand, the risk factors of cigarette smoking, hypertension, and obesity can be affected by the resident. Other factors to consider are hyperlipidemia, hyperglycemia (diabetes), low levels of high density lipoproteins, inactivity, and personality type. The changes brought about by this physical arteriosclerotic state are observable in physical as well as psychosocial symptomology.

Physically, the individual's ability to maintain health may be affected by this disease process. The client may have the knowledge necessary to care for self, but physical limitations may hamper the "will." Diminished cardiovascular circulation may contribute to the inability to ambulate and/or carry out activities of daily living.

Psychosocially, arteriosclerosis may also affect the ability to maintain health. Knowledge of basic health practices may be lost due to memory impairments. Problem-solving abilities may also be affected by this process. The individual's inability to communicate and interact with others hinders the ability to maintain a healthy social and physical environment.

With the aging process, there is an increased prevalence of mental disorders. Disorders which seriously affect the individual's ability to make sound health decisions include dementia, Alzheimer's disease, and affective disorders (depressions and elations).

As an individual ages, the frequency of loss of social supports and resources increases. Loss of material as well as personal supports affect the ability to cope effectively; this loss also contributes to an inability to seek out health assistance and resources. The will to maintain health may also be affected with the loss of spiritual and/or support systems.

ETIOLOGIES

◆ Lack of, or significant alteration in, communication skills (written, verbal, and/or gestural)

◆ Lack of ability to make deliberate and thoughtful judgments; perceptual/cognitive impairment (complete/partial lack of gross and/or fine motor skills)

◆ Ineffective individual coping/dysfunctional grieving [depression or elation]

◆ Unachieved developmental tasks

◆ Ineffective family coping: disabling spiritual distress [despair with dying]

◆ Lack of material resources [housing, financial, insurance]

ALTERED HEALTH MAINTENANCE

◆ Nursing Diagnosis

Health maintenance alteration as displayed by the inability to identify, manage, or seek help (self, other, or community) to maintain health.

DEFINING CHARACTERISTICS

◆ Demonstrated lack of knowledge regarding basic health practices

◆ Demonstrated lack of adaptive behaviors to internal or external changes

◆ Reported or observed inability to take responsibility for meeting basic health practices in any, or all, functional pattern areas

◆ Reported or observed lack of equipment, finances, or other resources for health maintenance

◆ Reported or observed impairment of personal support system

◆ History of lack of health-seeking behavior

◆ Expression of interest in improving health behavior

GOALS/OUTCOME CRITERIA

The resident becomes knowledgeable in basic and/or specific health practices.

The resident develops adaptive behaviors that maintain health.

The resident demonstrates health-seeking behaviors.

INTERVENTIONS

1. Assess factors contributing to lack of knowledge:

   a. pathophysiological (medical condition)

   b. situational (language differences, treatments, personal characteristics: motivational level, denial, coping patterns)

   c. maturational (sensory deficits) (RN)

2. Utilize information gained to target educational approach, specific to factors having contributed to knowledge lack (RN, SW)

3. Assess resident's learning capabilities

   a. subjective data—determine current knowledge of illness, prognosis, treatment regimen, and preventive measures, available resources

   b. objective data

      1. ability to read, write

      2. assess sensory functioning levels of hearing, vision, smell, taste, touch

      3. physical abilities and limitations including circulation, respiratory status, nutritional status, ambulation (RN)

4. Establish Teaching Plan, specifically identifying goals to be achieved

   a. target approach to client's learning capabilities

   b. present education in clear, concise, relevant manner

   c. reinforce with visual display of information

   d. demonstrate and practice

    e. return demonstration and/or return of information shared

    f. evaluate effectiveness of education conducted (RN, STAFF)

5. Evaluate overall goal attainment.

1. Evaluate *client's ability* to control behaviors as they relate to status of met needs as identified by Maslow's Hierarchy of Needs: (RN, SW)

    a. Biologic integrity

- physiologic needs
- life support needs
- comfort needs
- drugs

    b. Safety and Security

- sensory awareness
- environmental safety
- legal/economics

    c. Belonging

- relationships
- intimacy
- affiliation
- social integration

    d. Self-esteem

- control
- useful roles
- cultural and cohort supports
- cognitive awareness
- psychosocial supports

    e. Self-actualization

- mastery and creativity
- legacies
- meaningful death

2. For those controllable behaviors identified: (RN)

    a. assess causative internal/external environmental changes

    b. assess individual's present ability to change behavior

    c. teach constructive problem-solving techniques

    d. assist client in developing appropriate adaptive behaviors

    e. follow up to augment client's adaptive success

3. For those uncontrollable behaviors identified: (RN)

    a. educate client in stress reducing activities to aid in adjustment

    b. draw upon and accentuate successful activities

    c. educate client as to available resources

    d. make appropriate referrals

    e. follow-up to evaluate status of behaviors

INTERVENTIONS

Assess client's status of health, as it relates to all functional areas. See Table 4–1: (RN)

    Establish Care Plan which identifies the achievement of all basic health practices. (RN, LPN)

    a. Establish teaching plan to empower client to take responsibility in basic health practices where able (RN, LPN)

    b. Establish system of resources (family and community)

        1. Assess factors contributing to lack of health-seeking behaviors

            a. Lack of knowledge or compliance:

                1) memory loss

                2) lack of written instructions

                3) environmental hazards (weather, physical facilities)

                4) sensory deprivation

                5) personality patterns of denial (RN)

        2. Establish plan of care specific to contributing factors.

        3. Evaluate effectiveness of plan

INTERVENTIONS

    1. Assess client need for resources necessary to:

        a. Identify health needs—equipment, financial, other

        b. Manage health needs—equipment, financial, other

        c. Seek help to maintain health—equipment, financial, other (RN)

    2. Establish plan to meet necessary resource needs of client (RN, LPN, SW)

    3. Establish network of available community resources (RN, SW)

    4. Educate client as to effective and efficient utilization of resources. (RN, STAFF)

    5. Follow up with full evaluation of effectiveness of plan. (RN)

INTERVENTIONS

    1. Conduct social history to ascertain presence of family, as well as client's attitude toward significant others. (RN, SW)

    2. Identify avenue for family assistance to client, i.e.,

        a. Taking client places

        b. Help with personal finances

TABLE 4–1 ◆ OARS Social Resource Scale

Now I'd like to ask you some questions about your family and friends.

Are you single, married, widowed, divorced, or separated?

1	Single	3	Widowed	5	Separated
2	Married	4	Divorced	__	Not answered

If "2" ask following

Does your spouse live here also?

   1 Yes
   2 No
   __ Not answered

Who lives with you?
(Check "yes" or "no" for each of the following.)

Yes	No	
_____	_____	No one
_____	_____	Husband or wife
_____	_____	Children
_____	_____	Grandchildren
_____	_____	Parents
_____	_____	Grandparents
_____	_____	Brothers and sisters
_____	_____	Other relatives (does not include in-laws covered in the above categories
_____	_____	Friends
_____	_____	Nonrelated paid help (includes free room)
_____	_____	Others (specify) _____

In the past year about how often did you leave here to visit your family and/or friends for weekends or holidays or to go on shopping trips or outings?

   1 Once a week or more
   2 1–3 times a month
   3 Less than once a month or only on holidays
   4 Never
   __ Not answered

How many people do you know well enough to visit with in their homes?

   3 Five or more
   2 Three to four
   1 One to two
   0 None
   __ Not answered

Table continued on following page

TABLE 4–1 ◆ *Continued*

About how many times did you talk to someone—friends,
relatives or others—on the telephone in the past week (either
you called them or they called you)? (If subject has no phone,
question still applies.)

3 Once a day or more
2 Twice
1 Once
0 Not at all
__ Not answered

How many times during the past week did you spend some
time with someone who does not live with you, that is, you
went to see them, or they came to visit you, or you went out
to do things together?

*How many times in the past week did you visit with someone, either
with people who live here or people who visited you here?*

3 Once a day or more
2 Two to six
1 Once
0 Not at all
__ Not answered

Do you have someone you can trust and confide in?

2 Yes
0 No
__ Not answered

Do you find yourself feeling lonely quite often, sometimes, or
almost never?

0 Quite often
1 Sometimes
2 Almost never
__ Not answered

Do you see your relatives and friends as often as you want to, or
are you somewhat unhappy about how little you see them?

1 As often as wants to
2 Somewhat unhappy about how little
__ Not answered

Is there someone *(outside this place)* who would give you any
help at all if you were sick or disabled, for example, your
husband/wife, a member of your family, or a friend?

1 Yes
0 No one willing and able to help
__ Not answered

a. If "yes" ask a and b.

a. Is there someone *(outside this place)* who would take care
of you as long as needed, or only for a short time, or only

TABLE 4–1 ◆ *Continued*

someone who would help you now and then (for example, taking you to the doctor, or fixing lunch occasionally, etc.)?

   1 Someone who would take care of subject indefinitely (as long as needed)

   2 Someone who would take care of subject for a short time (a few weeks to six months)

   3 Someone who would help subject now and then (taking him to the doctor or fixing lunch, etc.)

   __ Not answered

  b. Who is this person?

    Name _____

    Relationship _____

Rating Scale

Rate the current social resources of the person being evaluated along the 6-point scale presented below. Circle the *one* number that best describes the person's present circumstances.

1. **Excellent Social Resources:** Social relationships are very satisfying and extensive; at least one person would take care of him (her) indefinitely.

2. **Good Social Resources:** Social relationships are fairly satisfying and adequate and at least one person would take care of him (her) indefinitely, *or*
Social relationships are very satisfying and extensive, and only short-term help is available.

3. **Mildly Socially Impaired:** Social relationships are unsatisfactory, of poor quality, few; but at least one person would take care of him (her) indefinitely, *or* \
Social relationships are fairly satisfactory and adequate, and only short-term help is available.

4. **Moderately Socially Impaired:** Social relationships are unsatisfactory, of poor quality, few; and only short-term care is available, *or*
Social relationships are at least adequate or satisfactory, but help would only be available now and then.

5. **Severely Socially Impaired:** Social relationships are unsatisfactory, of poor quality, few; and help would be available only now and then, *or*
Social relationships are at least satisfactory or adequate, but help is not available even now and then.

6. **Totally Socially Impaired:** Social relationships are unsatisfactory, of poor quality, few; and help is not available even now and then.

Note: Italicized questions apply to those living in institutions.
(From Duke University Center for the Study of Aging and Human Development. *Multidimensional Functional Assessment: The OARS Methodology.* Durham, NC: Duke University Press, 1978.)

    c. Household chores

    d. Errands

    e. Emotional support

    f. Inclusion of client in family rituals (RN, SW)

  3. In cases where there are no available family members:

    a. Assess and make home care referral.

    b. Identify and utilize available "secondary relationships"

      1) Informal groups—senior citizens activities, parks, etc.

      2) Formal groups—day care, organized groups at need related sites, i.e., nutrition, disabilities, etc. (RN, SW)

    c. Establish links with appropriate organizations:

      1) Religious

      2) Fraternal/social

      3) Patriotic/veteran

      4) Aged

      5) Social/expressive

      6) Hobby

      7) Professional/work related

      8) Service

      9) Other

      10) Charitable/Health

      11) Political (RN/SW)

POTENTIAL FOR SUFFOCATION

◆ Nursing Diagnosis

The ability to maintain adequate air inhalation is an essential for life. This air supply may be accidentally disrupted by internal (individual) occurrences, as well as external (environmental) stimuli. In the case of the internal stimuli, the individual may have control over some of the occurrences and be victim of other uncontrollable situations. All external environmental stimuli are controllable, although some may be controlled only by the society, not by the individual.

◆ Assessment

A nurse, practicing in a nursing home/community environment would carry out a full assessment to arrive at the diagnosis of "Potential for Suffocation." As part of this assessment, the internal occurrences should be suspected if the individual is found to be a smoker, is immobile, or has chronic allergies. Additionally, the individual may be ineffective in airway clearance, breathing patterns, or gas exchange. As part of this assessment, the clues to an external stimuli creating a suffocation potential include habits increasing one's suffocation risk.

AGE-RELATED PHENOMENON

As an individual ages the potential for suffocation, known to exist in children, is no less present. Changes in the pulmonary system increase the risk of suffocation. Included are changes in airflow rates, gas exchange, and lung volumes. Alveolar ducts become enlarged and alveoli flattened, therefore creating a decrease in the internal surface area of the lung. In these altered air spaces, elastic recoil due to tension is lessened. Men have greater lung recoil during youth but lose it more rapidly than women, as they age. With age the chest wall adapts to lung changes by becoming more rigid. Because of loss of tone and substance in the abdominal wall, the diaphragm is additionally lower. It is not clear to what extent normal aging precipitates this process, versus the pulmonary stress created by atmospheric and/or industrial pollutants. Regardless of origin, mechanical pulmonary alternative occurring from the aging process increases suffocation risk. This may manifest itself not only in the increased production of mucous, but in the inability to clear the airway of that material.

The general increase in forgetfulness, as well as the decreased sensory/motor speed and acuity, precipitates risks for the elderly, from situations that may not have existed in younger years. Safety precautions once known and practiced may be forgotten as the elderly focus on daily living. Lack of a keen olfactory sense may increase risk of suffocation from things like gas leaks, smoking in bed, suffocation from fire. These mental changes, coupled with the inability to effectively carry out full pulmonary function, makes the suffocation risk very high.

ETIOLOGIES

◆ Interactive conditions between individual and environment which impose a risk to the defensive and adaptive resources of the individual

   a. Internal factors (host)

   ◆ Biological—decreased ability to effectively clear respiratory passages

   ◆ Chemical—effects of medication in decreasing respirations, increasing grogginess

   ◆ Physiological—lung diseases precipitating inelasticity

   ◆ Psychological perception—memory loss, creating suffocation hazards

   ◆ Developmental—increased time alone, diminishing availability of immediate assistance

   b. External environment

   ◆ Biological—lack of complete mastication of large mouthfuls of food

   ◆ Chemical—environmental pollutants increasing chronic lung disease

- ◆ Physiological—lack of mobility
- ◆ Psychological—lack of complete instructions to elderly regarding use of gas heaters, automobiles, etc.
- ◆ People/provider—lack of frequent turning and repositioning in the bedridden elderly

◆ Nursing Diagnosis

Potential for suffocation related to the presence of risk factors for accidental interruption in available air for inhalation.

DEFINING CHARACTERISTICS

- ◆ Reduced olfactory sensation
- ◆ Cognitive impairment or emotional difficulties
- ◆ Mobility impairment (bed mobility or ambulation)
- ◆ Lack of safety education or safety precaution
- ◆ Vehicle warming in a closed garage
- ◆ Household gas leaks
- ◆ Use of fuel burning heaters not vented to the outside
- ◆ Eating large mouthfuls of food

GOALS/OUTCOME CRITERIA

The resident's potential risk for suffocation is eliminated or minimized.

    The resident utilizes appropriate behavior and/or adaptive techniques in coping with decreased motor functions that could compromise airway integrity.

    The resident demonstrates knowledge of safety factors amid positive health behaviors.

INTERVENTIONS

1. Assess resident for diminished olfactory sense. (RN, MD)
2. Educate client regarding
   a. effects of specific drugs on smell
   b. toxic chemicals in home and effects of breathing fumes and/or mixing
   c. general safety precautions to avoid fires and poisonings.
3. Ensure home installation of and maintenance of smoke detector with audible and visual alarm. (NHA)
4. Ensure system for regular furnace maintenance. (NHA)

1. Assess client for degree of diminished motor abilities. (RN, MD)
2. Decrease suffocation risk by maximizing pulmonary function through:

    a. encouraging ambulation

    b. encouraging repositioning

    c. turn from side to side regularly if bedridden

    d. educate and encourage deep breathing exercises and coughing.

        1) Teach effective coughing techniques. (RN, PT, RT)

3. Position on right side after eating to minimize regurgitation and aspiration. (RN, LPN, NA)

4. For bedridden, elevate head of bed when feasible. (RN, LPN, NA)

5. Maintain adequate hydration to decrease viscosity of secretions. (RN, LPN, NA)

1. Assess level of knowledge of safety factors and various preventative measures. (RN)

2. Teach factors to aid in stinging insect avoidance:

    a. wear less bright colors

    b. keep hair tied back (avoid fragrances)

    c. wear shoes and socks

    d. avoid yard work during insect season

    e. have insect spray available

    f. move slowly from a stinging insect

    g. have professional exterminator inspect for nests (RN, LPN)

3. Teach instructions for dealing with unknown potential allergens

    a. Inform prescribing physician of medications currently being taken, as well as past allergies

    b. Take first medication dose in the presence of others

    c. List common food allergens. (RN)

4. Teach avoidance of eating/drinking/talking situation where regurgitation likelihood would be increased. (RN, LPN)

5. Teach proper positioning for eating and drinking.

6. Teach effective methods for swallowing pills (RN, LPN)

7. Teach Heimlich Maneuver, or usage for others as well as self (RN, LPN, NA)

8. Discuss need for annual immunizations (flu, etc.) (RN, LPN)

Assess level of risk associated with client's cognitive and/or emotional difficulties as they accentuate risk of accidental suffocation.

    a. Developmental level—may be such that knowledge of safety precautions is unable to be enhanced.

    b. Anxiety level—may be high due to unfamiliar environment, lack of understanding of diagnoses, difficulty breathing, fear of pulmonary obstruction, and/or death associated with obstruction. (RN)

Implement measures to reduce anxiety

   a. provide calm environment

   b. accompany client during respiratory distress

   c. decrease suffocation provoking stimuli

      1) open curtains, drapes

      2) approach client from side rather than front-on

      3) limit visitors

      4) unclutter room

      5) admin. O_2 via cannula (vs. mask)

   d. teach client about anxiety control techniques

   e. encourage verbalization of fear

   f. explain tests and procedures

   g. respond to calls expeditiously (RN, SW)

Assess client for effect of pain or respiratory effectiveness (RN, LPN). Implement measures to decrease pain's effect on decreasing respiratory effectiveness and increasing risk of suffocation.

   a. assist with nonpharmacological pain relief

      1) positioning

      2) guided imagery

      3) relaxation techniques

      4) diversional activities

   b. monitor for mild (non-narcotic) analgesic need. (RN, LPN)

Initiate efforts to minimize effects of disease as they increase suffocation risk.

   a. Proper positioning

      1) elevate head of bed

      2) position on side

      3) position tongue if necessary

   b. Maximize cough effectiveness

      1) teach how to cough

      2) keep airway clear of secretions

   c. Control pain (2 above)

   d. Dilute secretions

      1) increase hydration (2–3 quarts/day)

      2) humidity on

   3. Plan rest (RN)

1. Assess client's habits associated with vehicle usage.
   a. Does he/she drive?
   b. Does he/she have own vehicle?
   c. How does he/she warm car?
   d. Does he/she have electric garage door opener? (RN, LPN, SW)
2. Instruct client to
   a. Open garage door (manually or automatically) before starting vehicle.
   b. Allow car to idle only if out-of-doors (out of proximity to building air intake, doors, windows, etc.).
   c. Always leave car window open to a small degree.
   d. Have car checked routinely for properly functioning exhaust system. (RN, LPN, SW)

Teach client fully regarding rationale for *not* idling car in closed-in area. (RN, LPN, SW)

Assess client's susceptibility to this risk factor

a. Is there gas usage in the home?
b. How does the client cook?
c. How does the client heat?
d. Where is furnace vented?
e. Does client stay at other dwellings. (cottage, relatives, etc.) (RN, SW)

Teach client to

a. compensate for potential lack of smell by routinely asking guests if they smell anything peculiar.
b. report any suspicious odors immediately (remove self from dwelling immediately)
c. have gas connections, furnace, etc., checked routinely
d. set stove timer when turning on stove gas for any reason
e. suspect gas leak if unexplained symptoms appear (tightening of throat, air hunger, headaches, drowsiness, sore throat) and report
f. vent house regularly, regardless of season (open windows and doors for short time) (RN)

1. Assess client's smoking habits.
   a. Do they smoke?
   b. Do they ever smoke in bed?
   c. Does anyone in their dwelling smoke?
   d. Does anyone in their dwelling smoke in bed? (RN, LPN, SW)

2. Observe for signs of smoking (odor of smoke, stained teeth, fingers, cough) (RN, LPN)
3. Teach client, and client's significant others, to never smoke in bed, along with rationale. (RN, LPN)
4. If client is bedridden:
   a. remove cigarettes and matches
   b. erect signs for guests, etc.
   c. allow client to smoke only if attended. (RN, LPN)
5. Teach client the general hazards associated with smoking.
   a. heart disease
   b. lung disease
   c. hypertension
   d. vasoconstriction (RN, LPN)

Provide smoking cessation therapy. (RN)

1. Assess client's heating methods
   a. What is his or her primary heating method?
   b. Does client supplement heating with any other heating method?
   c. Does the supplemental heater require outside venting?
   d. Does client temporarily inhabit other dwellings and how are they heated? (cottage, etc.) (RN, SW)
2. Educate client as to need to vent fuel burning heaters to the outside. (RN, SW)
3. If questionably competent, remove heater from environment until client is able to independently make sound decisions. (RN, SW)
4. Instruct client not to use makeshift heaters (gas grills, charcoal, etc.) (RN, LPN, SW)
5. Instruct client to have existing venting checked routinely. (RN)

1. Assess client's eating habits.
   a. subjectively
      ◆ ask about size of mouthfuls usually eaten?
      ◆ ask about frequency of denture fittings?
   b. objectively
      ◆ obseve client eating, chewing
      ◆ observe denture and/or teeth for proper fit. (RN, LPN)
2. Teach clients to
   a. eat small mouthfuls of food
   b. chew mouthfuls fully before attempting to swallow
   c. not talk when food is in mouth

    d. sit up straight when eating

    e. have regular dental checks. (RN)

  3. If client is incompetent:

    a. cut food into small pieces

    b. observe client while he or she is eating

    c. position upright to aid in swallowing. (RN)

NONCOMPLIANCE

◆ Nursing Diagnosis

Noncompliance: A resident that decides not to follow the prescribed health care regime or advice is diagnosed and identified as a noncompliant individual. Compliance improves health care and noncompliance places the resident in jeopardy. Noncompliant behaviors cannot be attributed to any one specific group of people; individuals across all age and socioeconomic levels have the potential to be non-compliant in their health care needs.

ETIOLOGIES

Value conflict. Health regime is in direct or indirect opposition to personal beliefs and values.

Cultural conflict. Health regime is in direct or indirect opposition to cultural heritage and/or customs.

Spiritual conflict. Health regime is in direct or indirect opposition to religious beliefs and/or customs.

Knowledge or skill deficit. The resident cannot comply because of lack of understanding or inability to perform tasks, or both.

Perceived therapeutic ineffectiveness. The resident does not perceive the health care regime as effective, and therefore does not comply.

Perceived nonsusceptibility/invulnerability. Resident does not view health regime as necessary because she or he believes they are not in danger or afflicted by the illness or noncomplying with regime.

Denial of illness. Resident does not acknowledge illness and therefore does not comply with prescription.

Family Pattern Disruption. The elderly individual may not follow health regime if it is perceived as a dysfunctional component to the family homeostasis.

AGE-RELATED PHENOMENON

Noncompliance is seen more readily in the community than in the nursing home. Individuals in the community have greater control over their actions (or inactions) than those who are in the more externally controlled environment of an institution. Studies regarding noncompliance among the elderly offer conflicting definitions of the term, making accurate data assessment difficult. However, some theorists suggest that specific noncompliant behaviors, such as medicine taking, may be as high as 50 percent.

The older individual may be affected by limited resources (intellectual, financial, or social), alterations in thought patterns, alteration in energy and mobility, and isolation—all of which make compliance difficult. Also, elders in their seventh, eighth, or ninth decade or beyond have been socialized into belief patterns and customs that may be in opposition to the desired compliance. Changing behaviors may prove difficult. It is important to remember that behavioral change occurs prior to attitudinal change.

The elderly may also find compliance difficult, if not impossible, if the regime requires multiple actions.

Often overlooked in the noncompliant elder is the simple assessment of physical ability to perform the necessary tasks in order to follow the health regime. The elder may have decreased visual acuity, fine motor function deficit of impaired hearing—to cite a few—that affect their ability to comply.

The elder in a nursing home faces great difficulty in complying due to discontinuities in health care providers. In institutions without primary nursing model team conferences, individual compliance guidelines should be established. It is vital that the elder receive consistent and correct information.

ASSESSMENT

The nurse should assess for noncompliance as part of the daily resident evaluation. Specific events may provide cues as to a resident that is not following the prescribed health care regime. These include poor chronic disease control, unexpected failure of acute illness to resolve, and frequent exacerbations.

The resident may state noncompliance, directly or indirectly. The nurse should question the resident in a nonthreatening but probing manner.

The resident may not perform the required tasks in order to comply.

◆ Nursing Diagnosis

Noncompliance with prescribed health care regime.

DEFINING CHARACTERISTICS

- ◆ Direct observation of noncompliance
- ◆ Statements by resident or significant others describing noncompliance
- ◆ Objective tests revealing noncompliance (physiological measures, detection of markers)
- ◆ Evidence of development of complications
- ◆ Evidence of exacerbation of symptoms
- ◆ Failure to keep appointments
- ◆ Failure to progress

GOALS/OUTCOME CRITERIA

The resident complies with prescribed regime.

Resident or significant other* demonstrates accurate performance of required skill.

Resident or significant other verbalizes or otherwise communicates understanding of the process.

Implementation of social and support services as necessary.

INTERVENTIONS

◆ Access resident's level of cognitive functioning (RN)

◆ Assess for any sensory and/or motor impairment (RN)

◆ Obtain social, family, and cultural history (RN)

◆ Explain health care regime clearly and correctly (note that additional explanations by others should be consistent with the initial communication)

◆ Enhance explanation with appropriate pacing and visual clues

◆ Demonstrate necessary skill with observed return performance. Make corrections/alternates as necessary to accommodate the elder

◆ Fit the health care regime into the resident's daily pattern, if possible

◆ Provide and learn stress reduction techniques and exercise

◆ Assist resident with value clarification if necessary

◆ Routinely reassess and examine behavior for compliance to regime

◆ Encourage self-monitoring (i.e., journal writing)

POTENTIAL FOR INJURY

◆ Nursing Diagnosis

Potential for Injury: The elderly are at high risk for injury due to decreases in mental alertness, psychomotor functioning, and the senses and due to the presence of chronic disease conditions.

NANDA defines the diagnosis as "presence of risk factors for bodily injury." The potential for injury is environmentally dependent. The care setting (the environment) is a potential source of injury to the older person. The concept of injury differs from that of accident. An accident occurs by chance, whereas an injury is an energy force from the environment that is beyond the body's resiliency. Elders, because of their already decreased resiliency, are at high risk for injury.

---

*A significant other may assume the responsible role in seeing that the health care regime is being maintained. This would occur in the community more often than in a nursing home. However, strong relationships between roommates may develop, and the roommate can become instrumental in the compliance regime.

ETIOLOGIES

- ◆ Sensory Impairment
- ◆ Cognitive dysfunctions
- ◆ Osteoporsis
- ◆ Muscle weakness or atrophy
- ◆ Gait and balance problems
- ◆ Decreased insurance
- ◆ Anxiety and affect disorders
- ◆ Polypharmacy
- ◆ Poor lighting (even during daylight)
- ◆ Numerous stairs—lack of handrails
- ◆ Poverty
- ◆ Poor or unsafe storage of poisonous chemicals
- ◆ Lack of opportunity or ability to learn about medications and their side effects
- ◆ Health care and family providers

AGE-RELATED PHENOMENON

Twenty-three percent of all deaths of people over age 65 are the result of injury. Women experience injury from falls more than men. Males have a higher rate of injury from auto accidents and burns. In general, however, the injury rate is higher for males 65 or over than for females.

Due to age related changes in physical and cognitive functioning, older people have an increased potential to negatively interact with their environment and cause tissue damage or injury. Elders newly admitted to a nursing home, or transferred to an acute care facility, are placed in unfamiliar surroundings and should be observed for potentially harmful occurrences.

The more a person's competence is compromised or limited, the more at risk they are. This is an interesting paradox. Elders who are restrained because they have an ataxic gait (or for some other reason) may experience a decrease in competence and be more at risk for injury. Anything that places an unfamiliar barrier between the individual and the environment can result in injury.

◆ Nursing Diagnosis

Potential for injury due to interaction with the environment beyond the individual's bodily resilience.

DEFINING CHARACTERISTICS

- ◆ Sensory impairment: visual, auditory, vestibular, peripheral, sensation
- ◆ Cognitive impairments, especially judgment

◆ Altered blood profiles, especially leukopenia, leukocytosis, thrombo-cytopenia, altered clotting factors, anemia

◆ Physical findings: broken skin, multiple ecchymoses, reduced muscle mass, impaired balance, ataxia

◆ History of falls, family violence, affective disorder, drugs with low therapeutic index or those associated with falls

◆ Recent major environmental change

◆ Presence of nosocomial agents

SOCIOCULTURAL FACTORS

◆ Lack of awareness by significant others

◆ Lack of safety education

◆ Fatalistic attitude about injuries

◆ Lack of knowledge of developmental stages

◆ Presence of family stress (marital, financial, health)

◆ Inadequate community emergency medical services response

◆ Lack of public education (first aid and CPR)

◆ Lack of community safety programs (water safety, lifeguards, crossing guards, building codes)

ASSESSMENT

Assessment for the diagnosis of resident should include both individual and environmental assessments. The nurse should assess how individuals relate to their environment. Good interaction will help decrease the likeness of injury.

The health history should identify any previous falls, existing medical conditions and their treatments, any drug (prescription, OTC, and/or illicit) use, and any vertigo episodes.

The physical assessment should include (but not be limited to): atypical pulse or rate and system (an EKG may be needed if irregularities noticed); blood pressure; posture and gait evaluation, and visual and auditory acuity.

Environmental assessment should be on-going. Assess the nursing home for any item or factor that puts residents at risk. Such conditions include scatter rugs, inadequate lighting, clutter, wet floors, non-skid bath mats, and the like. Remember that the number one injury sustained in a nursing home is a fall.

GOALS/OUTCOME CRITERIA

◆ The resident remains injury free.

◆ The resident becomes familiar with his or her environment.

◆ The resident is able to identify factors that increase the potential for injury.

INTERVENTIONS

◆ Introduce resident to their environment via a short tour. Concentrate on their immediate living space (RN, STAFF)

◆ Perform injury assessment—individual and environmental (RN)

◆ Inform resident of any health condition or treatment that may predispose them to injury, i.e., medications that may cause orthostatic changes (RN)

◆ Provide appropriate adaptive strategies to help the individual cope with his or her environment (RN, PT, TO, RT)

◆ Identify any habits (i.e., nightly walks) that may place resident at risk and incorporate them into plan of care

◆ Remove physical risks from the environment (RN, STAFF)

◆ Provide education to the resident and their family on injury prevention (RN, LPN)

POTENTIAL FOR INFECTION

◆ Nursing Diagnosis

Potential for Injury: The elder is at risk for the potential of infection. NANDA defines this as "the state in which an individual is at increased risk for being invaded by pathological organisms." Nursing home residents are at increased risk because of their environment, and the presence of nosocomial infections.

ETIOLOGIES

◆ Chronic diseases

◆ Decreased functioning of immune system

◆ Malnutrition

◆ History of smoking

◆ History of alcohol and/or drug abuse

◆ Immobility

◆ Breaks in skin integrity

◆ Poor handwashing by residents and care givers

◆ History of decreased mental function (i.e., dementia)

AGE-RELATED PHENOMENON

The older individual because of the normal aging process has a lower defense against infection. For the individual in the nursing home, the three most common sites of infection are urinary tract, skin, and the respiratory tract. Nearly 75 percent of all nursing home residents develop at least one nosocomial infection. Also, the older the individual, the more likely they are to become infected.

ASSESSMENT

Assessment for potential of infection is performed as a general physical assessment, noting any irregularities in the body systems, and by careful history taking.

Physical assessment should pay close attention to the condition of the skin. Note any breakdown, edema, contractures, or obesity. Check for capillary refill action, warmth, and moisture. Also note the condition of the respiratory tract. Ask the resident to cough and deep breathe. Assess the elder's ability to clear his or her airway, and note the status of the gag reflex. In examining the urinary tract palpate the empty bladder for any urine residual which could be a potential source of infection. Always check any indwelling catheter for date of insertion and any discharge.

The detailed health history should specifically ask for the presence of any conditions such as diabetes mellitus, COPD, cancer, and immobility. Note all drugs (including alcohol) with dose and frequency. Check on immunization history—when was their last tetanus vaccine? Have they ever been immunized for "the flu"? List any allergies and any previous infections.

◆ Nursing Diagnosis

The potential for infection due to increased risk for being invaded by pathogenic organisms.

DEFINING CHARACTERISTICS

- ◆ Interrpution of skin integrity
- ◆ Abnormalities of white blood cells, lymph glands
- ◆ Low immunization level of individual or a community
- ◆ Factors influencing immune mechanism (immunosuppressive drugs, malnutrition, etc.)
- ◆ Inadequate waste disposal
- ◆ Presence of viruses, bacteria, rickettsiae, fungi, or animal parasites

GOALS/OUTCOME CRITERIA

- ◆ The resident remains free from infection.
- ◆ The resident demonstrates knowledge about specific conditions that may place him or her at risk for infection.
- ◆ The resident demonstrates skills necessary to alter the environment (or seek assistance with) when the threat of infection exists.

INTERVENTIONS

- ◆ Provide for immunization against influenza and pneumonococcal pneumonia (RN, MD)
- ◆ Provide for tetanus vaccine (This should be administered every ten years) (RN, MD)

◆ Resident should cough and deep breathe Q2H if potential respiratory infection exists (RN, LPN)

◆ Encourage fluids < 2000 cc daily (unless contraindicated by cardiac or renal disease) (RN, LPN)

◆ Develop increased mobility program—regular walking or some other physical exercise (RN, LPN, PT)

◆ If gag reflex is impaired—supervise at meal time and examine mouth for any unchewed food that could obstruct the airway (RN, LPN, NA)

◆ Examine skin's integrity daily (RN, LPN, NA)

◆ Provide meticulous skin care (RN, STAFF)

◆ Turn and reposition Q2H with massage of bony prominances (RN, LPN, NA)

◆ Examine feet daily for any pressure points, corn, callus (RN, LPN, NA)

◆ Check in-dwelling urinary catheter for patency and any discharge (RN, LPN)

◆ Change catheter as per nursing home protocol (RN, LPN)

◆ Perform catheter care daily (RN, LPN, NA)

◆ For the resident without a catheter

  ◆ Encourage voiding Q3-4 W to prevent urinary stasis (RN, LPN, NA)

  ◆ Encourage fluids (RN, LPN, NA)

  ◆ Employ crede' to further empty bladder (RN, LPN)

  ◆ Assess nutritional history and status (RN, RD)

◆ Develop appropriate diet plan (if necessary) to ensure proper nutrition (RN, RD)

References

Andres, R, Bierman, EL, Hazzard, WR. *Principles of Genetic Medicine.* New York: McGraw-Hill; 1985.
A text relaying the knowledge of human aging, health care of the elderly specific to diseases of the various organ symptoms.

Burgess, A. (ed.) *Rape and Sexual Assault.* New York: Garland Publishing Co.; 1985.

Burnside, I. *Nursing and the Aged.* 3rd ed. New York: McGraw-Hill; 1988.

Carpenito, LJ. *Nursing Diagnosis: Application to Clinical Practice.* New York; J.B. Lippincott; 1983.
A text providing a condensed, organized outline of clinical nursing practice designed to communicate creative clinical nursing.

Ebersole, P, Hess, P. *Toward Healthy Aging.* St. Louis: C.V. Mosby; 1981.
A text outlining the process for the identification of human needs and appropriate nursing responses.

Hurley, ME. *Classification of Nursing Diagnosis.* St. Louis: C.V. Mosby; 1986.
A text of material covering the proceedings of the Sixth Conference of the North American Nursing Diagnoses Association.

Ledray, L. *Recovering from Rape.* New York: Henry Holt; 1986.

Libow, LS, Sherman FT. *The Care of Geriatric Medicine.* St. Louis: C.V. Mosby; 1981.
A text for the students in geriatric medicine, this material presents a basic care approach to the management of the geriatric patient.

Matterson, M, McConnell, E. *Gerontological Nursing.* Philadelphia: W.B. Saunders; 1988.

Thompson, JM, et al. *Clinical Nursing.* St. Louis: C.V. Mosby Company; 1986.

Ulrich, SP, Canale, SW, Wendell, SA. *Nursing Care Planning Guides.* Philadelphia: W. B. Saunders Co.; 1986.

5

Nutritional-Metabolic Pattern

♦

NUTRITIONAL MANAGEMENT

The elderly patient presents the clinician with unique factors, which must be addressed in order to maintain and/or restore nutritional status. The nutritional status of the elderly patient is influenced by physiological and psychosocial factors, which will be addressed in this chapter. Since it is now well-accepted that proper nutrition is a vital component in maintaining health and preventing complications in the elderly person, the clinician must be able to identify nutritional problems and provide appropriate nutritional care.

◆ Nursing Diagnosis

Altered nutrition: potential for more than body requirements or potential obesity. This diagnosis applies to the individual who is getting more calories than his or her metabolic requirements. This could be either from an inappropriate intake of calories or from low-energy requirements. The diagnosis includes the actual occurrences as well as the potential for this problem.

ASSESSMENT

The key to assessing a patient for this problem is to obtain the following information:

1. weight
2. usual weight
3. diet history
4. caloric requirements

You must get an accurate measurement of the patient's current weight. Information given by the patient in this population may not be completely accurate. It would also be important to obtain the patient's usual weight so that you will be able to note how this weight has changed over time. The patient's diet history will give you an idea of his or her usual caloric intake over a specified time period. The information obtained may only cover a limited period of time.

From this information you can estimate the patient's usual caloric intake. Then using the person's age, height, sex, weight, and activity level, you can estimate the patient's total caloric needs. A caloric intake greater than the person's energy requirements has the potential for causing weight gain over time.

AGE-RELATED PHENOMENON

Obesity in the elderly person is a multifactorial problem resulting from socioeconomic and physiological factors. The aging process itself is associated with changes in body composition, i.e., lean body mass is known to steadily decrease with age with accompanying increase in body fat. Another change that occurs as the person ages is a drop in the basal metabolic rate. Therefore, weight and caloric requirements must be interpreted carefully in the elderly person. Overweight patients are generally more difficult to manage. They are more likely to develop complications secondary to their weight (pulmonary or cardiovascular), decubitus and arthritis.

A sensible approach to weight reduction involves dietary restriction of approximately 500 calories per day to promote a one pound per week weight loss. This could be achieved by decreasing the portion sizes of the usual diet and results in a safe weight loss.

The definition of overweight and obesity is arbitrary and there are not clear standards for the elderly person.

ETIOLOGIES

- ◆ Hereditary predisposition
- ◆ Excessive intake relative to energy requirements
- ◆ Dysfunctional eating patterns
- ◆ Sedentary life style
- ◆ Loss of financial resources (selection of low cost, high calorie foods)

◆ Nursing Diagnosis

Altered nutrition: potential for more than body requirements or potential obesity

- ◆ related to lack of knowledge of effects of hereditary disposition

GOALS/OUTCOME CRITERIA

- ◆ Verbalizes understanding of relation of hereditary disposition to weight gain
- ◆ Maintains desirable weight
- ◆ Loses weight to achieve desirable level

INTERVENTIONS

◆ Nutrition counseling
◆ Behavior modification counseling
◆ Exercise counseling

ACCOUNTABILITY

RN, RD

ALTERED NUTRITION: potential for more than body requirements or potential obesity related to excessive intake relative to energy expenditure

GOALS/OUTCOME CRITERIA

◆ Decreases caloric intake
◆ Increases activity

INTERVENTIONS

◆ Nutritional counseling
◆ Exercise program

ACCOUNTABILITY

RN, RD

ALTERED NUTRITION: potential for more than body requirements or potential obesity related to dysfunctional eating patterns

GOALS/OUTCOME CRITERIA

◆ Verbalizes understanding of why existing meal patterns or habits are inappropriate
◆ Follows regular, appropriate meal patterns

INTERVENTIONS

◆ Nutrition counseling, emphasizing behavior modification

ACCOUNTABILITY

RN, RD

ALTERED NUTRITION: potential for more than body requirements or potential obesity related to sedentary life style

GOALS/OUTCOME CRITERIA

◆ Increases activities in home, if homebound
◆ Increases involvement in outside activities
◆ Decreases or compensates for weakness that limits activities

INTERVENTIONS

◆ Nutritional counseling
◆ Exercise program counseling
◆ Referral to community groups

ACCOUNTABILITY

RN, RD, PT

ALTERED NUTRITION: potential for more than body requirements or potential obesity related to lack of financial resources and selection of low cost, calorically dense foods

GOALS/OUTCOME CRITERIA

◆ Has adequate resources to purchase needed food
◆ Selects fewer calorically dense foods; selects nutrionally dense foods that fit into financial resources

INTERVENTIONS

◆ Nutritional counseling
◆ Refer to financial assistance programs, community food programs
◆ Establish contact with appropriate social services

ACCOUNTABILITY

RN, RD, SW

◆ Nursing Diagnosis

Altered nutrition: more than body requirements or exogenous obesity. This diagnosis would include those individuals who are taking in more calories than needed for energy expenditures. This excess might be related to inappropriate intake or to a sedentary life style.

ASSESSMENT

The patient assessment should include height and weight. This should be compared to sets of norms for the patient's height and frame. Information should be obtained on the patient's usual meal patterns and intakes so as to obtain information on the usual caloric intake. The patient should be assessed to see if there are signs of complications secondary to excess weight (cardiovascular changes, skin integrity problems, or glucose regulation problems). The activity level of the patient should also be assessed. With the formation obtained, the patient's total caloric needs can also be estimated and compared with their usual caloric intake.

ETIOLOGIES

- ◆ Food intake-energy expenditure imbalance:
- ◆ Dysfunctional eating patterns (reported or observed):
    - **A.** pairing food with other activities
    - **B.** concentrating food intake at the end of the day
    - **C.** eating in response to external cues (time of day, social situation)
    - **D.** eating in response to internal cues other than hunger (anxiety, depression)

◆ Nursing Diagnosis

ALTERED NUTRITION: more than body requirements or exogenous obesity, related to food intake imbalance with energy expenditure and to dysfunctional eating patterns (reported or observed)

GOALS/OUTCOME CRITERIA

- ◆ Decreases weight to level appropriate for height and frame
- ◆ Increases activity according to individual tolerance
- ◆ Verbalizes understanding of effects of dysfunctional eating patterns
- ◆ Demonstrates decrease in dysfunctional eating habits
- ◆ Maintains weight loss

INTERVENTIONS

- ◆ Caloric restriction emphasizing balanced meal patterns, and adequate intake of necessary nutrients
- ◆ Monitor weight
- ◆ Nutritional counseling, including behavior modification
- ◆ Activity counseling
- ◆ Counsel about elimination of dysfunctional eating habits
    - **a.** Pairing food with other activities
    - **b.** Concentrating food intake at end of day
    - **c.** Eating in response to external cues (time of day, social situations)
    - **d.** Eating in response to internal cues other than hunger (anxiety, depression)

ACCOUNTABILITY

RN, RD, PT

◆ Nursing Diagnosis

Altered nutrition: less than body requirement, or nutritional deficit. This diagnosis would relate to the problem of a patient who is unable to consume adequate amounts of calories or individual nutrients into their diet. This would include those who are unable to meet their energy requirements, and those patients who have increased needs. This may be related to a physical condition or unavailability of foodstuffs.

ASSESSMENT

The patient must be assessed for information on their usual food intake. This would include not only the types of food, but the quantities consumed. The patient's weight and weight change over time should also be assessed. In addition you must assess the patient's caloric requirements, which are related to his or her age, sex, weight, height, and activity level. Information should also be obtained on how the patient provides himself or herself with food and by what means they are paying for this food.

AGE-RELATED PHENOMENON

Poor dietary intakes and changes in eating habits seen in elderly patients can result from social, medical, and economic factors. Psychosocial changes affecting the elderly can increase their risk for nutritionally deficient diets. The elderly person living alone frequently consumes a poor diet. Poor dietary habits may result from loneliness to inability to meet energy required for meal preparation. There are also a significant number of older persons who have limited income, limiting their ability to purchase food. These factors have important implications for the dietary quality in terms of protein, vitamins, and minerals.

Older persons with poor dentition may be at risk for inadequate nutritional intake. Meats and vegetables are usually limited in their diets and soft carbohydrate foods such as white bread, cake, and jelly, which require less chewing, are often substituted. Many elderly persons develop lactose intolerance due to a deficiency in the enzyme lactase that occurs with the aging process. Elderly persons with this problem frequently avoid milk and dairy products to avoid the discomfort of the experience. Avoidance of these foods can lead to calcium and protein deficiencies. Other nutritional problems may be related to the fact that elderly people are often taking multiple medications that can affect their appetite.

Side effects such as nausea, vomiting, and diarrhea will affect the ability to maintain an adequate nutritional status. The overall effect of these physiological changes suggest that the elderly person can be at risk for poor nutritional status.

ETIOLOGIES

- ◆ anorexia
- ◆ early satiety
- ◆ decreased or altered taste sensitivity
- ◆ decreased ability to detect odor
- ◆ decreased gastrointestinal tract absorption

◆ muscle weakness (mastication/swallowing)
◆ side effects of medications
◆ buccal cavity discomfort or pain
◆ difficulty in preparing or procuring food
◆ edentulous
◆ financial limitations
◆ social isolation

◆ Nursing Diagnosis

ALTERED NUTRITION: less than body requirements related to

◆ anorexia
◆ early satiety
◆ decreased or altered taste sensitivity
◆ decreased ability to detect odors
◆ lack of teeth
◆ buccal cavity discomfort
◆ muscle weakness (mastication/swallowing)

GOALS/OUTCOME CRITERIA

◆ takes in adequate food relative to minimum daily requirements (reported or observed)
◆ increases caloric intake
◆ maintains appropriate weight
◆ improves nutritional status

INTERVENTIONS

◆ Eliminate or alleviate physical barriers to adequate intake
◆ Limit foods with little or no caloric value
◆ Increase amounts and types of nutritious foods in diet. Identify nutritious foods that are well-liked and tolerated.
◆ Provide high calorie, high protein nutritional supplements as prescribed
◆ Adjust interval of feedings to patient's desires. Small frequent feedings may be taken best and reduce discomfort and fatigue.
◆ Provide assistance as needed for preparation of food and eating. Provide assistive devices and proper positioning. Keep surroundings as pleasant as possible during meals.

ACCOUNTABILITY

MD, RN, RD

ALTERED NUTRITION: less than body requirements related to

◆ decreased GI absorption as evidenced by abdominal cramps or diarrhea

◆ side effects of medication as evidenced by abdominal cramps or diarrhea

GOALS/OUTCOME CRITERIA

◆ Decrease in abdominal cramps and diarrhea

INTERVENTIONS

◆ Change consistency and texture of diet
◆ Insure appropriate temperature of foods served
◆ Refer to physician for changes in medication

ACCOUNTABILITY

MD, RN, RD

> *ALTERED NUTRITION:* less than body requirements related to

◆ Financial limitations
◆ Social isolation

GOALS/OUTCOME CRITERIA

◆ Obtains adequate financial resources for nutritious diet
◆ Increases social contacts and social support

INTERVENTIONS

◆ Refer to community agencies
◆ Refer to social worker

ACCOUNTABILITY

SW, RD, RN, MD

◆ Nursing Diagnosis

Impaired Swallowing. Definition: The state in which an individual has decreased ability to voluntarily pass fluids and/or solids from the mouth to the stomach. The patient with this problem has difficulty with the stage of the swallowing process in which the bolus of food is moved from the mouth to the esophagus. There are a variety of conditions in which this problem may develop, such as hemi- and supra-laryngectomy patients, stroke patients, and situations in which there is a physical impairment in the swallowing mechanism.

ASSESSMENT

This patient requires a very close assessment of their ability to swallow solids and liquids. This would involve preparations to help the patient if they should encounter any difficulty during the assessment (i.e., suction equipment). The assessment process would involve testing the patient to establish his or her ability to swallow. This is usually done with endoscopic or radiologic evaluation, along with a qualified swallowing therapist.

Dysphagia places the elderly at risk for nutritional deficiency, because they simply cannot ingest essential nutrients. Typically, solids are more easily swallowed than liquids.

AGE-RELATED PHENOMENON

There are several age-related factors that will impact on the swallowing process. With age the amount of saliva produced decreases and can impair the ability to swallow. Side effects of many medications taken by the elderly produce xerostomia (dry mouth), as well as taste changes, and can also produce detrimental effects on the ability to swallow. Along with this decrease in saliva seen in the elderly patient, there is often an increase in damage to the oral mucous membrane. This problem may render the elderly patient unable to wear dentures.

Another problem with decreased saliva is an impairment of the tongue and teeth to function in their normal capacity. Dental caries and candidiasis can also be potential age-related problems. Other changes that occur with age include the drifting of teeth, which will affect chewing ability, and subsequent nutritional intake.

ETIOLOGIES

- ◆ Uncompensated muscular weakness
- ◆ Decreased saliva
- ◆ Compression
- ◆ Uncompensated paralysis

◆ Nursing Diagnosis

Impaired Swallowing related to uncompensated muscular weakness

GOALS/OUTCOME CRITERIA

- ◆ Maximizes ability to swallow and tolerate diet

INTERVENTIONS

- ◆ Refer to swallowing therapist for intervention

ACCOUNTABILITY

Speech/swallowing therapist

Impaired swallowing related to uncompensated paralysis, decreased saliva

GOALS/OUTCOME CRITERIA

- ◆ Increase in ability to chew/or swallow foods
- ◆ Improve nutritional status

INTERVENTIONS

◆ Change texture of diet. Starting with thick liquids, then carbonated beverages, which may stimulate the swallowing mechanism

◆ Make diet changes to include easy to swallow foods. Well-cooked or ground foods are easier to swallow and should replace tough foods. Add puddings and nutritional supplements.

ACCOUNTABILITY

RN, RD, DDS

◆ Nursing Diagnosis

Altered oral mucous membranes. This diagnosis would involve situations where there is some change in the oral cavity that produces pain and discomfort. This change could be in the structure of the oral cavity or in the type and amount of secretions that are produced.

ASSESSMENT

The patient should have a very careful history and physical examination of the oral cavity performed. It should include a careful study of all the oral cavity structures. The patients should be questioned as to the problems they have encountered with their oral cavity. They should also be asked what medications they are taking and what treatments they received in the recent past. This will give you information on drugs or treatments that have caused the problem or may cause a problem in the future.

AGE-RELATED PHENOMENON

The oral mucous membrane involves the smooth tissues of the cheeks and the gingiva around the teeth. The smooth oral mucous membrane that covers the soft palate, cheeks, floor of the mouth, and the undersurface of the tongue is the lining mucosa and is composed of thick epithelium. The tongue is a specialized mucosa that is covered by small papillae and taste buds. The tongue has a slight whitish band called the linea alba along the lateral margin where it interferes with the teeth. During aging the alveolar mucosa becomes thin and may be more susceptible to trauma.

Sometimes there is increased fibrosis and degeneration of collagen fibers. The gingiva can experience more keratinization appearing whitish as a result.

Age-related tongue changes include atrophy of the papilla resulting in a smooth grazed appearance. The taste buds can also atrophy with age. The mouth can also change with age. The progressive loss of teeth leading to an edentulous condition is another result of the aging process. As a consequence of the above conditions, eating habits of the elderly persons may change with the result being inadequate nutrient intakes.

◆ Etiologies

◆ ineffective oral hygiene

◆ malnutrition
◆ dehydration
◆ restricted intake
◆ decreased salivation
◆ chemical irritants (acid foods, medications)
◆ mechanical irritants (ill-fitting dentures)
◆ surgery to the oral cavity
◆ trauma
◆ radiation to the oral cavity
◆ infections

ALTERED ORAL MUCOUS MEMBRANES RELATED TO

◆ ineffective oral hygiene as evidenced by halitosis, oral plaque, or carious teeth
◆ mechanical irritants (ill-fitting dentures), as evidenced by irritation to oral mucous membranes or edema of membranes

GOALS/OUTCOME CRITERIA

◆ Increase in oral hygiene practices to level patient is capable of
◆ Decrease in halitosis, oral plaque, and carious teeth
◆ Decrease in oral mucous membrane irritation

INTERVENTIONS

◆ Patient teaching about oral hygiene practices
◆ Referral to dentist
◆ Nutritional counseling

ACCOUNTABILITY

RN, MD, RD, DDS

ALTERED ORAL MUCOUS MEMBRANES RELATED TO

◆ Malnutrition as evidenced by decreased weight and nutritional status
◆ Dehydration as evidenced by poor skin turgor, decreased weight, coated tongue, xerostomia
◆ Decreased salivation as evidenced by dry mouth, thirst, and decreased saliva

GOALS/OUTCOME CRITERIA

◆ Improved nutritional status
◆ Improved hydration
◆ Decrease in oral discomfort

INTERVENTIONS

◆ Nutritional counseling
◆ Hydration (po, IV)
◆ Include foods easy to chew in diet

ACCOUNTABILITY

RN, RD

ALTERED ORAL MUCOUS MEMBRANES RELATED TO

◆ chemical irritants (acid foods, medications)
◆ effects of surgery to oral cavity
◆ effects of trauma to oral cavity
◆ effects of radiation to oral cavity
◆ effects of infections in oral cavity

GOALS/OUTCOME CRITERIA

◆ Decrease in irritation to mouth
◆ Decrease in pain
◆ Proper healing occurs in mouth

INTERVENTIONS

◆ Medical information. Referral to physician for changes in medication.
◆ Nutritional counseling
◆ Pain therapy as prescribed; therapy for infections as prescribed.
◆ Mouth care

ACCOUNTABILITY

RN, RD, MD, RPh

◆ Nursing Diagnosis

Fluid volume deficit, potential. This diagnosis describes someone who is at risk for developing a deficit in their total body fluid volume.

ASSESSMENT

The patient must be assessed for the presence of risk factors. They must be carefully assessed for total body fluid volume. The patient's weight must be measured as well as the change in weight over time. Fluid intake and output must be measured. The patient's vital signs must also be monitored.

AGE-RELATED PHENOMENON

Elderly persons may have problems in maintaining their fluid balance. This maintenance of balance may be difficult because of problems with mobility, which limits the person's abilities to obtain fluid. There may also be a decreased ability to respond to the stimulus of thirst. The elderly person may limit their fluid intake to prevent or limit the incidence of incontinence.

The elderly person may also be on a medication regimen that includes the use of diuretics. With age, there is a reduction in the efficiency of the heart with a decrease in cardiac output. This will result in a decrease of perfusion to such organs as the kidneys.

ETIOLOGIES

- ◆ impaired regulatory mechanisms
- ◆ loss of body fluid
- ◆ inadequate intake of fluid

FLUID VOLUME DEFICIT, POTENTIAL: related to

- ◆ effects of extreme age
- ◆ effects of extremes of weight
- ◆ deviations affecting access to fluids, intake of fluids, or absorption of fluids (e.g., physical immobility, unconsciousness)
- ◆ change in fluid requirements (e.g., hypermetabolic states; hyperthermia; dry, hot environment)
- ◆ lack of knowledge about fluid volume requirements
- ◆ effects of medications (e.g., diuretics)
- ◆ increased fluid output ·
- ◆ urinary frequency
- ◆ thirst
- ◆ effects of impaired regulatory mechanisms

GOALS/OUTCOME CRITERIA

- ◆ Fluid imbalance is prevented

INTERVENTIONS

- ◆ Monitoring of intake and output (RN, RD, MD)
- ◆ Nutritional counseling

◆ Nursing Diagnosis

Fluid volume deficit, (actual). This diagnosis would include those individuals who have an increased loss of body fluid due to a physical inability to regulate water balance.

ASSESSMENT

The patient must be checked carefully for total body fluid volume. The patient's weight must be measured as well as the change in weight over time. A review of the patient's intake and output must be done to find areas of excess fluid loss. The patient's medications must be checked to see what may be contributing to the total fluid loss. The vital signs must be checked and a physical examination done to see the total extent of the fluid volume deficit.

AGE-RELATED PHENOMENON

Elderly persons may have problems in maintaining their fluid balance. This maintenance of balance may be difficult because of problems with mobility, which limits the person's abilities to obtain fluid. There may also be a decreased ability to respond to the stimulus of thirst. The elderly person may limit their fluid intake to prevent or limit the incidence of incontinence.

The elderly person may also be on a medication regimen that includes the use of diuretics. With age, there is a reduction in the efficiency of the heart with a decrease in cardiac output. This will result in a decrease of perfusion to such organs as the kidneys.

ETIOLOGIES

◆ Failure of regulatory mechanisms.

◆ Nursing Diagnosis

Fluid volume deficit (actual), related to effects of failure of regulatory mechanisms, as evidenced by

◆ dilute urine
◆ increased urine output
◆ sudden weight loss
◆ hypotension
◆ decreased venous filling
◆ increased pulse rate
◆ decreased pulse volume pressure
◆ hemoconcentration
◆ dry skin, mucous membranes
◆ decreased skin turgor
◆ increased body temperature
◆ edema, possible weight gain
◆ thirst
◆ weakness

GOALS/OUTCOME CRITERIA

◆ Fluid balance is attained
◆ Future episodes of fluid imbalance are prevented

INTERVENTIONS

◆ Fluid volume replacement (po, IV)
◆ Monitoring of intake and output
◆ Nutritional counseling

ACCOUNTABILITY

RN, RD, MD

◆ Nursing Diagnosis

Fluid volume deficit, (actual). This condition would involve the loss of a greater amount of body fluid than is replaced through oral or IV intake. This active loss could be facilitated by loss from drains, wounds, diaphoresis or by the effect of medications (diuretics).

ASSESSMENT

The patient must be carefully assessed for total body fluid volume. The patient's weight must be measured as well as the change in weight over time. A review of the patient's intake and output must be done to find areas of excess fluid loss. The patient's medications must be checked to see what may be contributing to the total fluid loss. The vital signs must be checked and a physical examination done to see the total extent of the fluid volume deficit.

AGE-RELATED PHENOMENON

Elderly persons may have problems in maintaining their fluid balance. This maintenance of balance may be difficult because of problems with mobility, which limits the person's abilities to obtain the fluid. There may also be decreased ability to respond to the stimulus of thirst. The elderly person may limit fluid intake to prevent or limit incontinent episodes. The elderly person may also be on a medication regimen that includes the use of diuretics. With age, there is a reduction in the efficiency of the heart with a decrease in cardiac output. This will result in a decrease of perfusion to such organs as the kidneys.

ETIOLOGIES

◆ Active loss of body fluid.

◆ Nursing Diagnosis

Fluid volume deficit (actual), related to active loss of body fluid as evidenced by

◆ decreased urine output
◆ concentrated urine

◆ output greater than intake
◆ sudden weight loss
◆ decreased venous filling
◆ hemoconcentration
◆ increased serum Na, BUN
◆ hypotension
◆ thirst
◆ increased pulse rate
◆ decreased skin turgor
◆ decreased pulse volume and pressure
◆ change in mental state
◆ increase in body temperature
◆ dry skin and mucous membranes
◆ weakness

GOALS/OUTCOME CRITERIA

◆ Attains fluid balance
◆ Further episodes of fluid volume deficit are prevented

INTERVENTIONS

◆ Fluid volume replacement (po, IV)
◆ Monitoring of intake and output
◆ Nutritional counseling on fluid maintenance

ACCOUNTABILITY

RN, RD, MD

◆ Nursing Diagnosis

Fluid volume excess. This diagnosis would indicate the condition in which the patient has an increased amount of total body fluid. The condition would indicate those who have received an excess of fluid or have been unable to excrete the excess fluid absorbed.

ASSESSMENT

The patient should be assessed for signs of fluid volume overload. This assessment would include weight and weight change over time. The patient's daily intake and output must be carefully obtained and assessed for imbalances. A physical examination should be done to assess for signs of fluid retention such as pulmonary edema, distended neck veins, or pitting edema. The patient's vital signs (including blood pressure) should be carefully monitored.

AGE-RELATED PHENOMENON

Elderly persons may have problems in maintaining their fluid balance. This maintenance of balance may be difficult because of problems with mobility, which limit the person's abilities to obtain the fluid. There may also be a decreased ability to respond to the stimulus of thirst. The elderly person may limit their fluid intake to prevent or limit the episodes of incontinence. The elderly person may also be on a medication regimen that includes the use of diuretics. With age, there is a reduction in the efficiency of the heart with a decrease in cardiac output. This will result in a decrease of perfusion to such organs as the kidneys (Ebersole, Hess, 1981).

ETIOLOGIES

- ◆ compromised regulatory mechanisms
- ◆ excess fluid or sodium intake

◆ Nursing Diagnosis

Fluid volume excess, related to compromised regulatory mechanisms and/ or related to excess fluid or sodium intake, as evidenced by

- ◆ edema, effusion, anasarca, sudden weight gain
- ◆ restlessness and anxiety, change in mental status
- ◆ intake greater than output
- ◆ oliguria
- ◆ shortness of breath, dyspnea, orthopnea
- ◆ abnormal breath sounds
- ◆ pulmonary congestion by CXR
- ◆ changes in BP, venous pressure
- ◆ jugular vein distention
- ◆ altered electrolytes
- ◆ decreased hemoglobin and hematocrit

GOALS/OUTCOME CRITERIA

- ◆ Decrease in total body fluid volume

INTERVENTIONS

- ◆ Fluid restriction
- ◆ Diuretics
- ◆ Diet counseling
- ◆ Restrict fluid and sodium in diet
- ◆ Increased potassium may also be required if patient is on diuretics
- ◆ Regular physical assessment

ACCOUNTABILITY

RN, RD, MD

◆ Nursing Diagnosis

Potential impaired skin integrity. This diagnosis would apply to individuals who have risk factor for skin breakdown. Age-related changes contribute to risk factors. Other risk factors include inadequate or inappropriate nutritional intake, dry skin, pressure points, immobility, or decreased activity.

Impaired skin integrity. This diagnosis relates to breaks in the skin. These could be decubitis ulcers, abrasions, tears involving any part of the skin. It would include breaks in the skin but would not apply to breaks that occur through surgical or medical interventions.

ASSESSMENT

The patient should be examined thoroughly to locate potential areas for skin impairment. All skin surfaces are assessed. Any signs of impaired circulation, pressure points against the skin, signs of breakdown, lesions, or redness are assessed. A nutritional assessment is done to determine the patient's daily nutrient intake.

Skin assessment is a major critical factor influencing the elder's health. Physical assessment should include past history and current status of the skin. (See Table 5–1.)

Any ulcer, lesion or other skin condition should be fully described, using specific measurements, not just estimates. It is much preferred to state that an ulcer is 2 cm in diameter, rather than "size of a quarter." All areas of redness or ulceration should be assessed on a regular and continuous basis, for example, every Tuesday and Thursday. Regular documentation by the taking of instant color photographs is an excellent method of recording the skin condition. Be sure to obtain any necessary releases from the patient and to record the time, date, person taking the photograph, and the skin treatment for each photograph.

Skin assessment should also include the risk level for developing pressure sores. The Norton Score Chart (see Fig. 5–1) is a simple, yet efficient, method of determining risk.

AGE-RELATED PHENOMENON

The skin consists of three distinct departments (epidermis, dermis, and subcutaneous fat). Age-related changes occur in the epidermal and dermal skin layers. There is also atrophy of the sebaceous glands. Decreased amounts of sebum decrease the outer lipid film of the skin and allow more rapid evaporation. The subcutaneous fat layer diminishes with age in most areas and is replaced with adipocytes.

The major aging changes in the skin include dryness, wrinkling, and pigmentation. The most striking and consistent change is flattening of the dermo-epidermal junction. This subsequently results in a considerably

TABLE 5–1 ◆ Skin Assessment

History
Past and present skin conditions:
  Onset, development, pattern, duration, symptoms
Past and present systemic diseases:
  History and treatment
Drug history:
  Topical, systemic, prescription, nonprescription, allergies
Nutrition:
  Malnourished, obese, diet and eating habits
Functional status:
  Mobility, mental status, activities of daily living capacity
Environment:
  Physical (temperature, climate, use of soaps or other drying agents)
  Social (support systems, work, family interactions)
Physical Assessment
Color:
  Red, jaundiced, brown, gray, cyanotic, pale, blotchy
Temperature:
  Hot, warm, cool
Moisture:
  Dry, oily, or combination of both; moist, clammy
Texture:
  Rough, smooth, scaly, flaky
Edema:
  Location, extent
Thickness:
  Differences among various parts of the body, relationship to itching or redness
Mobility and turgor:
  Supple, pliable, flexible, creases and folds
Lesions:
  Color, size, texture, identifying characteristics, distribution
Hair:
  Amount, distribution, texture, color, dandruff or scaling, odor
Nails:
  Color, length, cleanliness, thickness, splitting, swelling, accumulations

From Matteson and McConnell, *Textbook of Gerontological Nursing*. Philadelphia: W.B. Saunders; 1988; 167.

smaller surface between the two compartments. Less nutrient transfer may result and less resistance to forces, so less pressure can be withstood.

ETIOLOGIES

◆ altered circulation, metabolic state
◆ hyperthermia or hypothermia
◆ physical immobilization

FIGURE 5–1 ◆ Norton Score Chart

Name of Patient _____ Room No. _____

Dates

General physical condition:	Good	4		
	Fair	3		
	Poor	2		
	Bad	1		
Mental state:	Alert	4		
	Apathetic	3		
	Confused	2		
	Stuporous	1		
Activity:	Ambulant	4		
	Ambulant with help	3		
	Chair-bound	2		
	Confined to bed	1		
Mobility:	Full	4		
	Slightly limited	3		
	Very limited	2		
	Immobile	1		
Incontinence:	Not incontinent	4		
	Occasionally incontinent	3		
	Usually incontinent of urine	2		
	Doubly incontinent	1		
	Totals			

(From Norton, D., McLaren, R.S. and Exton-Smith, A.N. Pressure sores. In *Investigation of Geriatric Nursing Problems in Hospitals.*

FIGURE 5–1   The Norton Score for measuring the risk of pressure sore formation. Rate the patient for each of the categories. Patients scoring 15 to 20 have little risk of pressure sore development, whereas patients with scores between 12 and 15 have a moderately high risk of developing a pressure sore, and patients scoring below 12 are at high risk. Pressure sore prevention methods should be instituted for those with scores less than 15.

- ◆ humidity
- ◆ alteration in turgor (elasticity)
- ◆ altered nutritional status (obesity, emaciation)
- ◆ altered sensation, pigmentation
- ◆ immunological deficit
- ◆ medication
- ◆ psychogenic factors

Loss of dermal thickness occurs in almost 20 percent of elderly persons. This may account for the paper thin quality of the skin. The aging skin is increasingly rigid and less capable of responding to stress. The functions of the human skin that decline with age include decreased sensory perception, decreased immune responsiveness, thermoregulation, and injury response. Therefore, the older patient with a history of a debilitating disease and in poor nutritional status is likely to be at risk for disorders of skin integrity.

◆ Nursing Diagnosis

Potential (or actual) impaired skin integrity, related to

- ◆ altered circulation or altered metabolic state
- ◆ hyperthermia or hypothermia
- ◆ physical immobilization
- ◆ effects of altered nutritional status (obesity; emaciation)
- ◆ effects of altered sensation
- ◆ effects of immunological deficit
- ◆ effects of medication
- ◆ psychogenic factors
- ◆ developmental factors

GOALS/OUTCOME CRITERIA

- ◆ Disruption of skin surface is prevented or minimized
- ◆ Wounds heal
- ◆ Complications of skin disruptions are prevented or reduced

INTERVENTIONS

- ◆ Frequent skin assessment and observation
- ◆ Protective devices and measures to prevent skin damage
- ◆ Wound care
- ◆ Nutritional counseling to emphasize high protein, calorically balanced diet, multivitamins, especially vitamin C and zinc
- ◆ Frequent changes in position

ACCOUNTABILITY

RN, RD, MD

◆ Nursing Diagnosis

Impaired Skin Integrity (Decubitus Ulcer: specify stage). A decubitus ulcer is damage to integumentary tissue, usually occurring over a bony prominence. It is commonly associated with increased pressure on these sites in a person whose mobility is limited. *Impaired Tissue Integrity* is a possible diagnosis when damage is extensive.

ASSESSMENT

The patient should be assessed carefully for signs of skin impairment or injury. When a decubitus ulcer is present, the size and depth of the wound is recorded. The patient's nutritional status must also be assessed in order to determine whether it is adequate.

All dermal ulcers should be accurately classified as to their size, shape, depth, presence of granulation or necrotic tissue, drainage, odor, inflammation, and any other significant factors. Staging of ulcers can be done as follows:

Stage I: reddened area, no break in skin.

Stage II: Reddened area, small ulceration

Stage III: Deep ulceration, with drainage; no necrosis, with slough or eschar

Stage IV: Deep ulceration, necrotic area with slough or eschar

AGE-RELATED PHENOMENON

Decubitus ulcers or pressure sores occur commonly in the elderly person who is confined to bed or the wheelchair. The lesion itself is usually classified as a systemic rather than a cutaneous disorder. Chronic disease and debility seen in the elderly make them particularly vulnerable to this problem.

The decubitus ulcer usually occurs over bony prominences. Prolonged directive pressure produces tissue anoxia with necrosis of the epidermis and superficial dermis. There are several predisposing factors in the elderly. These include reduced blood flow in large vessels, reduced subcutaneous fat resulting in greater pressure on the skin over bony prominences. Older persons also can manifest a greater variation in pressure of the sitting surface. The older individual experiences greater pressure when seated or lying on a firm surface than does a younger individual of the same size and weight. This is possibly due to loss of skin tone and integrity.

Once a decubitus ulcer forms, healing may be slow in the elderly. This is due to a variety of reasons, including general poor nutritional intake, contamination of the ulcer area, or inadequate vascular supply of the area affected.

Although decubitus ulcers are difficult to manage in the elderly patient, prevention is much easier than treatment. Maintaining proper nutritional status is essential in the patients in order to help in the healing process.

ETIOLOGIES

◆ Prolonged pressure
◆ Friction, shear injury
◆ Immobility
◆ Incontinence
◆ Undernutrition (protein, Vit. C)
◆ Sensory-motor loss
◆ Cognitive impairment

IMPAIRED SKIN INTEGRITY related to

◆ Prolonged pressure
◆ Friction, shear injury
◆ Effects of incontinence on skin
◆ Undernutrition (protein, vitamin C)
◆ Effects of sensory-motor loss
◆ Effects of cognitive impairment

As evidenced by

◆ Reddened area
◆ Verbalization of pain, discomfort, or numbness over bony prominence without exterior skin destruction (deep decubitus)
◆ Reddened area, small ulceration, no necrosis (Stage III)
◆ Deep ulceration, necrotic area (Stage IV)

GOALS/OUTCOME CRITERIA

◆ Wounds heal
◆ Further injuries are prevented
◆ Nutritional status is improved
◆ Complications are prevented

INTERVENTIONS

◆ Wound care (RN, LPN)
◆ Nutrition support (MD, RD, RN)
◆ Nutrition counseling (RD, RN, MD)
◆ Skin care teaching (i.e., cleaning, positioning, prevention of injury) (RN, LPN)
◆ Physical therapy (PT)

ACCOUNTABILITY

LPN, RN, RD, MD, PT

References

Bowman, BB, Rosenberg, IH. Assessment of the nutritional status of the elderly. In *American Journal of Clinical Nutrition.* May 1982; 35:1142–1151.

Ebersole, P, Hess, P. *Toward Healthy Aging.* St. Louis: The C. V. Mosby Company; 1981; 75.

Munro, HN. Nutrition and the elderly: A general overview. In *Journal of the American College of Nutrition.* 1984; 3:341–350.

Nelder, KH. Nutrition, aging, and the skin. In *Geriatrics.* February 1984; 39:69–88.

Nutrition needs for the elderly. In *Iowa Medicine.* January; 76:32.

Vin, SC, Lone, AHG. Anthropometric measurements in the elderly. In *Gerontology.* 1980; 26:1.

Yearick, ES, Wang, ML, Pieseas, SJ. Nutritional status of the elderly: Dietary and biochemical findings. In *Journal of Gerontology.* 1980; 35:663.

Bates, B. *A Guide to Physical Examination.* 3rd edition. Philadelphia: J.B. Lippincott; 1983.

6

Elimination Pattern

Judith Conway

◆

CONTINENCE PROBLEMS

◆ Nursing Diagnosis: Stress Incontinence

This diagnosis refers to involuntary urination related to physical activity.

◆ Assessment

The assessment should consist of physical examination, urinalysis, and patient interview.

A history should be obtained either by patient interview or review of the nurses' notes. Information about the onset is important in planning the course of treatment. For example, it would be helpful to know if the problem was longstanding and had been treated previously, or if this problem presented recently. The resident should provide information about what types of physical activity are associated with the episodes of stress incontinence: sneezing, coughing, laughing, bending over, or other changes in position. It would also be important to know if the resident has had a history of multiple urinary tract infections or trauma to the area.

Physical assessment should include palpation of the abdomen to rule out retention or presence of abdominal mass. The perineal area should be inspected for signs of irritation or tissue breakdown. Presence of cystocele or rectocele should also be identified at this time. Urinalysis should be obtained to rule out presence of infection.

◆ Age-Related Phenomena

Stress incontinence is a condition resulting from a weakening of the pelvic floor muscles due to atrophy. Support for the lower bladder becomes less reliable and any undue pressure on the bladder, such as that exerted during coughing or sneezing, will result in a release of at least a small amount of urine.

It is believed that stress placed upon the pelvic floor muscles, such as that which occurs during traumatic or multiple delivery, coupled with a decline in estrogen levels, will result in loss of muscle tone and stress incontinence. Thus, the condition is seen mainly in older women and may be more prevalent in obese women.

Other conditions, such as prolapsed uterus or cystocele, enterocele, and rectocele, will cause pressure on the bladder directly or indirectly. These conditions may influence the occurrence of stress incontinence.

Stress incontinence may also be seen in women who have experienced multiple urinary tract infection. Scarring or adhesions may form inside the bladder and interfere with the ability of the bladder to hold the urine.

ETIOLOGIES

INTERNAL

◆ Infection
◆ Sphincter weakness
◆ Prolapsed uterus
◆ Cystocele
◆ Rectocele
◆ Enterocele
◆ Loss of tone of pelvic floor muscles

◆ Nursing Diagnosis

Stress incontinence related to one or more etiologies.

DEFINING CHARACTERISTICS

Involuntary passage of urine during varied physical activities.

GOALS/OUTCOME CRITERIA

Episodes of incontinence are reduced.

NURSING INTERVENTIONS

◆ Assess for causative factors: (see internal etiologies), and treat as appropriate. (RN/LPN)
◆ Teach importance of fluid intake to assist in maintenance of detrusor muscle integrity. (RN/LPN)
◆ Teach Kegel exercises, and exercises to strengthen abdomino-perineal muscles. (LPN)
◆ Maintain skin integrity: Provide hygiene after each incontinent episode including application of skin barrier cream. (NA)
◆ When appropriate, offer the patient a choice of using protective undergarments (for use during outings, etc., to reduce the chance of an "accident" causing embarrassment). This will assist in eliminating self-isolation. (LPN)

◆ Nursing Diagnosis

Alteration in urinary elimination pattern.

This diagnosis refers to any change in the individual's pattern of voiding.

ASSESSMENT

The focus of the nursing assessment includes examination of the patient (subjective and objective), examination of the urine, and documentation of the voiding pattern.

The nursing notes should be reviewed to determine the onset of the problem. The resident should be interviewed, if appropriate, to discover whether there is agreement about symptoms or if they have additional information to contribute. The resident should be asked about what type of symptoms he or she may be experiencing: frequency, urgency, dysuria, hesitancy, incontinence. The male resident should be asked if he has noticed increased difficulty initiating voiding. The female resident should be questioned about urethral or meatal irritation or vaginal discharge.

If the resident's mental status is such that an interview would not yield any data, observation for changes in behavior at voiding time may provide important information. For example, a nonverbal patient may suddenly start to cry after voiding or become very restless before an incontinent episode.

Intake and output should be recorded in order to document whether a change in a pattern exists, frequency of voiding, and amount voided. If the resident is already on I&O, a retrospective look at the sheets may show whether intake or output has decreased or demonstrate other recent changes.

The abdomen should be palpated for bladder distension or discomfort. The perineal area should be checked for irritation or signs of tissue breakdown. Urinary meatus may be inspected for signs of irritation or bleeding. The nurse or resident should look for the presence of blood on the toilet tissue after voiding.

A screening analysis should be obtained. At this time, appearance of the urine should be examined and documented for color, cloudiness, odor, sediment, mucus, and blood. Culture and sensitivity may then be ordered if appropriate.

Finally, a rectal examination should be performed in order to eliminate the possibility of constipation as the contributing factor to a sudden change in elimination pattern. The presence of a large fecal mass in the rectum may cause frequency or incontinence.

AGE-RELATED PHENOMENA

The bladder is composed primarily of the detrusor muscle, which is capable of contracting and forcing urine out through the urethra. As we age, the shape of the bladder changes from round to funnel, due to changes in the supporting connecting tissue and weakening of the pelvic floor muscles. The detrusor muscle elongates, and the capacity of the bladder becomes diminished. Additionally, what is thought to be the "internal sphincter" is actually more closely woven connective tissue. As this becomes weaker, more pressure is brought to bear downward, and there may be a tendency to lose control of the external sphincter.

The kidney slowly loses its ability to concentrate urine, and the older person may experience nocturia more frequently.

Females experience two changes. First, loss of the estrogen hormone may result in frequent irritation to the lining of the urethra, placing them at risk for infection. In addition, the uterus may tip forward on the bladder. This will further diminish the capacity of the bladder to hold urine.

The elderly male may experience an alteration in urinary elimination due to prostate enlargement. A great majority of men will discover that as the prostate enlarges and places pressure on the neck of the bladder and urethra, it becomes more difficult to initiate a stream. They may also experience increasing urinary frequency.

Frequently, in an attempt to deal with the symptoms that occur as a result of these body changes (especially frequency), the elderly will voluntarily decrease fluid intake. Unfortunately, this only further irritates the detrusor muscle, which needs at least 200 cc of urine in order to be stimulated and maintain tone.

ETIOLOGIES

EXTERNAL

Positioning: A non-upright position contributes to bacteria traveling upward from anus to urethra.

Hygiene: Lack of hand washing. Failure to wipe front to back: (see above).

INTERNAL

Infection: kidney/bladder

Hormonal insufficiency

Detrusor muscle instability: neuromuscular disease

Detrusor muscle irritability: reduced fluid intake (vol.)

Confusion

Habit: establish pattern of frequent voiding.

Sphincter weakness

Uterine prolapse

Enlarged prostate

Constipation

Immobility: cannot reach bathroom in time

Medications: (Side effects) Nocturnal incontinence from sedatives (deep sleep).

Retention: anticholinergic

Depression or Apathy: Grieving process or change in environment

Alzheimer's Disease: Later stages

Diabetes

Congestive Heart Failure

◆ Nursing Diagnosis

Alteration in urinary elimination related to one or more etiologies.

DEFINING CHARACTERISTICS

Dysuria, Frequency, Hesitancy, Nocturia, Retention, Urgency, Incontinence

GOALS/OUTCOME CRITERIA

Restoration of previously established pattern.

INTERVENTIONS

Assess for contributing etiologies, i.e. review medications (RN/LPN)

Obtain urine for analysis, or culture and sensitivity where appropriate. (RN/LPN)

Review voiding pattern. (RN/LPN)

Place on I&O. (NA)

Force fluids to 2000 cc unless contraindicated. Encourage high acid fluids (cranberry juice). (LPN)

Avoid natural diuretic type fluids: pineapple juice, coffee, tea. (NA)

Limit fluids after early evening. (LPN)

Provide loose-fitting garments that are easily removed. (NA)

Teach hygiene: hand washing, and wiping from front to back. (NA)

Teach resident to hold back urine if possible to increase bladder capacity. (LPN)

Position resident as upright as possible if voiding on bedpan. (LPN/ NA)

Teach Kegel exercises to strengthen pelvic floor muscles. (LPN)

Teach resident about relationship between fluid intake and detrusor muscle integrity. (LPN)

Provide toileting program: on awakening, ½ to 1 hour after meals, every 2 hours while awake, and before bedtime. (LPN)

Evaluate interventions in 2 weeks, and adjust as necessary. (RN/LPN)

◆ Nursing Diagnosis

(Alteration in bowel elimination: diarrhea.)

This diagnosis refers to a pattern of elimination that is associated with frequent, loose, or watery stools.

ASSESSMENT

The development of diarrhea may be due to many factors. In order to determine possible causes, the assessment should include several areas. First, the pattern should be observed via accurate record keeping. Onset and frequency of diarrhea can be important in determining the cause. For example, acute diarrhea may be caused by an infection (i.e., food poisoning), or an ulcerative condition (i.e., diverticulitis). If an infectious process is the cause, the onset is usually quick and dramatic. It is particularly dangerous to the frail elderly because dehydration may occur very quickly. Other causes of diarrhea (diabetic neuropathy or bacterial overgrowth) may present more slowly.

In addition to recording pattern, the consistency of stool should be noted: loose versus watery, presence of blood, undigested particles of food, or presence of mucous should be noted.

Physical assessment should include presence of bowel sounds, distension, flatulence, palpation of the abdomen for areas of pain or discomfort, peri-anal skin integrity, and the patient's subjective description of comfort. Rectal examination is appropriate as it could verify the presence of a large fecal mass that was allowing only the passage of liquid stool. The resident should be observed frequently for signs of dehydration: poor skin turgor and dryness of the oral mucous membrane (the resident might complain of inability to produce saliva).

Finally, diet and medication regimens should be reviewed at this time. Development of food allergies or intolerances may occur at any age, and side-effects to medications may also develop at an individual rate.

AGE-RELATED PHENOMENA

The elderly may be more at risk to develop diarrhea for many reasons. Thus, an understanding of circumstances that are specific to the aging population may be helpful in intervening with this problem.

While all age groups are certainly subject to many stressful life events, the elderly experience unique ones, such as changes in living arrangements and loss of loved ones. The occurrence of diarrhea due to events such as these may be of limited duration, but the possibility exists that it may be long-lasting and should be addressed.

Many elderly have developed the habit of using laxatives as a means of daily elimination. This stems from a belief that lack of daily bowel elimination could serve as a source of other health problems. The problem that results, of course, is the presence of diarrhea, insult to the intestinal tissue, and the risk of complications.

The elder's living conditions may lend itself to the risk of diarrhea. For example, if storage conditions such as refrigeration are not available, the possibility of foods such as potato salad "going bad" is high. Many people do not understand the relationship between conditions for bacterial growth and food storage conditions. If the resident is receiving nourishment through a nasogastric or gastrostomy tube, the formula should be stored according to the manufacturer's directions.

The presence of physical problems may indirectly cause diarrhea. For example, if the elder is being treated with long-term antibiotic therapy for infection, the medication may destroy normal intestinal flora and cause an overgrowth of pathogens. In addition, disease conditions such as diverticulitis or tumors may first present with symptoms that include diarrhea.

ETIOLOGIES

EXTERNAL

Contaminated foodstuffs

    a. Tube feeding formula

    b. Picnic foods (i.e., potato salad)

Medications

Parasitic Infections

Helminths

INTERNAL

Intolerance/Allergy to food

Medications: (Side effects)

Presence of disease:

    a. Colitis

    b. Diverticulitis

    c. Tumor

    d. Virus

    e. Hyperthyroid

    f. Diabetes

◆ Nursing Diagnosis

Altered bowel elimination: Diarrhea related to one or more etiologies.

DEFINING CHARACTERISTICS

Frequent, loose, watery stool

Abdominal pain, cramping, distension

Urgency

Increased frequency of bowel sounds.

GOALS

Return to normal pattern of elimination

INTERVENTIONS

Assess patient: pattern, consistency. Keep accurate record. (LPN/NA)

Culture stool if appropriate. (RN/LPN)

Observe for signs of dehydration: notify MD if patient is unable to tolerate replacement fluids. (RN/LPN)

Assess and record: bowel sounds, pain, distension. (RN/LPN)

Review medication and diet. (RN/LPN)

Review food storage facilities. (LPN)

Provide special skin care to perineal area after each episode. (NA)

Promote hygiene for both patient and staff. (LPN)

◆ Nursing Diagnosis

(Impairment of urinary elimination: incontinence.)
This diagnosis refers to uncontrolled urination.

ASSESSMENT

Nursing assessment includes observation and documentation of the voiding pattern, and physical and psychosocial examination.

First, changes in voiding pattern should be observed for onset and frequency of the problem. If the nurse accompanies the resident to the toilet, the amount of urine passed should be documented. If the resident is immobile, episodes of incontinence including measurement of amounts should be recorded.

Physical assessment should include palpation of the bladder before and after urination to determine if the patient is retaining urine and only voiding overflow volume. The perineal area should be inspected for irritation or early tissue breakdown, and evidence of discharge from either bladder or vagina. Temperature should be taken daily since low-grade fever may indicate the possibility of infection. A rectal examination should be included in the physical assessment to eliminate the possibility of constipation as a contributing factor.

Mental status must be considered within the nursing assessment. Is the incontinence an outward sign of "giving up"? Or, is the patient suddenly or gradually unaware that this has occurred. This may be the first sign of a problem the resident has that has not been noticed. It may also be the side effect of a medication regimen. For example, if medication has been given that may cause confusion, the incontinent episode may be indirectly related.

Assessment of incontinence should also include an assessment for pattern development. The nurse should be examining any pattern to identify the repetitive factors, such as time of day, environment, and relationship to meals. Several incontinence diaries have been developed. Figure 6–1 is one example of an incontinence monitoring form. This tool may need to be maintained from a few days to several weeks in order to determine any pattern.

Finally, screening urinalysis and culture should be obtained.

INCONTINENCE MONITORING RECORD

INSTRUCTIONS: EACH TIME THE PATIENT IS CHECKED:
1) Mark *one* of the circles in the BLADDER section at the hour closest to the time the patient is checked.
2) Make an X in the BOWEL section if the patient has had an incontinent or normal bowel movement.

𝄙 = Incontinent, small amount Ø = Dry		X = Incontinent BOWEL
𝄙 = Incontinent, large amount 𝝙 = Voided correctly		X = Normal BOWEL

PATIENT NAME _____ ROOM # _____ DATE _____

| | BLADDER | | | BOWEL | | | |
	INCONTINENT OF URINE	DRY	VOIDED CORRECTLY	INCONTINENT X	NORMAL X	INITIALS	COMMENTS
12 am	● ●	○	𝝙 cc ___				
1	● ●	○	𝝙 cc ___				
2	● ●	○	𝝙 cc ___				
3	● ●	○	𝝙 cc ___				
4	● ●	○	𝝙 cc ___				
5	● ●	○	𝝙 cc ___				
6	● ●	○	𝝙 cc ___				
7	● ●	○	𝝙 cc ___				
8	● ●	○	𝝙 cc ___				
9	● ●	○	𝝙 cc ___				
10	● ●	○	𝝙 cc ___				
11	● ●	○	𝝙 cc ___				
12 pm	● ●	○	𝝙 cc ___				
1	● ●	○	𝝙 cc ___				
2	● ●	○	𝝙 cc ___				
3	● ●	○	𝝙 cc ___				
4	● ●	○	𝝙 cc ___				
5	● ●	○	𝝙 cc ___				
6	● ●	○	𝝙 cc ___				
7	● ●	○	𝝙 cc ___				
8	● ●	○	𝝙 cc ___				
9	● ●	○	𝝙 cc ___				
10	● ●	○	𝝙 cc ___				
11	● ●	○	𝝙 cc ___				
TOTALS:							

c 1984

FIGURE 6–1   Incontinence monitoring form (From Greengold, B.A., and Ouslander, J. Bladder retraining. *J. of Gerontological Nursing.* 1986; 12:31–35.

AGE-RELATED PHENOMENA

Several changes in the body occur as we age that contribute to the possibility of episodes of incontinence. First, changes in the shape of the bladder contribute to the decrease in capacity. The muscle tone of the detrusor decreases, and the result is usually an increase in the amount of residual urine.

Changes in the abdominal and perineal muscles that assist in voiding will also contribute to incomplete emptying of the bladder. Coupled with these changes is a decrease in inhibition to void. This will cause more of an urgency to urinate and may also cause incontinence in the elderly who have limited mobility.

Changes in the endocrine system may also affect the risk of incontinence indirectly. For example, the female loses hormones within the lining of the urethra, and experiences a shortening of the urethra itself. Both of these factors, in addition to the possibility of residual urine in the bladder, may place the older woman at greater risk to infection and resultant incontinence. The elderly male may experience enlargement of the prostate gland, which may also contribute to residual urine, the possibility of infection, and incontinence.

Since many elderly experience at least one chronic condition that requires drug therapy, they are at risk to develop incontinence as a result of the side effects of medications. For example, resident's requiring diuretic therapy will complain of incontinent episodes. This problem is directly related to the changes in the bladder and the voiding process previously discussed.

Environmental changes, such as institutionalization, may contribute to episodes of incontinence in several ways. First, the availability of toilet facilities may be limited due to sharing by several residents. Secondly, the elder's ability to utilize the toilet due to changes in mobility may be a factor. Finally, adjustment to a new environment may cause temporary confusion with resultant incontinence.

The most difficult type of incontinence to address from a nursing standpoint may be that which results from neuromuscular disease. Damage to the cerebral cortex that causes a loss in the inhibition or early awareness to void presents a challenge to attempts to provide a toileting program. Yet, these residents are at great risk for infection due to the high residual volume.

ETIOLOGIES

EXTERNAL

Facilities: Shared, unavailable

Medications: (Side effects) i.e., sedatives, anticholinergics

INTERNAL

Mobility: decreased (cannot get to the toilet in time)

Infection

Neuromuscular disease: Parkinson's, Muscular Dystrophy, stroke

Confusion

Mental Status: Depression/apathy, grieving, behavioral issue.

Decreased Cognitive Functioning: Alzheimer's Disease, Organic Brain Syndrome

◆ Nursing Diagnosis

Impairment of urinary elimination: incontinence related to one or more etiologies.

DEFINING CHARACTERISTIC

Uncontrolled urination.

GOALS

Establishment of controlled pattern of urination.

INTERVENTIONS

Assess pattern of incontinent episodes: record volume and frequency. (RN)

Review medication regimen. (RN)

Obtain urinalysis or culture if appropriate. (LPN/RN)

Force fluids to 2000 cc in 24 hours unless contraindicated. (LPN)

Limit fluids after 8 pm. (LPN/NA)

Provide toileting program if indicated: on awakening, every 2 hours while awake, and just before bedtime. (NA/LPN)

Hygiene: wash perineal area after every episode of incontinence and apply skin barrier cream. (NA/LPN)

Provide clothing that is easily removed. (NA/LPN)

Provide commode, if appropriate. (NA)

Review interventions in 2 weeks, and adjust program as necessary. (RN/ LPN)

Consult with psychiatric nurse, or other therapist as needed. (RN/LPN)

◆ Nursing Diagnosis

(Altered bowel elimination: incontinence.)
This diagnosis refers to involuntary bowel movements.

ASSESSMENT

An involuntary bowel movement may or may not be recognized by the resident. Therefore, the first clue to this problem may be when the nurse notices stool on the patient's clothing or recognizes a distinct fecal odor in the resident's presence. Another noticeable occurrence may be that of bed linen occasionally smeared with feces.

As in any other alteration in a normal or usual pattern, record keeping may assist when attempting to determine possible causes. For example, a gradual onset may refer to a decreased ability to recognize the need to move the bowels, while a sudden onset may refer to an infection, or impaction.

Physical assessment should include digital examination of the rectum to rule out fecal impaction. This examination should also provide information about the resident's ability to control the external sphincter. Color and consistency of the stool may be recorded at this time.

AGE-RELATED PHENOMENA

As the aging process progresses, the elder may notice a decreasing ability to control the external sphincter. The internal sphincter reflex, however, remains intact. The two sphincters do not function in their usual complimentary fashion as they do at a younger age.

In addition to a decrease in sphincter control, many disease processes such as Alzheimer's Disease or neuromuscular problems such as stroke, cause the elderly patient to lose or suffer a decreased awareness of rectal sensation. Presence of feces in the rectum may thus go unrecognized.

The overall decrease in muscle tone may also be a result of long-standing use of laxatives. A large percentage of elderly use elimination aids in the belief that a daily bowel movement is necessary.

ETIOLOGIES

EXTERNAL

Availability of facilities

Laxative abuse

INTERNAL

Decreased mobility: Unable to control sphincter long enough to get to the bathroom

Neurological deficit: i.e., stroke, Parkinson's Disease

Cognitive deficit: Unable to recognize the need to defecate

Psychological problem: Depression, behavioral situation, confusion

Infection: Viral, bacterial

◆ Nursing Diagnosis

Alteration in bowel elimination: incontinence

DEFINING CHARACTERISTICS

Involuntary bowel movements

GOALS

Return to controlled bowel evacuation

INTERVENTIONS

Assess for fecal impaction, sphincter control, presence of bacterial or viral infection: (obtain culture if appropriate). (RN/LPN)

Keep record to determine if pattern exists. (LPN/NA)

Assess diet: Adjust to insure appropriate amounts of fluid and fiber. (Dietitian)

Provide a toileting time that reflects the patient's past pattern. You may need to utilize a suppository in order to re-establish a toileting time. (LPN)

Place a commode at the bedside if needed. (NA)

Evaluate interventions and adjust as necessary. (RN/LPN)

◆ Nursing Diagnosis

(Alteration in elimination: constipation, or intermittent constipation.)

This diagnosis refers to a pattern of bowel elimination in which the resident experiences hard, dry stools that may be difficult to pass. There is usually a reported decrease in the frequency of bowel movements.

◆ Assessment

Assessment should include audit of the resident's record to determine frequency, amount, and consistency of bowel movements. The audit assists in identifying deviation in a previously established pattern. Bowel sounds and abdominal distension should be assessed. A digital examination of the rectum should be performed to determine the presence of hard stool. The resident should be assessed as to a feeling of fullness, headache, malaise, decreased appetite, presence of pain, dizziness, and sudden onset of confusion. A large fecal mass may cause episodes of incontinence: This may also serve as a clue to constipation, especially in the more severe state.

The nurse should attempt to elicit the resident's perception of constipation. Many elderly people are misinformed as to what constitutes a pattern of regularity. They may believe that daily bowel evacuation is necessary when indeed this is not always the case.

AGE-RELATED PHENOMENA

(Constipation, or intermittent constipation.)

The elderly are subject to several alterations in conditions necessary for optimum bowel functioning: the ability to chew, swallow and tolerate foods high in roughage, maintenance of a level of exercise conducive to bowel hygiene, and the ability to recognize the need to defecate, coupled with the strength to initiate the bowel movement.

In the oral cavity, a decrease in the production of saliva and the lack of proper dentures will greatly affect the ability to chew and swallow foods high in roughage.

After the food is swallowed, a decrease in esophageal peristalsis may result in a reflux of gastric contents or produce a feeling of fullness. This may cause self-imposed limitation to intake of food or fluids.

The stomach takes longer to empty, thus lengthening the feeling of fullness experienced after meals. Appetite may decrease. Presence of high acidity or gastric or duodenal ulcer may prohibit the use of added fiber in the diet.

In the lower intestine, there is a gradual decrease in the tone of the muscles needed to assist in defecation.

There may also be a loss of the internal sphincter reflex. The resident's mobility level will obviously affect the ability to exercise to a degree. There may be an inability to recognize the need to defecate due to disease (stroke) or changes in mental status (Alzheimer's disease).

Many elderly have developed a ritual of frequent laxation over the years in the belief that lack of a daily bowel movement could serve as a source of other health problems. Elimination aids that are utilized include suppositories, enemas, or oral medications. Prolonged use of elimination aids may result in chronic constipation due to atony of intestinal muscles. Another frequent need for laxative use may result from a regimen that includes constipating medications. The nurse should be aware of both possibilities when performing an assessment.

ETIOLOGIES

EXTERNAL

ENVIRONMENTAL: Change in living facilities: (institution)

a. shared toilet facilities: lack of privacy may cause suppressed defecation
b. availability of staff to assist to toilet: patient may suppress defecation

MEDICATIONS (CONSTIPATING)

Diuretics: Lasix

Iron preparations

Antipsychotics: Haldol, Thorazine

Antiparkinsonian: Cogentin

Antidepressants: Elavil

Calcium preparations

Antacids

DIET

Lack of income to purchase proper food

Lack of dentures

Restricted diet: i.e., Bland diet

Restricted fluid intake

Change in meal pattern

Restriction in choices of food

INTERNAL

Communication: Inability to communicate:

a. Language barrier
b. Disease: cannot speak or gesture due to stroke

Immobility:

a. Limited ability to ambulate due to arthritis, stroke, post-fracture

b. Unable to ambulate or sit on commode or toilet due to contractures

MENTAL STATUS

a. Depression or apathy may be due to side effect of medication or grieving due to institutionalization or loss of loved one.

b. Disease (Alzheimer's): cannot recognize need to defecate.

c. Changes in personality.

PRESENCE OF DISEASE

Hypothyroidism

Hypercalcemia

Diabetes

Diverticular disease

Tumor, polyps, hemorrhoids

◆ Nursing Diagnosis

Constipation related to one or more etiologies

DEFINING CHARACTERISTICS

Frequency less than usual pattern

Increase in hard-formed stool, with decreased quantity

Presence of palpable mass in rectum

Reported feeling of pressure in rectum

Complaint of backache

Reported feeling of fullness, bloating, malaise, headache, decrease in appetite

Straining pain or cramps

Sudden confusion

Incontinence of urine or stool

GOALS

Establishment of pattern of 2–3 soft, formed BM's per week

INTERVENTIONS

Assess for: Adequate fiber in diet (RN/LPN)
Adequate fluid intake
Exercise or mobility level
Over use of laxatives
Constipating medications
Presence of impaction (RN/LPN)

Consult with dietitian and resident to add fluid and fiber to diet.

Consult with P.T. and resident to develop exercise program.

Consult with Psychiatric Nurse if resident is depressed or grieving. (RN/ LPN)

Plan elimination time according habits: i.e., after breakfast or in the evening. (LPN/NA)

Use commode or toilet whenever possible. If bedpan must be used, position as upright as possible or lie on left side. (NA)

Keep an accurate record: of BM's—time, frequency, consistency. (NA)

Teach the residents not to ignore sensation to move their bowels. (NA)

◆ Nursing Diagnosis

Impairment of urinary elimination: retention.

This nursing diagnosis refers to the reduction or absence of urination.

ASSESSMENT

The nursing assessment should include physical examination, observation of behavior, and chart review, including the medication regimen.

The most obvious sign of urinary retention is that of the distended bladder. Palpation of the bladder coupled with the absence or dribbling of urine will confirm this suspicion. If appropriate, the resident may be catheterized after urination to measure the presence of residual urine.

Review of the nursing notes is important because it may reveal onset of the problem. If the resident's intake and output is being monitored, retrospective examination may show a pattern has developed with regard to increased frequency or decreased output. At a time, it would be prudent to review the medication regimen for those medicines that may cause urine retention.

Many who retain urine may be unable to communicate this problem. Therefore, observation is important in that the nurse may discover subtle changes in behavior around the urination pattern. For example, many people will become restless and/or diaphoretic if the bladder is distended and they are unable to verbalize the inability to void. If the resident is able to communicate, he or she may express the belief that complete bladder emptying is not occurring during urination.

AGE-RELATED PHENOMENA

Several factors influence the possibility of retaining urine. As we age, the rate at which the kidneys filter urine decreases gradually. If the elderly person limits the intake of fluid, urine is produced at an even slower rate than usual. As a result of this, the stretch receptors in the bladder wall do not necessarily activate. Thus, voiding will not occur because the reflex stimulation is absent.

In addition, the elderly may be more at risk to develop retention due to presence of chronic conditions requiring medications that cause retention as a side effect. They may also, by virtue of their mobility level, be prone to develop calculi. The calculi, in turn, may contribute to retention.

Finally, the risk of neuromuscular conditions such as stroke would damage or destroy the ability to recognize the need to void or initiate the voiding process.

ETIOLOGIES

EXTERNAL

Positioning

Immobility

Side effects of medications: Anticholinergics, antispasmodics, antidepressants, antipsychotics, antihistamines, Beta blockers, antihypertensives

INTERNAL

Neuromuscular disease

Enlarged prostate

Uterine prolapse

Infection

Fecal impaction

Bladder neck obstruction

Urethral stricture

Calculi

Fibrosis

Tumors

Psychological: i.e., anxiety

◆ Nursing Diagnosis

Impairment of urinary elimination: retention

DEFINING CHARACTERISTICS

Absence of urine, dribbling, restlessness, discomfort, distended bladder, diaphoresis, urgency

GOALS

Restoration of voiding pattern

Assistance to empty bladder

INTERVENTIONS

Assess for contributing etiologies and intervene as necessary. (RN/LPN)

Place on I&O. (LPN)

Strain urine if calculi are suspected. (NA)

Force fluids to 2000 cc, using high acid fluids unless contraindicated. (LPN/NA)

Provide toileting program: upon awakening, before meals, every 2 hours during the day, and before bedtime. (LPN)

Teach tips on bladder emptying: positioning by leaning forward; Crede maneuver. (RN/LPN)

Promote relaxation at toileting time: place hands in warm water, pour warm water over perineum, stroke inner thigh with light pressure to stimulate micturition reflex. (LPN)

Consult with MD to provide intermittent catheterization if necessary (i.e., every 8 hours). (RN/LPN)

Evaluate plan after 2 weeks, and consult with MD for feasibility of work-up. (RN/LPN)

References

Engel RME. Urinary tract infections. In Burevich I, Tafuro P, and Cunha BA. *The Theory and Practice of Infection Control.* 1984; Chapter 22.

Greengold BA and Ouslander JG. Bladder Retraining. In *Journal of Gerontological Nursing.* 1986; 12:31–35.

Luckmann J and Sorenson KC. *Medical Surgical Nursing: A Psychophysiological Approach.* 3rd edition. Philadelphia: W. B. Saunders; 1987.

7

Activity Exercise Pattern

Kathleen M. Nokes

◆

ACTIVITY EXERCISE PATTERN

Movement is one of the most important functional patterns because it permits people to control their immediate physical environment. It is the area of physical functioning that is most likely to affect that aged person's ability to cope. However, with aging, many people experience some limitation in mobility. Among persons 65 and older who live at home, 45 percent have some degree of limitation in activities of daily living and that percentage increases to 60 percent in persons 75 and older. Many factors impact on activity patterns. These factors include normal physical changes secondary to aging; chronic and acute disease processes; psychological status; and financial, environmental, and community resources.

The following section describes nursing diagnoses related to the activity-exercise pattern. The person's activity level is reflective of a synthesis of cardiac, respiratory, muscular, bone, and motivational influences. The person's home environment is also a strong factor impacting on one's mobility. Table 7–1 provides a list of nursing diagnoses and related medical diagnoses.

◆ Nursing Diagnosis

Activity Intolerance (Specify Level): Actual and Potential

Note: These three diagnoses are presented together to reduce repetition and to increase effectiveness.

Definition: Actual activity intolerance is the abnormal response to energy-consuming movements involved in required or desired daily activities. Potential activity intolerance is the presence of risk factors for abnormal responses to energy-consuming body movements. Diversional Activity Deficit results from decreased engagement in recreational or leisure activities.

Individuals may report a gradual decrease in activity tolerance secondary to the aging process or to a chronic disease, such as atherosclerosis; or they might experience a sudden inability to manage activities secondary to an acute change, such as a myocardial infarction. The person who adapts to a gradual decrease may not notice the problem until the weakness interferes with meeting essential needs. In contrast, the person whose intoler-

TABLE 7–1 ◆ Nursing Diagnoses and Associated Medical Diagnoses

Altered cardiac output, decreased	Congestive heart failure, arrhythmias, medication toxicity, e.g. Digoxin, myocardial infarction, angina, hypertension
Altered respiration 　Impaired gas exchange 　Ineffective airway clearance 　Ineffective breathing pattern	COPD, including bronchial asthma, bronchitis, emphysema, cancer of the lung, TB, pneumonia
Altered tissue perfusion	Atherosclerosis, peripheral vascular disease, diabetes
Total self-care deficit	CVA, neurological disease, e.g. Parkinson's disease, Alzheimer's disease, multiple sclerosis, brain tumor, severe depression
Activity intolerance	Arthritis, cardiovascular disease, respiratory disease
Potential joint contractures	Arthritis, neurological deficits, depression
Impaired physical mobility	Falls, fractures, arthritis: osteo and rheumatoid

ance is sudden will probably be more aware of his or her limitations and may be feeling anger and frustration at the restrictions.

There are four levels of activity intolerance. These are Level I: walk, regular pace, on level indefinitely; one flight or more but more short of breath than normally.

Level II: walk one city block 500 feet on level; climb one flight slowly without stopping.

Level III: walk no more than 50 feet on level without stopping; unable to climb one flight of stairs without stopping.

Level IV: dyspnea and fatigue at rest.

Nursing diagnoses and interventions will be directed toward the different levels.

ASSESSMENT

Ask aged people how they perceive their reactions to increased activity. Do they see a gradual decrease in abilities over the last 6 months, last year, last 5 years? What activities have been limited? Do the people think there is adequate energy to meet activities of daily living requirements? Is energy more plentiful at different times during the day, for example early morning? Do afternoon naps help the people to feel refreshed? Ask the older person to describe a picture of a common day including usual wake-up time; how long it takes to get dressed; how long it takes to prepare, eat, and clean up after meals; how does she or he pass the bulk of time—sewing, going for walks, gardening? When are meals usually eaten? How are evenings spent? What time is bedtime? Ask the older person if he or she leaves home—how is food shopping done; does he or she drive; how are food bundles handled; does he or she visit friends, family, attend religious ceremonies, senior citizen centers? Determine in an average week, how often the person leaves home. Who does the older person speak to during the day—does she or he have a telephone; do neighbors stop by; does the person live with someone? Identify if the client exercises regularly—how long does he or she exercise; what type of exercise; how many years has the client done this activity; how many times per week? If the client is in a nursing home, what activities does he or she participate in? Is the client willing to try something new? Who does the client relate to? What kind of activities cause shortness of breath or unusual fatigue?

Included in a activity history should be the kinds of activities in which the person would like to participate, the amount of time he or she would like to be involved, the present activities the person would like to continue, new activities he or she would like to learn, and the person's general attitude towards his or her current life style. Determine if the client is as active as possible within functional limitations. Recognize that if the musculoskeletal system is not used and the client is inactive, disuse osteoporosis can result. Discuss with the client if he or she is motivated to be more active.

AGE-RELATED PHENOMENON

Activity patterns reflect the person's physical ability to react to stress, the environmental parameters, and psychological attitudes. It is also a mirror of need. If the person is independent and not unusually depressed, she or he is more motivated to meet basic needs than if a significant other or nursing care staff is anticipating every need and fostering dependency. Activity patterns develop over the years and are difficult to change. In fact, these patterns should not be altered unless there are very important reasons. With aging, shortness of breath and fatigue and weakness increase and the individual will adapt the pattern to avoid distress. Actions are slower and activities take longer. A younger person may eat meals on the run because of time pressures but for an older person, lunch can be a high point of an otherwise routine day. There is more time to prepare and enjoy the meal at leisure. With advancing age, activities selected by the individual show a trend towards spectatorship, such as watching television, rather than participation. Activities are more often self-paced, such as gardening and reading.

The aged person may be reluctant to alter the activity pattern and may underestimate his or her ability to learn and so may others around the aged person. Although group activities are generally more successful than individual ones, older people frequently find groups threatening. It often takes time for them to relax and enjoy the group process and initially concentration may be low. Any alteration in pattern should be introduced only after the aged person expresses motivation and openness to something new or if the current activity pattern does not meet the person's basic needs.

ETIOLOGIES

INTERNAL

◆ Sedentary lifestyle

◆ Imbalance between oxygen supply and demand

◆ Generalized weakness.

EXTERNAL

◆ Bedrest, immobility

◆ Long term hospitalization

◆ Environmental lack of diversional activity

◆ Frequent lengthy treatments.

◆ Nursing Diagnosis:

Activity intolerance related to increasing shortness of breath (SOB) (Levels I and II)

DEFINING CHARACTERISTICS:

◆ Verbal report of fatigue or weakness

◆ Exertional discomfort or dyspnea

◆ EKG changes reflecting ischemia or arrhythmias

◆ Deconditioned status (prolonged bed rest, inactivity)

◆ Presence of circulatory or respiratory problems

◆ History of previous intolerance to activity

◆ Inexperience with the activity

◆ Intention or need to engage in energy-consuming body movement

◆ Boredom

◆ Usual hobbies or activities cannot be undertaken in hospital

◆ Wish for something to do, to read, etc.

GOALS/OUTCOME CRITERIA

1. Activity tolerance gradually improves
2. Participates in regular exercise program.

INTERVENTIONS

1. Discuss regular exercise program with client including:
   a. research showing that regular exercise programs increase cardio-vascular function including oxygen use, improve the size and strength of muscles, and decrease the amount of body fat. Also mention that regular exercise seems to slow the rate of physical and cognitive decline.
   b. exercise preferences and past history. (RN)

2. If a client is interested in exercise, get medical clearance. (RN/MD)

3. Determine if client is taking medications that may affect exercise tolerance, e.g. beta-blockers. (RN)

4. Working with a physical therapist, establish regular exercise program including:

    a. teach the client to check pulse at rest to get baseline.

    b. teach client normal pulse range in reaction to exercise.

    c. how to warm up with stretch exercises for 5 minutes before and after exercise to taper down.

    d. teach client exercises, which include both large and small muscle groups and ROM of joints.

    e. teach client to stop exercising if it is causing chest pain, excessive SOB, or pain. (RN/PT)

5. Instruct client to use good body mechanics. (RN/LPN/NA)

6. Warn client about postural hypotension and the need to change position slowly. Advise that falls are often associated with postural hypotension. (RN/LPN)

7. Offer client well organized activities and determine if interested in participating. (RN/OT)

8. Encourage client to continue those activities that he or she can tolerate, e.g. knitting, gardening. (RN/LPN/NA)

9. Determine interest in audiotapes if vision is impaired. (RN)

◆ Nursing Diagnosis

Activity intolerance related to inability to walk 50 feet without stopping (Level III)

DEFINING CHARACTERISTICS

See prior nursing diagnosis.

GOALS/OUTCOME CRITERIA

1. Client meets basic needs despite increased weakness.

2. Client continues to be as independent as possible.

INTERVENTIONS

1. Determine if environmental supports are available to assist client to meet basic needs such as food, especially food preparation, and hygiene. (RN)

2. Provide assistance to organize household, make necessary materials available. (RN/LPN/NA)

3. Encourage client to be as active as possible. (RN/LPN/NA)

4. Instruct significant others/staff not to over-anticipate client's needs. (RN/LPN/NA)

5. Check with MD about providing assistive devices as needed to improve independence. (RN/MD)
6. Adapt environment to client's increasing weakness. (RN/PT/OT)

◆ Nursing Diagnosis

Activity intolerance related to dyspnea and fatigue at rest (Level IV)

DEFINING CHARACTERISTICS

See prior nursing diagnosis.

GOALS/OUTCOME CRITERIA

1. Client does not get depressed.
2. Activities are paced so client doesn't develop acute distress.

◆ Nursing Diagnosis

Activity intolerance related to increasing SOB (Levels I and II)

DEFINING CHARACTERISTICS

◆ Verbal report of fatigue or weakness
◆ Exertional discomfort or dyspnea
◆ EKG changes reflecting ischemia or arrhythmias
◆ Deconditioned status (prolonged bed rest, inactivity)
◆ Presence of circulatory or respiratory problems
◆ History of previous intolerance to activity
◆ Inexperience with the activity
◆ Intention or need to engage in energy-consuming body movement
◆ Boredom
◆ Usual hobbies or activities cannot be undertaken in hospital
◆ Wish for something to do, to read, etc.

GOALS/OUTCOME CRITERIA

1. Activity tolerance gradually improves.
2. Participates in regular exercise program.

INTERVENTIONS

1. Organize day with client input to allow rest periods after each activity. (LPN/NA)
2. Encourage client to dress in everyday clothes. (LPN/NA)
3. Encourage client to stay OOB most of day. (LPN/NA)
4. Ask MD about prn oxygen. (RN)
5. Organize environment to minimize activities. (RN)

6. Give client time to ventilate feelings about increasing limitations. (RN/LPN/NA)

7. Monitor the client's weight to make sure weight loss or gain is not occurring. (LPN/NA)

8. Consult with MD about medications and diet to improve activity tolerance. (RN/MD)

◆ Nursing Diagnosis

Impaired Physical Mobility (Specify Level)

DEFINITION

This diagnosis refers to the limitation of ability for independent movement within the environment. Loss of mobility is a common problem for aging persons. Mobility is important not only in performance and independence but also in the way the persons define themselves. Decrease in mobility can be very threatening. Persons see themselves as aging and this process is resulting in lessened functioning. Instead of running up and down stairs, they have to curtail the number of trips. Nonessential but enjoyable activities are the first to be cut back. This makes the aging people even more fearful about how they will manage essential tasks. Independence and autonomy are important values to many people and immobility threatens them, creating situations of perceived dependency.

There are four levels of impaired physical mobility. These are the following:

Level I: Requires uses of equipment or device

Level II: Requires help from another person(s): assistance, supervision, or teaching

Level III: Requires help from another person(s) and equipment or device

Level IV: Is dependent and does not participate in activity.

Level appropriate nursing diagnosis and interventions will be identified.

ASSESSMENT

The initial meeting can reveal a great deal about a person's mobility status. What was the person doing right before the examination? Was he or she confined to bed, in a wheel-chair, walking to greet you, or sitting in a comfortable chair? Does the person rely on others to bring things into the room or does the person get up and get them himself or herself? When the person gets up from the chair, is it a quick movement or slow and painful? What kind of chair does the person choose to sit on? Pay attention to the quality of the person's handshake. This data can be gleaned within a few minutes after meeting the client and provides a sound foundation for more careful data collection. The client isn't aware that he or she is being watched and so is less likely to alter normal patterns.

Observe the individual's posture in a variety of positions. Posture is alignment of the body segments in relation to one another. Generally, as the person ages, the posture takes on a more hunchbacked appearance, consistent with spinal flexion due to wedging of the vertebrae and thinning of the intervertebral disks. Examine the back for kyphosis which is often associated with osteoporosis. Individuals often report a loss of height as they age. To estimate the amount of height loss accurately, the nurse should ask the client to raise her or his arms sideways to shoulder length. The nurse then measures the distance from longest fingertip on one side to the longest on the other side. A normal finding would be when the height equals the fingertip to fingertip measurement. If the fingertip measurement is more than the height, the amount of spinal compression is estimated as the difference between the two measurements. The increasing flexion can result in a shift in the center of gravity. The individual adapts to this shift by using more energy to maintain balance and a normal gait.

Much can be gained from watching a client walk. Is there a deviation from the midline during the swing phase of walking? Is the gait free and easy or is the base widened or the steps too small? Does the person lift the foot off the floor or is the gait shuffling? Does the client appear unsteady? Does he or she have difficulty getting started? Can the client turn and stop with ease? Gait may be affected by physical changes or it can reflect a depressed mood. Does the client touch furniture to stabilize herself or himself; does the client need assistive devices; can she or he manage steps. These are a few of the areas which must be assessed to determine if the client is experiencing impaired mobility.

The nurse observes the client's muscles for strength, tone, and flexibility. There may be some differences in the muscle strength of the upper extremities in that the dominant hand and arm are often slightly stronger, but the lower extremities should be of equal strength. Question the older client about any perceived changes in structure and function. Has the client noted any change in muscle bulk, tone, or strength? Clients will often report increased difficulty in opening doors. Both arm and leg muscles shrink and may have a flabby appearance. Assess muscle strength by observing the muscles' ability to overcome resistance. Does the client perceive himself or herself as weak or unable to perform some activities of daily living. How has the client adjusted to a permanent disability, such as after a CVA or amputation?

AGE-RELATED PHENOMENON

By retirement, 80 percent of the population has some type of rheumatic complaint. All patients older than 60 years have X-ray or physical evidence of arthritis but only 25 percent of the women and 15 percent of the men are symptomatic. Elastin which is a component of the connective tissue matrix becomes fragmented and calcified with age, and thus tissue elasticity is reduced. Cartilage becomes more brittle and easily disrupted. The long bones hollow out, the vertebral endplates thin and the skull becomes slightly enlarged. There is reduced bone mass, which is greater in women, approximately 25 percent, in comparison to 12 percent in men. This creates additional stress to the weight-bearing areas, which consequently are more susceptible to fracture. This process of bone loss starts at around 40 years. The older client fatigues more easily, has a slower reaction time due to a decrease in nerve conduction and muscle tone and may not display smooth, coordinated movement. Posture is characterized by increased flexion, and to compensate, the aged person widens the stance, lowers the height of each step, moves more cautiously, and tends to avoid hurrying.

The nervous system undergoes a steady loss of neurons, which affects the brain and the spinal cord, causing changes in motor and sensory function. Changes in the central nervous system lead to slowed reaction time and increased lateral sway, which makes balance more difficult to maintain. There may be some loss of muscle tone and the ankle jerk reflex. There is a loss of muscle mass, because muscle cells cannot regenerate and fibrous tissue replaces the contractile parts of the muscle. There is a decrease in muscle weight in relation to body weight. Reaction time is slowed, which makes the aged person particularly vulnerable in situations demanding quick response such as driving a car. On the other hand, in situations benefiting from experience, the older person can make valuable contributions.

ETIOLOGIES

- ◆ Intolerance to activity, decreased strength and endurance (Decreased Activity Tolerance)
- ◆ Pain, discomfort
- ◆ Perceptual-cognitive impairment
- ◆ Neuromuscular impairment
- ◆ Depression
- ◆ Severe anxiety

◆ Nursing Diagnosis

Impaired physical mobility related to need to use equipment or device (Level I).

DEFINING CHARACTERISTICS

Inability to purposefully move within the physical environment (mobility, be able to transfer, ambulation)

GOALS/OUTCOME CRITERIA

1. Use assistive devices safely.
2. Regain maximum function within activity restrictions.
3. Prevent falls and other accidents.

INTERVENTIONS

1. Assess posture, gait, muscle strength. (RN)
2. Ask client if he or she would agree to learn to use assistive device. (RN)

3. Consult with MD about physical therapy referral for appropriate assistive device. (RN/MD)
4. Instruct client to
   a. stand straight
   b. wear sturdy shoes with rubber sole, good heels
   c. sit in firm, straight-backed chair with arms
   d. sleep on firm mattress
   e. use good body mechanics
   f. avoid slouching especially of back (RN/NA)
5. Reinforce physical therapist's plan of care with client, staff, and significant others (RN/PT)
6. Assess environment and make adaptive changes (see impaired home maintenance) (RN)

◆ Nursing Diagnosis

Impaired physical mobility related to need for help from others (Level II).

GOALS/OUTCOME CRITERIA

1. Accepts that there is a mobility problem.
2. Accepts assistance
3. Adjusts behavior to reflect teaching.

INTERVENTIONS

#1,4,6 from above.

1. Determine who in client's environment is willing and able to provide assistance. (RN)
2. Teach person assisting client:
   a. body mechanics
   b. transfer techniques
   c. how to identify high-risk situations (RN)
3. Determine if client is eligible for telephone contact support services. (RN/SW)

◆ Nursing Diagnosis

Impaired physical mobility related to need for assistive devices and assistance from others (Level III).

GOALS/OUTCOME CRITERIA

1. Environment will be safe with the least possible restrictions.
2. Caretakers will respect the client, and care will be humanistic.

INTERVENTIONS

All of preceding.

1. Refer to social worker for
   a. long-term planning at home
   b. health-related facility placement (RN/SW)
2. Supervise home assistant or nurses' aide in how to best assist client. (RN)

◆ **Nursing Diagnosis**

Impaired physical mobility related to dependency (Level IV).

GOALS/OUTCOME CRITERIA

1. Skin remains free from breakdown
2. Muscle tone is maintained or strengthened
3. Residents can meet Activities of Daily Living (ADL)

INTERVENTIONS

1. Institute measures to prevent decubitus:
   a. supersoft mattress
   b. changing position every two hours, especially from side to side using oblique position and avoiding extreme lateral positions (Seiler and Stähelin, 1985)
   c. massaging with creams
   d. observing for red areas especially on bony prominences. (RN)
2. Instruct good fluid intake to prevent lung congestion, urinary tract infections, and constipation. (RN/NA)

◆ **Nursing Diagnosis**

Altered Cardiac Output: Decreased

DEFINITION

Presence of indicators of lowered cardiac output. Activity is hindered when the heart cannot pump enough blood to meet the body's needs. The individual may not notice the level of activity intolerance until it interferes with the ability to perform routine tasks.

ASSESSMENT

The nurse can assess decreased cardiac output indirectly by evaluating the pulse and determining if the client is growing tired more easily.

The nurse should assess the quality, rhythm, and strength of the pulse. Decrease in cardiac output is particularly noticeable after the heart is stressed as after increased activity or emotional trauma. The pulse of the aged person takes longer to accelerate to meet the body's increased demand for oxygen and longer to return to a baseline level. The "safe activity" pulse is derived by using the resting baseline pulse and multiplying it by 60 percent to get the safe lower increased activity range and by 80 percent to get the safe upper range, and then adding each number to the resting pulse. For example, if the resting pulse is 76, multiply by 60 percent and add the result (46) to the base line to get the lower limit (122) and then multiply the baseline by 80 percent and add this result (60) to get the safe upper limit (136). However, the nurse should recognize that a rapid pulse or pounding of the heart persisting longer than ten minutes after activity is indicative of pathology and the physician should be contacted.

If the nurse palpates an irregular pulse it should be further investigated, since there is no change in rhythm normally associated with aging. In listening to heart sounds, the nurse may discover a systolic murmur, which is present in about 20 percent of the older clients. This murmur is not usually treated, but other irregular patterns need to be medically investigated if the client denies knowledge of any pre-existing cardiac disease. The strength of the pulse relates to fluid balance and a change in strength should also be investigated further.

Because 48 percent of the aged population have some degree of congestive heart failure, the nurse should routinely check for signs of cardiac insufficiency secondary to this pathology. Increases in weight, swelling of dependent parts, tight-fitting clothing and shoes, and increasing SOB are all consistent with the conclusion that the heart is not functioning adequately. A thorough assessment can lead to early intervention and prevent serious failure. The normal heart does not increase in size with aging so the nurse should not expect normal changes in the location of the point of maximum impulse (PMI).

Blood pressure should be checked regularly even in the absence of known problems. Hypertension is reported if the blood pressure is greater than 140/90. Hypotension should also be investigated. It may be due to decreased potassium or, more commonly, the use of medications that either directly or indirectly affect blood pressure. Intolerance to activity or increasing fatigue are signs of decreasing cardiac output, which will be addressed elsewhere in this chapter.

AGE-RELATED PHENOMENON

The changes in the heart associated with aging result in the heart's need to work harder but at the same time it accomplishes less. The cardiac output decreases at a rate of about 1 percent per year, beginning in the mid-30's. The valves get thicker and more rigid. The endocardium thickens and scleroses and the amount of subpericardial fat increases. The left ventricular wall may be 24 percent thicker at age 80 than at age 30. The maximum cardiac rate and stroke volume are decreased, and therefore cardiac output is reduced.

The cardiac rate is impaired due to increased connective tissue in the sinoartrial and atrioventricular nodes and in the bundle branches. The stroke volume is impaired by changes in the valves, decrease in the size of the left ventricle, and decrease in resiliency of the arteries. Cardiac oxygen use is less efficient in the older adult. With increasing vascular rigidity associated with aging, the systolic blood pressure increases. The diastolic pressure may also increase to compensate for increasing peripheral resistance. Pathologies exacerbate these normal aging processes.

ETIOLOGIES

INTERNAL
- ◆ Aging changes in heart
- ◆ Inadequate fluid volume

EXTERNAL
- ◆ Emotional stress
- ◆ Physical activity

◆ Nursing Diagnosis

- ◆ Decreased cardiac output related to aging-associated changes.

DEFINING CHARACTERISTICS

- ◆ Variations in BP readings
- ◆ Changes in mental status
- ◆ Weakness
- ◆ Fatigue

GOALS/OUTCOME CRITERIA

1. Cardiac output is sufficient to meet activity needs.
2. Client adjusts to age-related changes.

INTERVENTIONS

1. Check pulse rate before and after activity. (RN/LPN)
2. Ask client if he or she feels increasingly tired. (RN/LPN)
3. Ask client if he or she has given up any activity within the past six months. (RN/LPN)
4. Check BP both arms in a sitting, lying down, and standing position. (RN/LPN)
5. Refer for medical evaluation if assessment findings suggestive of pathology:
   a. rapid pulse
   b. irregular pulse rate
   c. weak or bounding pulse
   d. increase in BP three times sequentially greater than 140/90 (RN/LPN)

6. Ask client if he or she has noticed increasing forgetfulness. (RN/LPN)
7. Consult with significant others about client's ability to remember significant things. (RN/LPN)
8. Instruct client to change position slowly. (RN/LPN/NA)
9. Instruct client to slightly increase salt intake in hot weather if he or she is sweating profusely and feels weak. (RN/RD)
10. Review with client how to pace activities. (RN)
11. Encourage client to achieve or maintain ideal weight. (RN/LPN)

◆ Nursing Diagnosis

Decreased cardiac output related to effects of pathology (i.e., congestive heart failure, pulmonary edema, life-threatening arrhythmias).

DEFINING CHARACTERISTICS

- ◆ Jugular vein distension
- ◆ Cold, clammy skin
- ◆ Oliguria
- ◆ Rales
- ◆ Dyspnea/SOB
- ◆ Orthopnea
- ◆ Restlessness
- ◆ Cough/frothy sputum
- ◆ Edema
- ◆ Arrhythmias
- ◆ Gallop/vertigo
- ◆ Syncope/vertigo
- ◆ Decreased peripheral pulses
- ◆ Color changes in skin and mucous membranes

GOALS/OUTCOME CRITERIA

1. Pathology will be stabilized and irreversible changes prevented
2. Cardiac output increases in proportion to body's needs.
3. Client will receive nursing and medical care at an acute care level.

◆ Nursing Diagnosis

Altered Tissue Perfusion

DEFINITION

This diagnosis refers to chronic deficit in blood supply to a part relative to metabolic needs. Circulatory problems are endemic to the aging population. So long as the demand does not overtax the system, a fine balance is maintained.

ASSESSMENT

The nurse assesses the adequacy of the circulation by checking the color and warmth of the body part. The color of a particular part should not be different from the overall body color. In a light-skinned person, paleness and mottling are consistent with circulatory impairment. In both light and dark-skinned persons, there may be redness especially when the extremity is dependent. There may also be greyish pallor on elevation of the foot or the limb may have a deep purple color which is unaffected by position. The temperature of the part can be evaluated either by comparing it to other parts and noting if there is asymmetry in temperature or by noting if the part is unusually cool. Some examples are cool feet in summer or if the person is wearing shoes and warm socks. Ask the person if he or she has a history of coolness in particular areas.

Tissue perfusion is further assessed by observing hair growth patterns. Sparse hair growth may be suggestive of decreased tissue perfusion, but should be assessed within the normal expectation of hair loss in the aging process. The older person also may report muscle cramps occurring in the upper and lower extremities at night or after activity; but this symptom is also non-conclusive, as it may occur without physiologic reason, or it may be consistent with intermittent claudication. Medical evaluation is necessary for a differential diagnosis.

Inadequate tissue perfusion may create changes in the nail beds such as thickening. It needs to be determined if the nail changes are due to circulation or another process such as fungus growth. The nurse assesses peripheral pulses bilaterally and notes differences in strength, regularity, and presence. The dorsalis pedis, pedal, and popiteal pulses should be compared to each other and also to the radial pulse. The client should be questioned as to the presence of altered sensations in the affected extremities such as numbness or tingling or pain. The location of the pain may help to locate the level of the obstruction. The nurse should also identify the presence of precipitating factors, such as exercise leading to claudication, and determine the client's activity tolerance.

AGE-RELATED PHENOMENON

Elastin, which normally occurs within the connective tissue in the body, gives arteries their resiliency and this process diminishes with aging. Arteriosclerosis appears to be a normal consequence of age-related changes in the arterial walls and results in decreased compliance and increased stiffening of the blood vessels. On the other hand, atherosclerosis—fatty plaque deposits—is considered to be pathological. The systolic blood pressure may increase due to a less distensible aorta. There is also an increased disposition of calcium in many arteries including the coronary arteries. Veins and lymphatics probably undergo changes similar to those occurring in the arteries, but to a lesser extent since they are under less stress. The overall result is a compromised circulation, which causes decreased oxygen to the tissues and leaves higher levels of carbon dioxide. This becomes problematic especially in areas further away from the heart such as the lower extremities.

ETIOLOGIES

INTERNAL

◆ Decreased resiliency in arteries/veins

◆ Decreased oxygen/carbon dioxide exchange at tissue level.

EXTERNAL

◆ Smoking

◆ Wearing tight or restrictive clothing

◆ Extremes of temperature such as frost-bite.

◆ Nursing Diagnosis

Alteration in tissue perfusion related to normal age-related changes.

DEFINING CHARACTERISTICS

◆ Cold extremities

◆ Shiny skin surfaces

◆ Loss of lanugo hair

◆ Slow growing, dry, thick brittle nails

◆ Blood pressure changes in extremities

◆ Diminished arterial pulsations

GOALS/OUTCOME CRITERIA

1. Skin surfaces remain intact.

2. Circulation to extremities improves.

INTERVENTIONS

1. Assess for circulatory changes including:
   a. monitor dorsalis pedis, pedal pulses
   b. compare bilaterally and to radial
   c. monitor BP
   d. monitor temperature, color of extremity
   e. ask if pain, altered sensation, and have client describe thoroughly. (RN)

2. Assist the client in smoking cessation. (RN)

3. Instruct client to cut down or stop drinking alcohol. (RN)

4. Instruct client to avoid wearing restrictive clothing, for example, knee-highs, garter belts, truss. (RN)
5. Instruct client/staff to use warm water and test temperature of water before applying to skin. (RN/LPN)
6. Instruct client/staff to use caution with heating pad. (Use of heating pads and/or hot water bottles is strongly discouraged. Many older people have reported burns and other injuries due to prolonged or incorrect use.) (RN/LPN/NA)
7. Instruct client to see podiatrist regularly to have toe nails and calluses cut. (RN)
8. Advise client that walking on level surfaces can improve circulation. (RN)
9. Instruct client/staff to wash feet every day and dry thoroughly, especially between each toe, and apply soothing lotions. (RN/LPN/NA)

◆ Nursing Diagnosis

Altered tissue perfusion related to circulatory impairment.

DEFINING CHARACTERISTICS

◆ Extremities blue or purple when dependent; pale on elevation and color does not return on lowering leg.
◆ Round scars covered with atrophied skin.
◆ Gangrene
◆ Slow healing of lesions
◆ Claudication
◆ Bruits

GOALS/OUTCOME CRITERIA

1. Skin breakdown area heals.
2. Client remains free of infection.
3. Amputation will be unnecessary.

INTERVENTIONS

1. #1 through 9 are relevant from prior interventions.
2. Assess break in skin for:
   a. extent—measure length
   b. depth—identify if superficial, deeper
   c. areas involved—draw pictures if helpful. (RN)
3. Consult with MD for prescription about wound care. (RN/MD)
4. Instruct client/significant others/staff in wound care. (RN)
5. Evaluate effectiveness of wound care at least weekly. (RN)

6. Check temperature and report elevation. (LPN/NA)
7. Instruct client to rest after activity, if claudication is problem. (RN)
8. Use stethoscope to check for bruits and report. (RN)
9. Advise client to keep extremity dependent, if arterial compromise is a problem. (RN/LPN)
10. Obtain bed cradle to keep covers off feet. (RN)
11. Provide analgesia by appropriate nursing interventions (see alteration in comfort). (RN)
12. Give prescribed medications to improve circulation, for example, trental, persantine, ASA. (RN/LPN)

◆ Nursing Diagnosis

Total Self-care Deficit (Specify level)

DEFINITION

This diagnosis refers to the inability to complete feeding, bathing, toileting, dressing, and grooming of self. This client is completely dependent upon others for the activities of daily living (ADL). Level of consciousness is possibly altered due to pathology such as a CVA. This degree of dependency may also result from neuromuscular deterioration, which can occur without intellectual impairment such as in Parkinson's disease. There are four levels of self-care deficit:

Level I: Requires use of equipment or devices

Level II: Requires help from another person(s): assistance, supervision, teaching.

Level III: Requires help from another person(s) and equipment or device.

Level IV: Is dependent and does not participate in self-care.

Total self-care deficit can also be broken down into self-grooming deficit; self-bathing deficit; self-feeding deficit; and self-toileting deficit.

ASSESSMENT

Demands of daily living arise from self-expressions, the demands and expectations of others, and even material possessions. There are many ADL assessment tools, but one that is widely used is the Older American Research and Service Center Instrument (OARS). This instrument yields information about functional ability in five domains including: 1) social resources; 2) economic resources; 3) mental health; 4) physical health; and 5) activities of daily living. The advantage of using a standardized instrument, such as OARS, is that it focuses on functional abilities or impairment rather than on the severity of disease. It is comprehensive and helps to identify the extent of assistance needed by the client.

In assessing ability to achieve ADL at a satisfactory level, the nurse must also consider the assistance that the client is willing to accept. The client might perceive that help is unnecessary, while the nurse sees trouble signs such as weight loss, disordered environment, and confusion about details, including medications. The emphasis needs to be on how patients see the situation as well as on objective reality, how they have been managing until this point, how satisfied or frustrated they are with their adjustments, and what they see their needs to be. Clients with total ADL deficits need continual assistance.

The nurse needs to determine who in the client's environment is willing and able to give the necessary assistance. A significant other might be willing to assist but unable because of physical disabilities or emotional burdens. On the other hand, a significant other might be able to assist but unwilling because of strained interpersonal relationships, other responsibilities, or generalized distaste for giving physical care. If a significant other is giving care, the nurse must assess its effectiveness.

AGE-RELATED PHENOMENON

Self-care deficits are not a result of the normal aging process. Rather, physical and psychological disease processes that the individual experiences cause increasing dependency on others. However, over 90 percent of those classified as elderly manage not only their ADL but also their own health care at some level within non-institutional settings. Families and friends often act as facilitators to help the aged persons maintain their independence. However, with aging come losses, death, and illness that affect support systems. These natural passages can precipitate a situation whereby the aged person needs more than casual assistance.

ETIOLOGIES

INTERNAL

◆ Intolerance to activity; decreased strength and endurance
◆ Pain, discomfort
◆ Perceptual-cognitive impairment
◆ Neuromuscular impairment
◆ Musculoskeletal impairment
◆ Severe anxiety, depression

EXTERNAL

◆ Loss of support systems
◆ Multiple environmental stressors

◆ Nursing Diagnosis

Self-care deficit related to self-dressing/grooming deficit.

DEFINING CHARACTERISTICS

◆ Impaired ability to put on or take off necessary items of clothing
◆ Impaired ability to obtain or replace articles of clothing
◆ Impaired ability to fasten clothing
◆ Inability to maintain appearance at a satisfactory level.

INTERVENTIONS

1. Assess kinds of clothing client has not been paying attention to including:
   a. fit
   b. ease of dressing, undressing
   c. cleanliness
   d. adequacy of quantity (RN)
2. Ask client if he or she is having difficulty dressing or undressing herself (RN/LPN)
3. Refer client to occupational therapist for assistive devices and teaching. (RN/OT)
4. Ask significant other or client to use adhesive substances rather than buttons, purchase clothes that are loose-fitting, and that close in the front (LPN)
5. Encourage client to keep hair clean and combed (LPN/NA)
6. Positively reinforce client when she wears make-up and dresses attractively or when he shaves. (RN/LPN/NA)
7. Encourage client to wear street clothes rather than pajamas (LPN/NA)
8. Give game prizes or gifts of toileting articles (OT/PT/RN)
9. Ensure that client can wash clothes regularly or provide necessary assistance. (RN)

◆ Nursing Diagnosis

Self-care deficit related to self-bathing, hygiene deficit.

DEFINING CHARACTERISTICS:

◆ Inability to wash body or body parts.
◆ Inability to obtain or get to water source.
◆ Inability to regulate temperature or flow.

GOALS/OUTCOME CRITERIA

1. Client remains clean and free from odor.

INTERVENTIONS

1. Assess bathing facilities (RN)
2. Determine how client usually handles hygiene needs:
   a. frequency
   b. time of day
   c. shower versus bath
   d. sponge bath (RN)
3. Request assistive devices such as:
   a. shower seat
   b. shower attachment
   c. safety rails
   d. non-skid mat for tub
   e. wash basin (RN/MD/PT)
4. Instruct client to bathe with assistance when feeling weak. (RN)
5. Instruct client never to lock bathroom door (RN/LPN/NA)

◆ Nursing Diagnosis

Self-care deficit related to self-feeding deficit.

DEFINING CHARACTERISTICS

Inability to bring food from a receptacle to the mouth.

GOALS/OUTCOME CRITERIA

1. Client maintains or achieves ideal weight.
2. Client eats balanced diet and enjoys normal bowel functioning.

INTERVENTIONS

1. Determine client's likes and dislikes. (RN/LPN/RD)
2. Determine if client has adequate resources to make food available. (RN/Social Service)
3. Make referral to Meals on Wheels if appropriate. (RN/SS)
4. Weigh client to get baseline. (NA)
5. Speak with dietitian and/or MD about nutritional supplements. (RN/RD/MD)
6. Determine if teeth are adequate to chew food and make dental referral, if inadequate. (LPN/RN)
7. Review with client/significant others well-balanced dietary requirements. (RN/RD)
8. Discuss need for vitamin supplements with dietitian and/or MD. (RN/RD/MD)

9. Refer to occupational therapist for assistive devices such as non-skid plates, padded knives and forks. (OT/RN)
10. If totally dependent, check with MD about tube feedings, if client can't swallow. (RN/MD)
11. Make sure client is being fed slowly and in a pleasant environment with tasteful foods. (LPN/NA)

◆ Nursing Diagnosis

Self-care deficit related to self-toileting deficit.

DEFINING CHARACTERISTICS

◆ Unable to get to toilet or commode
◆ Unable to sit on or rise from toilet or commode
◆ Unable to manipulate clothing for toileting
◆ Unable to carry out proper toilet hygiene
◆ Unable to flush toilet or empty commode
◆ Toileting facilities not available
◆ Doesn't know when needs to defecate, urinate.

GOALS/OUTCOME CRITERIA

1. Client has regular bowel movements.
2. Client urinates without incontinence.

INTERVENTIONS

1. Assess bathroom facilities (RN/PT/OT)
2. Request elevated toilet seat, especially if client has difficulty getting up from sitting position. (RN)
3. Request commode, if bathroom facilities are not readily available. (RN)
4. Make urinal/bedpan available if client is too weak to stand. (LPN/NA)
5. Request incontinent pad and bed protectors to control incontinence. (LPN/NA)
6. Instruct client to drink 6–8 glasses/day. (RN)
7. Instruct client to use prune juice, bran, other high fiber foods to regulate BM. (RN/RD)
8. Determine client's usual BM pattern and place on bedpan at that time, e.g. after breakfast. (LPN)
9. Advise client to limit fluids after 8 PM if urinary frequency at night. (RN)
10. Place call light/bell by bed so client can indicate when he or she needs assistance. (LPN/NA)

11. Discuss retention catheter with MD, if continual incontinence is causing skin breakdown and excessive burden on significant caretaker. (RN/MD)

◆ Nursing Diagnosis

Impaired home maintenance management (Mild, Moderate, Severe, Potential, Chronic)

DEFINITION

This diagnosis refers to the inability to independently maintain a safe, growth-promoting immediate environment. Impaired home maintenance can be mild when the individual is coping somewhat but not to the level at which she or he was able to previously. The home environment may not be at the level she or he was accustomed to, but basic needs are maintained. Moderate impairment would be characterized by uncertainty. When the client feels strong enough, tasks are completed, but there is not assuredness that the pattern will continue to improve. This situation is particularly difficult because it can either resolve or worsen, and the client may still be unwilling to recognize that a problem exists. Severe impairment requires intervention by others. The client may be dirty, undernourished, and the home disorganized. Either support services are provided in the home, or the client may need to be admitted to an institution. Potential impairment is those high risk situations where the client is coping but experience has shown that there is a strong possibility that actual impairment will occur. Chronic impairment may be associated with inadequate financial resources. The client has always made food decisions based on cost rather than on nutritional values, and home repairs are often neglected until they become major problems.

ASSESSMENT

Ask the client how long she or he has lived in this setting and why does she or he continue to live there. Ask if the client wants to continue to live there and why. If the client would like to move, ask about what kind of setting is preferred. Notice prized objects, especially pictures, and ask about the people depicted. Often wedding pictures, children, and grandchildren are displayed. See if there are many religious objects around the home; use their presence as a way of assessing importance of religion in the person's life and involvement with the church or synagogue.

A home assessment guide is given in Table 7–2. This guide is particularly valuable in assessing the home of the elderly client.

Explore the roles and relationships within the home. How many people live in the home? Are there adequate sleeping facilities for that many people? Does the elderly client have responsibility for a sick husband or wife or for a dependent child? How have the family dynamics evolved over the years—has the marriage been characterized by bickering or is mutual respect apparent? Are there available support systems outside the home? If there are children, do they live reasonably close and are they willing to be

TABLE 7–2 ◆ Home Assessment Guide

ROLES AND RELATIONSHIPS

Quality of relationships within the home

Available support systems outside the home

Responsibility for money management, household tasks

Pets

COMFORT AND CONVENIENCE

Home maintenance costs

Overall size of living quarters

Spatial arrangements

Decor

Heating and ventilation

SAFETY

Floors

Stairways

Electrical wiring and appliances

Exposed pipes or radiators

Lighting

Telephone

Particular rooms: Bathroom

Kitchen

Bedroom

Door and window locks

Smoke and fire detectors

Emergency plan

Safekeeping of valuables

Medications

Rauckhourst, L, Stokes, S, and Mezey, M. Community and Home Assessment. In Spradley, B. (ed) *Readings in Community Health Nursing.* Boston: Little, Brown and Co.; 1986; 163.

involved in their parent's care? Are they reliable or do they also have multiple responsibilities and can only lend telephone support? Are neighbors and friends willing to look in and bring items from the store, or are there no close neighbors? What are the community resources like—is there Meals on Wheels, support programs, senior citizen centers? Does the client want outside assistance or is the client specific about the kind of help he or she will accept? Assess who has primary responsibility for money management.

Are bills being paid regularly? Are family members giving assistance?

Are there pets in the home? Pets are important for the aged person and provide companionship, but they also have needs. Dogs must be walked; cat litter must be cleaned. Can the client manage these demands? Does the apartment smell from animals? If the nurse determines there is a problem, she needs to be diplomatic and give realistic suggestions.

Is the home comfortable? The furniture may reflect the styles of many years ago. Are possessions treasured and respected for their memories and still functional or are replacements imperative? Is the size of the living quarters consistent with needs. Are the maintenance costs consistent with the person's income? Has the person taken advantage of reduced rates for the elderly such as on heat and property taxes? The nurse should also assess the temperature of the environment. In cold winter weather, hot lines to call for emergency intervention are available, or perhaps the person will have to live with a friend or significant other for a few days until heating is adequate. Hypothermia is a particular problem for elderly people and every winter at least one person is found frozen to death in her or his apartment.

Safety is a particularly important factor for the elderly. They are often victims of crime, because they move more slowly and are less likely to be able to fight off an attacker. The neighborhood may have changed over the years and elderly people find themselves to be the last representatives of a particular cultural group in a totally changed neighborhood. Assess the home environment for safety hazards. Accidents are a leading cause of death in older persons, and falls are the leading cause of accidental death. Bathrooms and kitchens need to be examined for particular hazards. The elderly should have smoke detectors and then be assisted to replace the battery regularly so it is effective. If many different people are visiting the home, the client should be encouraged to put valuables, especially jewelry and money, out of full view. Aged people usually feel quite safe in their homes because they are familiar to them. The nurse has to alert the client to potential hazards without frightening him or her.

AGE-RELATED PHENOMENON

The concept of "home" is extraordinarily significant for many older persons because it is part of their identity. Home is that place where things are familiar and where the person can maintain some sense of autonomy and control. Home holds memories of the past that are part of one's history. Possessions symbolize interactions with significant others, birth of children, important occasions. Home is an escape from the outside world. Home equals independence for many elderly people and it is a familiar place.

Changing one's place of residence will result in many other changes— new stores, new place to worship, new neighbors, new transportation routes. The old residence might be too demanding, but the prospect of change is too frightening. The person feels trapped by two untenable choices. A precipitating factor, especially illness or death of a significant other, often results in the decision to move. This is a particularly stressful period for the aged person.

Women usually live longer than men, and so women are often left with the responsibilities of a home. Plumbing, boilers, windows, painting may have been the male's responsibility. Finances may also have been left to the man to manage. The elderly woman alone may be confused and sometimes victimized by service people. One 80-year-old woman was forced to sell her house after she developed a stress ulcer from trying to get a plumber to replace a broken oil burner. Some elderly people will say that they would have preferred to die first and not be faced by all these reponsibilities and decisions.

ETIOLOGIES

INTERNAL

◆ Impaired cognitive or emotional functioning
◆ Knowledge deficit
◆ Lack of role modeling

EXTERNAL

◆ Individual/family member disease or injury
◆ Insufficient family organization/planning
◆ Insufficient finances
◆ Unfamiliarity with neighborhood resources
◆ Inadequate or overstressed support systems

◆ Nursing Diagnosis

Impaired home maintenance management, related to inability to keep home organized.

DEFINING CHARACTERISTICS

SUBJECTIVE

◆ Household members express difficulty in maintaining their home in a comfortable fashion.
◆ Household requests assistance with home maintenance
◆ Household members describe outstanding debts or financial crises

OBJECTIVES

◆ Disorderly surroundings
◆ Unwashed or unavailable cooking equipment, clothes, or linen
◆ Accumulation of dirt, food wastes, or hygienic wastes
◆ Offensive odors
◆ Inappropriate family members (e.g. exhausted, anxious)
◆ Lack of necessary equipment or aids
◆ Presence of vermin or rodents
◆ Repeated hygienic disorders, infestations, or infections.

GOALS/OUTCOME CRITERIA

1. Home will be clean and organized
2. Client will be safe and accidents prevented.
3. Significant others will not be overwhelmed by client's needs and their responsibilities

INTERVENTIONS

1. Make social worker referral for:
   a. community resources
   b. eligibility for financial aid
   c. middle income assistance programs, e.g. property tax reduction
   d. long term planning (RN/MD/SW)
2. Speak with significant others about what they realistically can contribute to client's maintenance (RN/SW)
3. Evaluate input of significant others periodically, looking for:
   a. failure to complete agreed upon tasks
   b. symptoms of excessive stress
   c. interpersonal strain between client and significant other (RN)
4. Request assistive equipment, e.g. commode, walker, phone lifeline. (RN/PT/OT)
5. Assist client to investigate community resources, e.g. church, senior citizens center. (RN/SW)
6. Help client to organize his or her medications and:
   a. ensure that meds are being taken correctly
   b. any interactions are identified and changes made (RN/RPh)
7. Work with client in getting no-skid strips for throw rungs, wearing firm shoes. (RN/PT)
8. Speak with building superintendent, with client's persmission, about extermination, repairs. (RN/SW)
9. Request personal care worker to assist with housekeeping, personal care or encourage client to hire someone. (RN/SW)
10. If environment dirty and unsafe, confront client with reality and ask about client's perceptions and choices. (RN)
11. If environment unsafe and client acting in incompetent fashion, refer to adult protective services. (RN)

◆ Nursing Diagnosis

Altered Respiration.
   Consists of:

   a. Impaired gas exchange: disturbance in oxygen or carbon dioxide exchange in lungs or at cellular level.

b. Ineffective airway clearance: inability to effectively clear secretions or obstruction from respiratory tract.

c. Ineffective breathing pattern: respiration (respiratory compensations) inadequate to maintain sufficient oxygen supply for cellular requirements.

These three nursing diagnoses have been combined because of the goals of the setting where the client is living. In an acute care facility, many technological interventions would be appropriate. In contrast, the focus of this section is directed towards clients who are having normal respiratory changes associated with aging or chronic health care problems. The emphasis is not on pathology.

ASSESSMENT

Activity is often decreased because the individual is having difficulty with breathing. Ask the client if he or she has noticed any change in mobility patterns within the last six months. Also question if the client has been sleeping with more pillows at night. A positive response to this question is consistent with orthopnea. Observe the position that the client assumes naturally. Is he or she avoiding lying flat?

Breathing is controlled both voluntarily and involuntarily, but usually one is not aware of breathing patterns. Expected is an increase in rate after an activity such as walking upstairs, but routine activities such as walking across a room should not affect the rate. After activity it may take longer for the respiratory rate to return to baseline in the elderly client. An increased resting respiratory rate often appears prior to a rise in temperature consistent with infection and should be monitored carefully. The rhythm of the breathing should also be assessed. Insomnia may be related to Cheyne-Stokes respirations that appear in the older adult. Cheyne-Stokes repiration, apnea followed by shallow breathing, may be observed as a normal variation when the older client is asleep.

Depth of respiration should also be observed. Lung sounds do not normally change with aging but differences can be observed secondary to life-long patterns such as smoking. Question if the person is smoking or has ever smoked? For how long, and how many packs per day? If the client is still smoking, lung sounds may be diminished and the client is at higher risk for lung cancer and emphysema. Smokers often have coughs but all individuals should be assessed for cough including precipitating factors, past treatments that have been effective, and the presence of sputum. The color of sputum is particularly significant because it can give valuable clues to underlying pathology. Hemoptysis can be caused by many problems and always requires medical evaluation. Abnormal breath sounds such as rales or rhonchi also deserve further investigation, which usually includes a medical referral.

Look at the size and symmetry of the thorax. Differentiate changes in shape secondary to age-related changes from pathological processes. The anterior-posterior diameter of the chest increases with age. Kyphosis which often accompanies aging, especially in women, may interfere with lung expansion. Check nail beds and lips for cyanosis and observe if eating and speaking are causing respiratory distress. Listen for the speech pattern. Speech that sounds choppy or use of consistently short sentences or stopping to breathe during a sentence are all indicative of respiratory difficulty. Is the client losing weight because eating is causing shortness of breath? Ask the client if he or she feels SOB since dyspnea is a subjective symptom. Observe the amount of effort exerted during expiration. Presence of sufficient oxygen and removal of carbon dioxide affects every bodily system.

AGE-RELATED PHENOMENON

The aging lung shows a decrease in elastic recoil, which results in increased residual volume, or air trapping. The alveolar ducts enlarge, and the alveolar surface areas decrease with age. Airway resistance also increases. These changes are similar in effect to emphysema but are not to be confused with pathology. An outcome of age-related changes in the lungs is that healthy individuals in the ninth decade of life frequently will have lung function equal to only one half of that of their 30-year-old counterparts. However, these age-related reductions in pulmonary function don't result in dyspnea at rest or during standard exercise such as walking several blocks.

Although the pH of the arterial blood is essentially unchanged by aging, in that it remains between the parameters of 7.40 to 7.45, there are changes in the arterial pO_2. The oxygen component of arterial blood shows a small but steady decline with aging so that the normal pO_2 for a 70-year-old man is 75. The arterial CO_2 tension is unaffected by age. The nurse needs to remember these normal alterations when evaluating an individual's arterial blood gas results.

The thorax also develops changes related to the aging process. Both the internal and external costal muscles weaken, and kyphotic changes in the thoracic spine increase the size of the chest. The aged person may develop a barrel-like chest. A decrease in body fluids along with normal decrease of ciliary activity in the bronchial lining make expectoration of mucus more difficult. Effective coughing is impeded both by weakened chest muscles and thicker mucus. The aged person is at higher risk for pooling of secretions, which can lead to infection.

ETIOLOGIES

INTERNAL

◆ Ventilation–perfusion imbalance.
◆ Decreased energy/fatigue
◆ Tracheobronchial infection, obstruction, secretions
◆ Perceptual/cognitive impairment
◆ Musculoskeletal impairment
◆ Anxiety
◆ Pain

EXTERNAL
◆ Trauma
◆ Pollution
◆ History of working with carcinogens
◆ Smoking

◆ Nursing Diagnosis

Alteration in respiration related to ineffective breathing.

DEFINING CHARACTERISTICS

◆ Confusion
◆ Somnolence
◆ Restlessness
◆ Irritability
◆ Inability to move secretions
◆ Hypercapnea
◆ Hypoxia
◆ Abnormal breath sounds (rales, crackles, rhonchi, wheezes)
◆ Cough (effective/ineffective; with or without sputum)
◆ Change in rate or depth of respiration
◆ Tachypnea (rate increase)
◆ Dyspnea
◆ Cyanosis
◆ Use of accessory muscles
◆ Altered chest expansion
◆ Nasal flaring
◆ Assumption of three-point position
◆ Pursed lip breathing/prolonged expiratory phase
◆ Increase in anterior-posterior diameter.
◆ Fremitus
◆ Abnormal arterial blood gases.

GOALS/OUTCOME CRITERIA

1. Stressors such as infections and smoking are avoided.
2. Continued deterioration in breathing effectiveness is stabilized and, if possible, reversed.
3. Oxygen/carbon dioxide exchange is sufficient to meet bodily needs.

INTERVENTIONS

1. Assess rate, depth, symmetry of respirations (RN/LPN)
2. Follow-up on deviations in pulmonary function tests or arterial blood gas determination. (RN)
3. Strongly encourage client to stop smoking, assist in smoking cessation. (RN/LPN/STAFF)
4. Review with client/significant other how to use prescribed oxygen, including safety precautions. (RN/LPN)
5. Pace activities to avoid respiratory distress. (RN/LPN/NA)
6. Evaluate cough and help to identify ways to decrease. (RN/LPN)
7. Evaluate sputum. (RN/LPN)
8. Encourage increased fluids, but avoid milk if increased mucus. (RN/LPN)
9. Give prescribed anti-infectives, bronchodilators, and related medications. (RN/LPN)
10. Teach client how to:
    a. breathe deeply
    b. cough effectively
    c. increase airway pressure through pursed lip breathing. (RN)
11. Review use of nebulizers, humidifiers, steam. (RN/LPN)
12. Encourage client to achieve or maintain ideal weight. (RN)
13. Encourage client to use pillows as needed and make available or increase head of bed. (RN/LPN)
14. Insure that suctioning equipment is available and client/staff know how to use. (RN/LPN)
15. Instruct client in ways to use good posture. (RN)

◆ Nursing Diagnosis

Potential Joint Contractures

DEFINITION

This diagnosis refers to the presence of risk factors for shortening of tendons at movable joints (back, head, upper and lower extremities). When a person doesn't use a body part, contractures can develop. This usually happens in relationship to paralysis or altered neurological functioning, as in Alzheimer's disease or Parkinsonism. Contractures can also develop when the person is reluctant to move because of pain, such as from arthritis or from muscular spasticity. Psychological factors can lead to decreased use and development of contractures.

ASSESSMENT

Either passively, actively, or with assistance, each joint should be guided through its range of motion while observing for limitations. Watch the person's face for grimaces of pain or anticipated pain. Note if there is a deviation from normal motion and ask the person if she has noticed any change in size, shape, or ROM joints. One hundred percent ROM is not as critical as ability to perform normal living activities. Take a health history paying special attention to activity patterns and the presence of any neuromuscular disease. Reports of joint or back pain should be fully described as to location, temporal pattern, quality, intensity, and aggravating or relieving factors. The degree of joint limitation should be described in terms of percentage of free motion, for example shoulder achieves 180-degree rotation.

AGE-RELATED PHENOMENON

The surface of every joint is cartilage which often shows major deterioration as early as the third decade. These destructive changes probably result from accumulated trauma and result in fraying and chipping. There is loss of water from the cartilage, which results in narrowing of the joint spaces particularly of intervertebral disks. Calcification within the cartilage and crepitation, which is noise from bone touching bone, occurs. These age-related changes often result in compromised joint functioning and development of contractures.

ETIOLOGIES

INTERNAL

◆ Muscularskeletal impairment
◆ Neuromuscular impairment
◆ Perceptual-cognitive impairment
◆ Pain, discomfort
◆ Weakness

EXTERNAL

◆ Lack of assistance to do ROM exercises.
◆ Physical restraints

◆ Nursing Diagnosis

Potential joint contractures related to disuse.

DEFINING CHARACTERISTICS

◆ Maintenance of joint flexion in upright, sitting, or recumbent posture for long periods of time.

◆ Neuromuscular pathology associated with joint flexion (e.g. lack of voluntary postural muscle control, spasticity)

◆ Assumption of abnormal posture due to psycho-social factors or cognitive deficit.

GOALS/OUTCOME CRITERIA

1. Joint mobility will be improved or maintained.
2. Pain secondary to movement will be decreased.

INTERVENTIONS

1. Identify whether passive, active, or assistive help is appropriate. (RN/PT)
2. Grasp each limb by holding onto the distal and proximal joints. (NA)
3. Recognizing normal joint movement, put each joint through its normal motion. (NA)
4. Encourage the client to participate in regular exercise program. (RN)
5. Determine if swimming and/or social dancing is possible for client. (RN)
6. Instruct client to pace self so that exercise program doesn't result in pain in joints longer than two hours after activity. (RN)
7. Instruct client to achieve or maintain ideal weight. (RN)

References

Batehup, L, Squires, A. Mobility In Redfern, S. (ed). *Nursing Elderly People.* London: Churchill Livingstone; 1986; 95–124.

Carnevali, D, Enloe, C. Assessment in the elderly. In Carnevali, D, Patrick, M. (eds). *Nursing Management for the Elderly.* Philadelphia: J.B. Lippincott; 1986; 26–38.

Champlin, L. Functional assessment: A new tool to improve geriatric care. In *Geriatrics.* February 1985; 40:120–121, 124–125.

deVries, H. Physiology of exercise and aging. In Woodruff, D, Birren, J. (eds). *Aging: Scientific Perspectives and Social Issues.* Monterey, CA: Brooks/Cole Publishing Co.; 1983; 285–304.

Ebersole, P, Hess, P. *Toward Healthy Aging, Human Needs and Nursing Response.* St. Louis: C.V. Mosby Co.; 1981.

Gioiella, E, Bevil, C. *Nursing Care of the Aging Client: Promoting Health Adaptation.* CT: Appleton-Century-Crofts; 1985.

Goldman, R. Aging changes in structure and function. In Carnevali, D, Patrick, M. (eds). *Nursing Management for the Elderly.* Philadelphia: J.B. Lippincott; 1986; 73–101.

Gordon, M. *Nursing Diagnosis, Process and Application.* NY: McGraw-Hill Book Co.; 1982.

Hurley, M. (ed). *Classification of Nursing Diagnoses, Proceedings of the Sixth Conference.* St. Louis: C.V. Mosby; 1986.

Kane, R, Kane, R. *Assessing the Elderly.* MA: Lexington Books; 1981.

Larson, E. Assessment of the musculoskeletal system. In Eliopoulos, C. (ed). *Health Assessment of the Older Adult.* CA: Addison-Wesley; 1984; 199–218.

Lillington, G. Dyspnea in the elderly: Old age or disease? In *Geriatrics.* November 1984; 39:47–52.

Mezey, M, Rauckhorst, L, Stokes, S. *Health Assessment of the Older Individual.* NY: Springer, 1980.

Orem, S. Assessment of the cardiovascular system. In Eliopoulos, C. (ed). *Health Assessment of the Older Adult.* CA: Addison, Wesley; 1984; 47–79.

Ostrow, D. Managing chronic airflow obstruction: Part I. In *Geriatrics.* February 1985; 40:45–48.

Patrick, M. Characteristics of the aged population. In Carnevali, D, Patrick, M. (eds). *Nursing Management for the Elderly.* Philadelphia: J.B. Lippincott; 1986; 53–64.

Rauckhorst, L, Stokes, S, Mezey, M. Community and Home Assessment In Spradley, B. (ed). *Readings in Community Health Nursing.* Boston: Little, Brown and Co.; 1986.

Redfern, S. (ed). *Nursing Elderly People.* London: Churchill Livingstone; 1986.

Richards, M. Osteoporosis. In *Geriatric Nursing.* March–April 1982; 3:98–102.

Riffle, K. Falls: Kinds, causes and prevention. In *Geriatric Nursing.* May–June 1982; 3:165–169.

Rowe, J. Physiologic changes with age and their clinical relevance. In Butler, R, Bearn, A. (eds). *The Aging Process: Therapeutic Implications.* NY: Raven Press; 1984; 41–48.

Seiler, W, Stähelin, H. Decubitus ulcers: Preventive techniques for the elderly patient. In *Geriatrics.* July, 1985; 40:53–58,60.

Sigmon, H. Assessment of the respiratory system. In Eliopoulos, C. (ed). *Health Assessment of the Older Individual.* CA: Addison-Wesley; 1984; 81–97.

Simpson W Jr. Exercise: Prescriptions for the elderly. In *Geriatrics.* January 1986; 41:95–98, 100.

Stokes-Roberts, A. Maintaining activities and interests. In *Nursing Elderly People.* London: Churchill Livingstone; 1986.

Weg, R. Changing physiology of aging: Normal and pathological. In Woodruff, D, Birren, J. (eds). *Aging: Scientific Perspectives and Social Issues.* Monterey, CA: Brooks/Cole Publishing Co.; 1983; 242–284.

Wild, L. Cardiovascular problems. In Carnevati, D, Patrick, M. (eds). *Nursing Management for the Elderly.* Philadelphia: J.B. Lippincott; 1986; 361–378.

Wolff, H. Musculoskeletal problems In Carnevali, D, Patrick, M. (eds). *Nursing Management for the Elderly.* Philadelphia: J.B. Lippincott; 1986; 492–581.

Yurick, A. The nursing process and the activity of the elderly person. In Yurick, A, Spier, B, Robb, S, Ebert, N. (eds). *The Aged Person and the Nursing Process.* CT: Appleton-Century-Crofts, 1984.

8

Sleep-Rest Patterns

Norma Anderson

◆

SLEEP-REST PATTERN

◆ Nursing Diagnosis

Sleep Pattern Disturbance

Sleep-Pattern Disturbance is the state in which an individual experiences disruption of the quality or quantity of sleep patterns, which causes discomfort. The disruption(s) may cause interference with desire, lifestyle, and activities. Without appropriate amount and quality of sleep the individual's daily functioning is compromised, resulting in memory difficulties, difficulty with concentration, poor fine motor skills, increased aggressiveness, and other neurological disturbances.

ASSESSMENT

Everyone sleeps. Sleep is a complex biological rhythm that all persons experience. Sleep is a normal, physiological patterned condition involving altered states of consciousness. The person when sleeping has temporarily resigned from the environment. When sleep ensues, the person can be aroused by appropriate sensory and other stimuli.

Numerous factors affect the quality and quantity of sleep and rest in all persons. Most people do not realize the many factors that can affect the quality and quantity of sleep and rest. What is considered by most individuals is setting aside some time (which varies) for this process to occur. Among these variables: sex, age, stress, general health status, nutrition, employment, economic, social, mental and physical status—all have a profound effect on the ability to adequately sleep and rest.

What is considered adequate sleep and rest varies from individual to individual. As with other biological processes, sleep and rest have been widely studied and have indicated significant changes in patterns of sleep and rest within the elderly population.

The process of sleep involves a predictable sequence of operating states within the central nervous system, which is characterized by specific behaviors and patterns. These patterns can be identified by electro-encephalogram (EEG) tracings and a clinical polysomnographer.

Researchers have identified two kinds of sleep. The two kinds of sleep are non-rapid-eye-movement (NREM), composed of four stages, and rapid-eye-movement (REM). Table 8–1 describes the physiology of sleep, human responses, and EEG tracings.

The number of cycles of NREM and REM sleep is related to the total time spent asleep, but individuals ordinarily have 4–5 complete sleep cycles each night. The early sleep cycles are dominated by NREM stages III and IV; as the night continues, NREM periods decrease and REM periods increase. About 20 percent of sleep time is present in REM.

Sleep serves as a restorative process. The synthetic processes of tissue repair and renewal of epithelial and specialized cells such as brain tissue occur during NREM sleep. During stage IV sleep, there is an increased production of growth hormone with resultant protein synthesis and tissue repair. Other anabolic hormones, such as prolactin and testosterone, are secreted. The metabolic rate is decreased.

Sleep provides protection from exhaustion. NREM is a time of energy conservation; i.e. skeletal muscles are not contracting and relaxing actively so that chemical energy is preserved and is available for cellular anabolism.

During sleep, the brain is not relied upon to continually process environmental stimuli. Voluntary assimilation of surroundings is decreased. Filtering of stored information occurs during REM sleep; the day's activities are reviewed and organized, important information retained, and trivial information discarded. It is during this time that problems may be solved and new insights gained.

Dreaming allows for the sorting of emotions and a clearing of the mind for inputs of the following day. However, an individual deprived of REM sleep tends to become irritable, apathetic, less alert, and increasingly sensitive to pain. Continued loss of REM sleep may lead to decreased coping ability and increased anxiety and confusion. A person deprived of NREM sleep undergoes a breakdown in the body's defenses, rendering him or her vulnerable to disease, which have significant implications for nursing practice.

Sleep patterns vary from individual to individual. What one individual requires may not be the same for another. These differences in sleep-rest patterns are a result of the aging process and the body's ability to adapt to these changes. Each person, at his or her own varying age adapts to these changes. However, age-related changes in sleep-rest patterns can lead to many sleep-rest complaints, particularly in the older person.

Knowledge and assessment of the sleep-rest pattern of individuals at a particular age is important in the planning of nursing care. Sleep-rest requirements differ for each individual throughout the life cycle. The nurse needs to understand these individual differences when nursing interventions must focus on sleep and rest.

A sleep assessment is always included in the nursing admission database and thereafter as monthly documentation requires. How thorough is that assessment? The usual question asked of residents is "How many hours of sleep do you get each night?" It is imperative that nurses make a complete sleep assessment for each elder client. The following represents a guide that should be used for sleep assessment upon institutionalization

TABLE 8–1 ◆ The Physiology of Sleep

STAGE	CHARACTERISTICS	HUMAN RESPONSES	EEG TRACINGS
NREM I	Transition between wakefulness and sleep, lasts only a few minutes.	Relaxed, drowsy, yet somewhat aware of surroundings.	Patterns show low voltage waves of 3–7 cycles/second.
II	True sleep begins. Generally lasts from 5–20 minutes.	Thoughts are short, mundane, and fragmented. The person is aware of surroundings but wakes easily.	Waves show sleep spindles (burst of 13-voltage sharp waves shaped like the letter K), known as K complex.
III	Deep sleep. If uninterrupted, the sleeper usually moves into the deepest NREM.	Muscles relax. Pulse rate slows and temperature decreases.	Slow delta waves 1–4 cycles/ second.
IV	Deepest NREM sleep occurs about 40 minutes after start of Stage I. Stages III and IV when combined, last about 15–30 minutes.	Little movement of the body, and arousal is difficult. This period is thought to relax and restore the body.	
REM	After about 90 minutes of sleep, the individual gradually returns through the lighter stages of sleep. Instead of reentering Stage I or awakening, the person enters REM. Lasts about 10 minutes. Thought to be important to learning, memory, and adaptation.	The pulse, respiration, blood pressure, and basal metabolic rate increase and fluctuate. The head, neck, and general skeletal muscle tone and deep tendon reflexes are depressed. Vivid dreams are reported frequently after arousal from REM sleep. More difficult to arouse than in NREM deep sleep	Appear similar to wakefulness.

and as a means of follow-up post-institutionalization. Ask the resident or his or her resourceful significant other:

◆ What time do you go to bed at night?

◆ Do you nap during the day? If so, how often? How long?

◆ What bedtime rituals, such as reading, snacking, or watching TV, do you have?

◆ What medication(s) do you take during the day? At bedtime?

◆ Do you take any sleep medications? How often? How soon prior to bedtime?

◆ Does your sleep medication help you to sleep? How long does it allow you to sleep?

◆ How do you feel upon awakening from sleep? From your sleep medications?

◆ What is your most comfortable position in bed?

◆ In what room temperature, ventilation, and lighting do you like to sleep?

◆ How often do you wake up at night?

◆ Do you know what awakens you once you are asleep?

◆ How do you feel when your sleep is disrupted?

◆ Once awakened, how long does it take you to return to sleep?

◆ What time do you get up in the morning?

◆ How much do you exercise?

◆ What kind of exercise do you do?

◆ Do you snore during sleep?

The results of this assessment should be included when planning nursing care for the older client.

In addition to a detailed interview, the nurse should perform a complete physical assessment to determine any organic causes of sleep-rest disturbance. Residents may complain of having difficulty in falling asleep or maintaining sleep because of pain, dyspnea, vertigo, or change in elimination patterns.

AGE-RELATED PHENOMENON

As a result of the age-related changes in sleep-rest patterns, the common sleep-rest complaints of older persons include the following:

◆ spending more time in bed

◆ taking longer to fall asleep

◆ awakening more often

◆ being sleepy during the daytime hours

◆ requiring more time to adjust to changes in the usual sleep-wake schedule.

Accompanying these sleep-rest changes and complaints is an increased prevalence of sleep-rest related disturbances such as insomnia, hypersomnia, nocturnal behaviors, snoring, sleep apnea, delayed sleep phase syndrome, and restless leg syndrome.

INSOMNIA

Stress related to emotionalism and anxiety are the great enemies of sleep and are considered the most common cause of insomnia. Insomnia is described as inadequate and poor quality sleep with daytime fatigue. Symptoms include inability to fall asleep and to return to sleep; once asleep, frequent and prolonged awakenings, and early morning arousal (often associated with clinical depression).

HYPERSOMIA

Hypersomia is described as excessive sleep, persistent daytime drowsiness, sleep "attacks," drug states, comatose states, and post-encephalitic drowsiness. Signs and symptoms of hypersomia include fatigue, weakness, blackouts, learning and memory problems, inappropriate sleep and sleep attacks, hallucinations, and lack of energy. The intake of alcohol may accentuate daytime napping.

NOCTURNAL BEHAVIOR

Nocturnal behaviors usually occur from late afternoon into evening hours. "Sundowner's Syndrome" includes wandering and disorientation. Other behaviors include screaming, talking, moaning, regurgitating, belching, incontinence, nocturnal ejaculation, scratching, tooth-grinding, and coughing.

SNORING

Snoring usually indicates upper airway function impairment, which has serious implications for the elderly. Heavy snorers may develop cardiovascular problems due to hemodynamic abnormalities. The prevalence of snoring may increase with age as a result of tissue relaxation. Abnormal behavior may result as the snorer struggles to breathe. Clinical symptoms also include loud snoring, enuresis, and morning headache. ·

SLEEP APNEA

Sleep apnea is manifested by abnormal breathing as a result of respiratory pauses and/or apnea. As indicated, snoring may be a precursor of sleep apnea. Sleep apnea disturbance is viewed as a terminal illness because death may be sudden during sleep. Three types of sleep apnea have been identified: central, obstructive, and mixed.

DELAYED SLEEP PHASE SYNDROME

In the delayed sleep phase syndrome, an individual has difficulty falling asleep but sleeps soundly while he or she is asleep. The body's inner clock is programmed for sleep to occur much later than the standard societal bedtime.

RESTLESS LEG SYNDROME

As implied, the individual has trouble keeping his or her lower extremities at rest for a period necessary to fall asleep. This occurs during the waking stage and is characterized by recurrent, rhythmic movements of the feet and legs.

Other factors specific to sleep-rest disturbance in older people include the use of medications (prescription and non-prescription) and lifestyle.

MEDICATIONS

The type of medication and/or their side effects may be responsible for interfering with sleep-patterns in the older adult. Tranquilizers, antidepressants, barbiturates, alcohol, and stimulants are known to suppress REM sleep. Withdrawal of these medications will trigger a rebound compensatory REM sleep. The rebound is characterized by intense dreaming, nightmares, and disturbed sleep. Sleeping pills decrease REM sleep and are effective only for approximately one week. After 5–7 consecutive days of therapy, a rebound effect occurs. The person experiences more difficulty initiating and maintaining sleep than before treatment.

Medications such as anti-hypertensives and diuretics can interfere with the sleep cycle. These medications act to eliminate excess body fluids and dilate blood vessels. The person, therefore, experiences frequency and urgency in elimination. This urgency to urinate can interfere with the sleep cycle.

The elderly are particularly at risk, since the number of medications an individual takes tends to increase with age. Thus, it is important, that when medications are prescribed for, and administered to, the elderly, one should start low and go slow.

LIFESTYLE

A person's lifestyle can affect the quality and quantity of sleep, which in and of itself has great implications for the institutionalized elderly.

Stress and the ability to cope with stress, manifested through emotionalism, anxiety, grief related to loneliness, and depression—all contribute to sleep disturbances.

A change of environment, such as transfers to hospitals (translocation shock), may also contribute to changes in sleep patterns, as well as other conditions.

When planning nursing care for the elderly, the nurse needs to consider the lifestyle and its changes as we age. If older people sleep six or seven hours per night, their institutional routines need to reflect this reality with longer, rather than shorter, days.

These, as well as other changes and factors in one's lifestyle, have implications when planning nursing care for the institutionalized elderly. It will certainly impact on the outcomes of nursing care.

ETIOLOGIES

◆ All conditions that cause discomfort or pain

◆ Hyperthyroidism tends to lengthen the pre-sleep period

◆ Nocturnal angina may awaken the sleeper without an awareness of pain

◆ Hypertension secondary to anxiety may precipitate early morning awakenings and non-refreshing sleep

◆ Gastric secretions increase during REM sleep, and may foster exacerbations of duodenal ulcer or reflux esophagitis

◆ Respiratory conditions interfere with breathing and impair restful sleep

◆ Nocturia disrupts sleep-rest and the sleep cycle

◆ Personal or family stress

◆ Daytime boredom or inactivity

◆ Fear

◆ Nursing Diagnosis

Sleep pattern disturbance

DEFINING CHARACTERISTICS

◆ Verbal complaints of difficulty falling asleep (sleep onset)

◆ Early awakening

◆ Interrupted sleep

◆ Sleep pattern reversal

◆ Verbal complaints of not feeling well rested

◆ Reduction (change) in performance (behavior)

◆ Increasing irritability

◆ Disorientation

◆ Lethargy

◆ Listlessness

◆ Mild, fleeting nystagmus

◆ Slight hand tremor

◆ Ptosis of eyelids

◆ Expressionless face

◆ Thick speech with mispronunciation and incorrect words

◆ Dark circles under eyes

◆ Frequent yawning

◆ Changes in posture

GOALS/OUTCOME CRITERIA

◆ Sleeps longer at night, preferably without the use of medications.

◆ Increases participation in activities.

◆ Decreases and rechannels anxiety and "acting out" behaviors.

◆ Expresses feelings of adequate sleep, rest, and activity.

◆ Maintains personal integrity and orientation to surroundings.

INTERVENTION

◆ Encourage and increase activities during the day (RN/LPN/NA)

◆ Plan short rest periods (15-minute intervals) between activities (RN/LPN/NA Resident/Family)

◆ Allow for rest/nap between 2–3 pm q. day (RN/LPN, Staff)

◆ Encourage walking with supervision (RN/LPN/NA/PT)

◆ Modify environment to develop a sense of routine at bedtime (RN/LPN/NA)

◆ Teach resident and family about sleep changes that older adults experience as normal (RN)

◆ Maintain bedroom environment for sleeping only (RN/LPN/NA)

◆ Reduce the number and frequency of daytime naps (RN/LPN/NA)

◆ Gradually increase activities during the day (RN/LPN)

◆ Use relaxation techniques/methods with resident (RN/SW)

◆ Plan monotonous activities for nighttime awakenings that the resident can perform (RN)

References

Bahr, Sr. RT. Sleep-wake patterns in the aged. In *Journal of Gerontological Nursing*. October 1983; 9:534–541.

Blackford, N. Waking patients up. rise and shine? In *Nursing Mirror*. May 1981; 151:19.

Brown, C, Hartmann, E, Usdin, G, et al. Help for the patient who can't sleep. In *Patient Care*. 1976; 10:98–133.

Busse, E, Blazer, D. (eds). *Handbook of Geriatric Psychiatry*. New York: Van Nostrand Co.; 1980.

Carotenuto, R, Bullock, J. *Physical Assessment of the Gerontological Client*. Philadelphia: F.A. Davis Co.; 1980; 127–8.

Clapin-French, E. Sleep patterns of aged persons in long-term care facilities. In *Journal of Advanced Nursing*. England; January 1986; 11:57–66.

Cohen, D, et al. Sleep disturbances in the institutionalized aged. In *Journal of the American Geriatrics Society*. February 1983; 31:79–82.

Colling, J. Sleep disturbances in aging: A theoretic and empiric analysis. In *ANS*. October 1983; 6:36–44.

Deni, L. The nightmare of sleep problems. In *Journal of Nursing Care.* 1980; 13:8–10, 27.

Hayter, J. Sleep apnea. In *Journal of Gerontological Nursing.* September 1984; 10:26–8.

Hayter, J. Sleep behaviors of older persons. In *Nursing Research.* July–August 1983; 32:242–6.

Hayter, J. To nap or not to nap? in *Geriatric Nursing.* March–April 1985; 6:104–6.

Hoch, C, Reynolds, C, 3rd. Sleep disturbances: Does it really work? In *Journal of Geronotological Nursing.* January–February 1986; 11:7–12.

Kaverely, N, Anderson, D. Why every patient needs a good night's sleep. In *R.N.* December 1986; 16–19.

Kramer, M, Kupfer, D, Pollack, C. When patterns of sleep go askew. In *Patient Care.* 1980; 14:122–174.

Lerner, R. Sleep loss in the aged: Implications for nursing research. In *Journal of Gerontological Nursing.* November 1982; 8:323–326.

Malasanos, L et al. *Health assessment* (2nd ed). St. Louis: C.V. Mosby Co; 1981.

Miles, LE, Dement, WC. Sleep and aging. In *Sleep.* 1980; 3:119–120.

Mitchell, CA. Generalized chronic fatigue in elderly people. In *Journal of Gerontological Nursing.* April 1986; 12:19–26.

Norris, C. Restlessness: A disturbance in rhythmicity. In *Geriatric Nursing.* November–December 1986; 7:302–6.

Schirmer, MS. When sleep won't come. In *Journal of Gerontological Nursing.* January 1983; 9:16–21.

Yurick, AG. *The Aged Person and the Nursing Process.* New York: Appleton; 1980.

Cognitive Perceptual Pattern

Jean A. Elmore

♦

KNOWLEDGE DEFICIT

Definition: Inability to state or explain information or demonstrate a required skill related to disease management procedures, practices, and/or self-care-health-care management.

Learning is inherent in the acquisition of knowledge. The process of learning information requires attention, perception (sensory and cognitive), memory, integration, and rehearsal. Functional integrity of the brain as evidenced by the ability to transfer knowledge from past experiences, problem solve, and recall recent and past events is necessary for learning to take place. An individual's readiness to learn can greatly influence the extent to which knowledge is acquired. Emotional and motivational status of the individual in learning play a significant role in readiness.

Although the cognitive ability to learn and motivation may be present, additional factors can act as barriers to learning. Lack of comfortable surroundings, fatigue, environmental disturbances, inadequate resources, and lack of time are major hindrances to learning.

AGE-RELATED PHENOMENA

In the elderly learner, those internal and external factors that may impact the learning process must be considered. Aside from the disease-related changes affecting the brain and sensorium, normal aging changes do not seem to alter the intellectual capacity of the elderly.

There are a number of physiologic, emotional, and developmental changes that commonly occur in the elderly, which impact on their ability to acquire knowledge. Included in these changes are

◆ extended response time
◆ decreased attention span (more easily distracted)
◆ delayed recall of recent events
◆ difficulty in identifying and organizing relevant data

◆ increasing concreteness of thought
◆ decreased stamina
◆ increased possibility for sensory impairment
◆ lack of motivation to change

Coupled with these age-related factors are environmental interferences often experienced by the aged, which present problems in acquiring new knowledge.

◆ inadequate lighting
◆ visual aids of inappropriate size and color
◆ distracting noise
◆ lack of physical comfort

Assessment of the elderly person to determine the presence of a knowledge deficit regarding a disease process, health practice, or procedure can be carried out through observation and/or inquiry. Observe the resident to determine if he or she is accurately following instructions, which were given, or performing a skill satisfactorily. Interview of the older individual will reveal information recall and application to his or her overall health situation. Merely asking if the information has been received is not enough. Comprehension is verified through verbalization, written communication, or demonstration.

ASSESSMENT

Once a deficit in knowledge has been determined, it is necessary to assess for the etiologic factors involved. The following areas are common causes of knowledge deficit in the elderly.

1. Altered Sensory Perception
   A. Visual
      ◆ Assess ability to read written instructions (be sure to provide good lighting, corrective lens).
      ◆ Check color discrimination
      ◆ Check ability to distinguish fine detail (syringe markings, thermometers)
   B. Hearing
      ◆ Acuity with respect to verbal communication at 3–5 feet with a normal tone of voice.
      ◆ Compare hearing in one ear versus the other
      ◆ Check function of hearing aids
   C. Tactile
      ◆ Assess person's ability to distinguish differences in temperature, texture, and pressure.
2. Emotional State

The emotional status of any individual influences their desire and ability to focus on change, learning, and factors outside themselves. Depression and excessive anxiety are two factors which can negatively impact on the elderly person's knowledge.

A. Moderate to Severe Anxiety

◆ Is this person fearful of new procedures, routines, people?

◆ Is the person's perception of sensory input distorted?

◆ Is the person disorganized and scattered in their thoughts and actions?

◆ Does the person have difficulty focusing attention for any length of time? Sitting still for more than a few minutes? Solving relatively simple problems?

B. Depression

◆ Does the person convey feelings of hopelessness, helplessness, powerlessness?

◆ Does the person demonstrate limited focus beyond self?

3. Cognitive Functioning

Altered cognitive functioning may be the result of physiologic deterioration, altered emotion state, or sensory deficit.

A. Intellectual processing of information. (Refer to section on Thought Impairment)

Does the person have the ability to:

◆ Follow 1, 2, and 3 step instructions?

◆ Read (person may not be literate)?

◆ Comprehend written material?

◆ Respond appropriately to questions in expected time frame for an older person?

◆ recognize similarity in ideas, concepts, and procedures?

4. Memory (Refer to section on Memory Deficit)

A. Short-term

◆ What is person's ability to recall recent events, date, name, and current president?

B. Long-term

◆ Is the person able to recall own date of birth, marriage date, past occupations, residences?

5. Motivation

Assessment of motivation is essential in understanding not only why a person may not be motivated to learn but also how you can use those motivational factors present to encourage learning.

A. Does the person feel that he or she has some control of his or her situation?

B. Does the person understand the relationship between his or her condition and the proposed procedure, treatment, or approach?

C. Does the person want to change his or her condition, abilities or the approach to the situation?

D. What has been a motivating factor in the past?

◆ increasing level of independence

◆ increasing productivity

◆ increasing socialization

◆ increasing length of life

◆ increasing knowledge of self

◆ increasing own decision-making abilities

E. Is there a physical limitation that may interfere with performance of a skill and hence decrease motivation. (e.g. decreased strength, tremors)?

6. Resources

A. Availability, accessibility, and appropriateness

◆ Has information been made available?

◆ Is the material presented appropriately? (Language, reading level, cultural considerations)

B. Does the person know where to go to obtain information?

◆ Nursing Care Plan

ETIOLOGIES

EXTERNAL

1. lack of information made available

2. unfamiliarity with information resources

3. inability to use material/information resources (language, cultural, illiteracy)

INTERNAL

1. sensory limitations

2. cognitive limitations

3. uncompensated memory loss

4. lack of interest or motivation

5. low readiness for reception of information (altered attention span)

◆ A. Nursing Diagnosis with External Etiologies

Knowledge deficit regarding disease process, procedure, or health practice related to:

1. lack of available information

2. unfamiliarity with available resources
3. inability to use resources: language, cultural, or literacy barrier.

◆ B. Nursing Diagnoses with Internal Etiologies

Knowledge deficit regarding disease process, procedure, or health practice related to:

1. sensory limitations
2. cognitive limitations
3. uncompensated memory loss
4. lack of interest/motivation
5. low readiness for reception of information

DEFINING CHARACTERISTICS

1. verbalization and written feedback indicate less than adequate recall of information or inadequate understanding, misinterpretation, misconception
2. inaccurate follow-through on previous instruction
3. inadequate demonstration of a skill
4. inappropriate or exaggerated behaviors

GOALS/OUTCOME CRITERIA

The knowledge level of the elderly person will be appropriate regarding information about a disease process, or demonstration of a skill, practice, or procedure for health management.

This will be evidenced by the individual's ability to:

◆ adequately relate in writing and/or verbally the recall of information about and an understanding of a disease process and the related practices, skills, and procedures
◆ satisfactorily demonstrate a skill, practice, or procedure.

INTERVENTIONS AND ACCOUNTABILITY

EXTERNAL ETIOLOGIES

1. Provide an adequate amount of written or audio-visual material to address the topic (RN)
   ◆ use appropriate reading level
   ◆ develop own visual aids if needed
   ◆ adapt to patient's individual needs/abilities
2. Acquaint the older person with various resources. (RN) Pamphlets, brochures distributed by a variety of groups:
   1. AARP (American Association of Retired Persons)

    2. agencies on aging

    3. local pharmacies

    4. health departments and hospitals

    5. clinics, physicians offices

    6. libraries

3. Insure that instructional materials are appropriate for the educational level, language, and cultural background of the elderly person. (RN and LPN)

◆ obtain literature in native (or reading) language.

◆ use pictures to supplement verbal or written presentation.

◆ if illiterate, teach with pictures and diagrams. Have family/friend participate in learning as a support/resource. Refer to an adult literacy program; contact your local library for resource information.

◆ augment presentation and written materials to adapt to cultural differences.

◆ allow the elder to have input into how the material is to be presented, the pace of presenting, and his or her degree of active participation.

INTERNAL ETIOLOGIES

1. Present information in a format that accommodates the elderly person's sensory deficits (if any). (RN/LPN)

◆ use print of adequate size.

◆ provide sufficient lighting without glare.

◆ prevent interferences (noise, activity)

◆ use easily distinguishable colors

◆ provide multisensory educational materials.

2. Present information at the elderly person's cognitive level of complexity. (LPN, RN)

◆ explain in non-technical terms

◆ draw association with well known examples

◆ use demonstration when possible

◆ use repetition with differing methods of delivery (written, pictorial, auditory, experiential)

◆ validate whether or not the elderly person is understanding material as it is being presented. *Ask* for feedback

◆ decrease distracters

◆ present small pieces of information at a time

◆ allow enough time for processing, considering options, and decision-making. Pacing is essential.

3. Give the older person with uncompensated memory loss additional cues to facilitate recall, such as: (RN, LPN)
   ◆ charts, schedules
   ◆ pictorial reminders of demonstrations
   ◆ use of association
   ◆ use of acronyms (when teaching about control of Diabetes: Diet, Exercise, Emotions and Medication—DEEM)
   ◆ provide written material as reinforcement whenever possible
   ◆ tie new material to old concepts.

4. Identify motivational factors which will encourage the elderly to acquire knowledge. (LPN, RN/NA)
   ◆ establish rapport and trusting relationship with the elder
   ◆ give praise and supportive encouragement when learning takes place or an effort to learn is evident
   ◆ show relationship between acquired knowledge and ability to help self, increase independence, sense of control, productivity, and avoidance of further complications.

5. Alter setting and presentation to account for exaggerated anxiety or depression in the elderly. (RN, LPN)
   ◆ allow enough time for presentation; be relaxed.
   ◆ allow for questions, concerns, and feedback.
   ◆ use repetition and multisensory approach.
   ◆ allow learners to handle equipment, examine pictures.

SENSORY PERCEPTUAL ALTERATIONS: INPUT EXCESS (OVERLOAD) OR DEFICIT DEPRIVATION

Definitions: Sensory Overload: Environmental stimuli greater than habitual level of input and/or monotonous environmental stimuli. Sensory Deprivation: Reduced environmental and social stimuli relative to habitual (or basic orienting) level.

Both sensory overload and sensory deprivation result from a real or perceived change in the amount, type, or variety of environmental and social stimuli, which is not in keeping with the "norm" for that particular individual. Any person who is placed in a new environment due to a geographical move, employment move, or perhaps an institutional move is likely to experience some increase or decrease in environmental and/or social stimuli.

AGE-RELATED PHENOMENON

In the latter phase of development, the elderly are stereotypically viewed as withdrawing from the mainstream of social involvement with a preference for being alone. In actuality, this is most often not the case. Many elderly prefer to remain actively involved with others. Factors that may preclude that involvement, such as lack of physical stamina, disability, or sensory deficit, may lead to a degree of social isolation and hence sensory deprivation.

Sensory deficits, such as visual and hearing impairment, are often associated with the aging process (see section on Uncompensated Sensory Deficits) and may lead to isolation. Elders who do not wish to demonstrate their deteriorating senses or suffer embarrassment from miscommunication may prefer to limit their social contacts and "keep to themselves." With this decreased social contact comes decreased stimuli and possible sensory deprivation.

Elderly persons coming into a long-term care facility may be accustomed to a significant decrease in external stimuli because of isolation and decreased sensory perception. Upon entering the new environment, the variety and number of incoming stimuli are greatly increased. Not all stimuli are meaningful or understood and thus can pose a threat to the elderly person's self-concept, degree of control, and independence. As a result of this lack of control and independence, the individual may experience anger, frustration, difficulty concentrating, and disorientation.

Other alterations common to the elderly that may cause problems with interpreting and processing external stimuli include diminished short-term memory, decreased attention span, and easy distractibility. Most elderly can process new and varied stimuli; however, they may require additional time or assistance in processing that information.

ASSESSMENT

The effects of sensory overload and sensory deprivation can be manifested in a number of ways.

The individual suffering from *sensory overload* may experience:

◆ restlessness
◆ anxiety
◆ insomnia
◆ fatigue
◆ muscle tension
◆ difficulty problem-solving

All of these symptoms would be in contrast to the elder's past behavior and abilities.

The person experiencing *sensory deprivation* may display some of the following symptoms:

◆ anxiety and tension
◆ confusion
◆ hallucination, vivid sensory imagery
◆ inability to concentrate and organize thoughts

- ◆ disorientation
- ◆ somatic complaints
- ◆ apathy and tendency to sleep more

Because some of these symptoms of sensory overload and deprivation overlap with each other, it is necessary to thoroughly assess the possible etiologies.

ETIOLOGIES

The environment of the elderly individual as well as his or her ability to perceive that environment needs to be accurately assessed in dealing with sensory alterations.

EXTERNAL ETIOLOGIES

ENVIRONMENT

1. Recent change in environment
   - ◆ relocation within a facility
   - ◆ hospitalization
   - ◆ long-term care facility
2. Significant change within the same location
   - ◆ change in social contacts: increase, decrease
   - ◆ change in furnishings or activity
   - ◆ many new unfamiliar words
   - ◆ unpredictable schedule
3. An increase, decrease, or sameness in sensory stimuli
   - ◆ lighting changes
   - ◆ type and intensity of noise
   - ◆ lack of tactile variety or human touch
   - ◆ presence or absence of TV or radio
   - ◆ persistence of certain odors, lack of variety
   - ◆ positional sameness
   - ◆ dietary monotony in texture, taste, and color
4. Significant change in social interactions—both frequency and variety
   - ◆ increased social contact by a variety of unfamiliar people
   - ◆ decreased social contact and interaction due to:
     a. restricted physical activity
     b. decreased sensory perception
     c. isolation
5. Basic loss of control of the environment
   - ◆ recent disability such as a stroke, MI
   - ◆ institutionalization

INTERNAL ETIOLOGIES

SENSORY CHANGES

Is there actual sensory impairment?

◆ Vision: acuity, accommodation, sensitivity to light, cataracts, glaucoma, loss of glasses

◆ Hearing: presbycusis, total deafness, loss of high frequency hearing, loss of hearing aid, nonfunctioning hearing aid.

◆ Touch: decreased sensation due to deterioration, medication side effects, or neurological damage.

◆ Smell: decreased sensation with aging, nasal congestion.

◆ Proprioception: decreased awareness of body position, posture.

SPEECH DEFICITS

Is there an inability to relate to others socially due to speech deficits?

◆ aphasia

◆ laryngectomy

◆ tracheostomy

◆ paralysis

IMPAIRED PROCESSING OF SENSORY STIMULI

◆ impaired short-term memory

◆ difficulty integrating sensory data

Identification of these etiologies may require investigation into past records, interviewing the family and friends as well as thorough patient assessment.

◆ Nursing Care Plan

A. SENSORY OVERLOAD: NURSING DIAGNOSES WITH EXTERNAL ETIOLOGIES

1. Sensory-perceptual alterations: Sensory overload related to environmental complexity.

2. Sensory-perceptual alterations: Sensory overload related to environmental monotony.

DEFINING CHARACTERISTICS

◆ irritability and anxiety

◆ concern and excessive questioning regarding treatment

◆ restlessness

◆ sleeplessness

◆ disorientation (periodic or general)

◆ difficulty in solving problems

◆ decreased productivity in work

- complaints of fatigue
- complaints of muscle tension
- inappropriate interpretation of sensory stimuli
- increased sensitivity to pain

GOALS/OUTCOME CRITERIA

1. The sensory overload of the elderly person will be reduced as evidenced by:
   a. decreased anxiety and irritability
   b. decreased muscle tension and fatigue
   c. orientation and lack of confusion
   d. increased work productivity
   e. increased ability to problem solve
   f. decreased insomnia
   g. decreased suspicion about treatment, procedures
   h. greater sense of control of environment
   i. appropriate interpretation of sensory stimuli

INTERVENTIONS AND ACCOUNTABILITY

1. Reduce clutter in the elder's immediate environment. Place equipment and machines away from the individual, if possible. Maintain organization of materials and eliminate unnecessary items. (RN, LPN, Aide, Therapists)
2. Allow the elder some control of his or her environment, e.g. placement of articles, curtains open or closed, lights on or off, music or TV on or off. (All Staff)
3. Offer explanations for treatments, machines, procedures, and need for repeated monitoring. Allow time for processing and questioning. (RN, LPN)
4. Decrease monotonous machine and verbal noise. (RN, LPN)
5. Provide variety in lighting intensity, source, and possibly color. (RN, LPN, NA)
6. Outline the routine, the rationale for it, and unexpected interruptions. (RN, LPN)
7. Acquaint the elder with all new and unfamiliar faces and terminology. (RN, LPN)
8. Present explanations in simple terms, using some repetition in a reasonably short span of time. (RN, LPN)

B. SENSORY-PERCEPTUAL ALTERATIONS: NURSING DIAGNOSES WITH INTERNAL ETIOLOGIES

Sensory overload related to impaired thought processes and impaired memory.

DEFINING CHARACTERISTICS

◆ restlessness, agitation, anxiety
◆ loss of appetite
◆ increase in confusion and disorientation
◆ decreased attention span
◆ sleeplessness
◆ fatigue
◆ muscle tension
◆ reduced problem-solving ability
◆ decreased tolerance of stimuli

GOALS/OUTCOME CRITERIA

The elder with sensory overload related to thought and memory impairment will be able to perceive stimuli appropriately and experience less overload as evidenced by:

◆ decreased anxiety, agitation (decreased need for PRN anti-anxiety drugs)
◆ less muscle tension
◆ less confusion and disorientation
◆ better dietary intake
◆ appropriate response to stimuli

INTERVENTIONS

1. Maintain a consistent routine. (RN, LPN, NA)
2. Provide familiar staff. (RN)
3. Wear name tags, other easily identifiable clothing or symbols. (RN, LPN, NA)
4. Maintain eye contact when speaking. (All Staff)
5. Use touch when speaking to demonstrate acceptance and put the person at ease. (All staff)
6. Speak slowly, using simple short sentences with visual cues. (All staff)
7. Maintain a relaxed environment. Move slowly. (All staff)
8. Decrease noise and visual clutter. (All staff)
9. Listen carefully. (All staff, family)

SENSORY DEPRIVATION: NURSING DIAGNOSES WITH EXTERNAL ETIOLOGIES

1. Sensory-Perceptual Alterations: Sensory Deprivation related to restricted environment.

2. Sensory-Perceptual Alterations: Sensory Deprivation related to therapeutic environmental restriction (bed rest, isolation, intensive care, traction, ventilator).

3. Sensory-Perceptual Alterations: Sensory Deprivation related to socially restricted environment (debilitated, immobility, homebound, institutionalization).

DEFINING CHARACTERISTICS

◆ alert with periods of confusion, forgetfulness, and disorientation
◆ hallucinations
◆ apathy and excessive sleeping
◆ auditory, visual, olfactory, gustatory, or tactile reality orienting or time orienting input is absent or reduced.

GOALS/OUTCOME CRITERIA

The sensory deprivation of the elderly individual will be diminished or absent as evidenced by:

◆ alertness, orientation to time, person, and place
◆ lack of hallucinations
◆ demonstration of interest in activities outside self and immediate needs
◆ regular, nonexcessive sleeping patterns.

INTERVENTIONS AND ACCOUNTABILITY

1. Provide multi-sensory stimuli in the resident's environment. (RN, LPN, NA, family, therapists)
   a. Visual stimulation
      ◆ mobiles
      ◆ plants
      ◆ games
      ◆ drawing/painting
      ◆ clock, calendar
      ◆ photographs
      ◆ wall hangings
      ◆ flowers
      ◆ seasonal decorations
      ◆ mirrors
      ◆ crafts
      ◆ colorful clothes
      ◆ keep glasses clean and available

b. Auditory stimulation
- ◆ decrease background noise
- ◆ use of telephone
- ◆ music of various types and volumes
- ◆ TV, radio
- ◆ tapes
- ◆ outside activities
- ◆ verbal interaction with others on various topics
- ◆ use gestures and demonstration to emphasize and reinforce information
- ◆ allow time for response

c. Touch stimulation
- ◆ provide various textures for the elderly person to feel
- ◆ provide contact with animals—stuffed and real
- ◆ use massage, back rubs, hair brushing to stimulate
- ◆ allow elder to care for self as much as possible

d. Taste stimulation
- ◆ provide multiple flavors, seasonings, textures, and temperatures of food
- ◆ allow the elder some control of food selection
- ◆ encourage family to bring in favorite foods
- ◆ keep mouth clean and dentures in place

e. Olfactory stimulation
- ◆ allow elder to smell various foods, flowers, scented candles, cologne, pot pourri
- ◆ eliminate offensive odors

2. Periodically change sensory input.
- ◆ change the resident's furniture arrangement (with consent)
- ◆ change routine (with consent)

3. Acquaint the elder with new staff, familiarize the elder with new activities outside his or her immediate environment.

4. Make a point of including the elder in social activities, e.g. bring others in to *his* or *her* environment if necessary.
- ◆ bring in entertainment—singing, instruments
- ◆ artistic display
- ◆ young children performing songs, reciting, presenting gifts (intergenerational programming).

5. Provide an opportunity for the elder to come in contact with his or her environment.
- ◆ water plants

◆ arrange his or her own articles on bedside stand
◆ create/make something
◆ write a letter

SENSORY DEPRIVATION: NURSING DIAGNOSES WITH INTERNAL ETIOLOGIES

1. Sensory-Perceptual Alterations: Sensory Deprivation related to uncompensated sensory deficits (vision, hearing, touch, taste, smell, proprioception)
2. Sensory-Perceptual Alterations: Sensory Deprivation related to impaired communication (aphasia, paralysis, tracheostomy, laryngectomy)

DEFINING CHARACTERISTICS

◆ limited proprioceptive input
◆ presence of uncompensated visual, hearing, olfactory, and gustatory deficits
◆ apathy, withdrawal
◆ isolation
◆ confusion
◆ disorientation
◆ somnolence

GOALS/OUTCOME CRITERIA

1. The elder with sensory deprivation will experience increasing awareness of sensory input and body locomotion.
2. The elder with sensory deprivation will be able to compensate for loss of verbal communication.

INTERVENTIONS AND ACCOUNTABILITY

1. Insure availability and operability of sensory-related prosthesis. (RN, LPN, NA)
   a. have glasses cleaned and within reach
   b. have hearing aid(s) cleaned and in place with operating batteries.
   c. have dentures cleaned and in place.
2. Insure that ear canals are not occluded with wax. (RN)
3. Compensate for deficits in vision and hearing. (All staff, family)
   a. provide large print materials
   b. attract the person's attention before speaking
   c. speak in "good" ear, if appropriate
   d. use eye contact when speaking
   e. speak in low tones, enunciate, and speak slowly

f. use gestures and facial expressions

g. allow time for response and questioning

h. warn of hazards and assist when necessary

i. use headphones for music, if needed

j. have patient use stethoscope for hearing if very hard of hearing. (see section on Uncompensated Sensory Deficits)

4. Stimulate proprioceptive receptors by changing the elder's position—sitting, reclining, lying, standing—throughout the day. Provide explanation before moving. Have the resident assist with the repositioning. Provide Range of Motion exercises—passively or actively—to assist in increasing body awareness. (RN, LPN, NA)

5. Provide alternate methods of communication for those elders with verbal/auditory impairment. (RN, LPN)

◆ write on message-paper, chalk board, magic slate

◆ pictorial messages on a board used for quick reference

◆ head and hand gestures, facial expressions

◆ do not interrupt

◆ listen patiently

PAIN; CHRONIC PAIN

Definition: Verbal report and presence of indicators of severe discomfort. (Demonstration of guarded behavior, distraction behavior, narrowing focus to self, look of pain-grimacing, change in muscle tone, autonomic responses)

Pain is a subjective symptom that is difficult to accurately assess. Every individual experiences and responds to pain differently. It is important to accept the individual perception of pain as valid for that person. There are basically three types of pain:

1. Physiologic Pain—A direct result of pathology of the body, i.e. tissue, bone, or organ injury or damage.

2. Pathologic Pain—Results from pathology of the nervous system, i.e. peripheral neuropathy associated with diabetes mellitus.

3. Psychologic Pain—A very poor pain tolerance and in some cases no stimulus need be applied for pain to be perceived.

Several non-physical factors can influence one's perception of the amount and quality of pain. A person's cultural and social background may instill certain values regarding pain and response to pain. Psychological conditions such as depression and anxiety are known to intensify or even cause the sensation of pain. Increased anxiety regarding one's physical condition and associated pain can bring about a more concentrated focus on self and the lack of well-being. This increased attention paid to the pain along with fatigue or poor health may intensify the sensation.

When speaking of a person's response to pain the terms threshold and pain tolerance are often used.

◆ Threshold refers to the intensity of the stimulus which is first perceived as being painful.

◆ Pain tolerance refers to the ability to maintain control over one's self despite pain.

ASSESSMENT

Pain can have a variety of characteristics. It can be continuous or intermittent, sharp or dull, localized or general, and predictable or unpredictable. Pain is often a symptom of some underlying disease process.

Because the pain may be caused by anything from emotional stress to metastatic cancer, the assessment may be very involved and must often be carried out over the period of days or even weeks. Data collection regarding the assessment of pain will include subjective information from the resident, and objective data regarding the patient's behavior, activity, and response to activity.

Specific information must be obtained regarding the character of the pain. Once this has been documented, it is necessary to determine how emotional, social, and spiritual factors may be influencing pain. Exploring with the elder their feelings and fears about the pain, why it is present, why and when it abates is important for establishing a plan of action.

Chronic pain may be a learned response. Are there positive outcomes which result from having pain? One theory developed by Wilbert Fordyce proposes that within the area of chronic pain, people can learn to perceive recurring or chronic pain because of the response that follows the occurrence of that pain. The person may receive pain medication, increased attention from others, special privileges, rest, or decreased work load and responsibility. Pain may provide an excuse for not carrying out certain activities, which the elder person is incapable of performing well due to sensory impairment or cognitive deficits. Because of these "positive" consequences, the pain behavior if reinforced, a pattern of behavior developed.

At the onset of evaluation of pain the nurse must acknowledge that pain does exist. Once this acceptance has been established, the elder can be directed to describe in detail the characteristics of the pain. The nurse must guard against trying to describe the pain for the elder.

1. Location	Is it in a definite location or is it general?
2. Radiation	It is significant to note if the pain travels. Does it always go to the same location?
3. Intensity	Have the elder rate the pain on a scale of 1–10. Is this an ache or sharp stabbing pain? Is the elder incapacitated? Are ADLs possible with the pain?

4. Onset and Precipitating Factors	Does the pain coincide with certain activities, follow certain activities or situations, relate to emotional changes, intensity with an increase in emotions? Is the onset sudden or gradual?
5. Duration and Frequency	Is the pain intermittent or continuous? How long does it last? How often does it occur in 24 hours?
6. Relief	What brings relief? Pain medication, application of hot or cold treatments, massage, rest, etc.? To what degree is the pain relieved?
7. Sequelae	Are there other symptoms that occur with the pain or as a result of the pain, i.e. nausea and vomiting, shortness of breath, inability to move a certain part of the body, numbness and tingling, loss of vision, etc.? What emotional feelings are present at the time of pain (fear, anger, anxiety, embarrassment, depression)?

Often it is helpful for the elder person to keep a log of when pain occurs, its character, duration, etc. This will allow the elder to have input into the planning and intervention. The elder can also begin to see the patterns that develop and possible associated factors that cause pain. This should be maintained after the intervention is initiated to document the effects of those strategies.

It is essential that the nurse observe the pattern of pain occurrence and determine if the perception of pain may be a conditioned response.

AGE-RELATED PHENOMENON

In general the elderly have a decreased sensation of pain. In particular the neuro-receptors in the skin are not as sensitive to heat, cold, tactile and pressure stimulation, thus increasing their pain threshold. While this is true, it must also be noted that there are several degenerative aspects of aging that bring about discomfort and pain. Much of this pain is chronic in nature for the elderly but may fluctuate in intensity.

Health alterations common to the elderly that bring about pain/discomfort would include:

◆ deterioration of intervertebral discs

- osteoporosis
- arthritis
- neuritis
- peripheral arterial sclerosis
- herpes zoster
- angina pectoris
- vascular insufficiency
- inadequate foot care, nails, callouses
- dental and gingival problems
- urinary tract infections
- altered bowel activity
- allergic reactions, infections
- skeletal fractures

Not uncommonly, the elderly are subject to more than one of these problems. With this we see a complex picture involving several pains or discomforts.

ETIOLOGIES

EXTERNAL

1. Injuring agents—examples include:

   - Chemicals—allergens, irritating soaps, foods, urine, feces, tape, medications
   - Biologicals—bacteria, viruses
   - Physical—friction, pressure, blows, excessive heat or cold, obstacles causing falls

INTERNAL

1. Injuring agents—examples include:

   - Chemicals—toxins, increased production of HCL in stomach
   - Biologicals—infections
   - Physical—degenerative changes, cancer, other abnormal growth, vascular changes, unstable gait, dizziness
   - Psychological—depression, anxiety, stress, loss of control, need for attention, recognition

2. Knowledge Deficit:

   - Lack of knowledge about pain management techniques
   - Cognitive impairment, inability to learn or retain information

◆ Nursing Care Plan

NURSING DIAGNOSIS: PAIN

DEFINING CHARACTERISTICS

1. Communication (verbal or coded) of pain descriptors
2. Guarding behavior: protective of certain aspects of body, avoiding certain positions
3. Self-focusing: constantly commenting on body functions, own feelings, needs, and wants
4. Narrowed focus: altered time perception, withdrawal from social contact, impaired thought process
5. Distraction behavior: moaning, crying, pacing, seeking out other people and/or activities, restless
6. Facial mask of pain: eyes lack luster, "beaten look," fixed or scattered movement, grimace
7. Alteration in muscle tone: may span from listless to rigid
8. Autonomic responses not seen in chronic, stable pain: diaphoresis, blood pressure and pulse rate change, pupillary dilation, increased or decreased respiratory rate.

GOALS/OUTCOME CRITERIA

1. Will experience decrease or absence of perceived pain as evidenced through verbal communication, and demonstrated lack of crying, moaning, restlessness.
2. Will experience increased pain threshold as evidenced by increasing freedom of body movement, relaxed face, and maintenance of reality-based perspective on self and environment.

INTERVENTIONS AND ACCOUNTABILITY

1. Avoid contact with known allergens—soaps, perfumes, foods, and beverages. (RN, LPN, NA)
2. Avoid exposure to excessive heat—burners on stove, irons, heaters, heating pads. (Recognize decreased sensitivity to heat and cold.) Avoid exposure to cold—adequately dress for cold weather, apply warm stockings if peripheral circulation is impaired. (RN, LPN, NA, Resident)
3. Prevent friction/pressure when using braces, casts, supports, and restraints by applying padding and making necessary adjustments. Avoid ill-fitting shoes. Note pressure points, adjust if possible and replace if necessary.
4. Identify and eliminate hazards that could cause falls, resulting in fractures, concussions, and soft tissue injury:
   ◆ obstacles on the floor

- ◆ inadequate lighting
- ◆ inappropriate placement of furniture
- ◆ unstable furniture, poor height
- ◆ lack of assistive devices to compensate for sensory losses. (RN, LPN, NA, Resident)

5. Place grab bars and hand rails in locations where patient might be unsteady. (bathroom, halls)

6. Practice sound hygiene in respect to toileting and handling of food. (RN, LPN, NA, RD, Resident)

7. Maintain adequate nutrition and rest habits. (RN, LPN, NA, RD, Resident)

8. Decrease intake of caffeine if elder is predisposed to high acidity in stomach.

9. Decrease focus on pain:
   - ◆ decrease talk of pain
   - ◆ increase diversional activities that appeal to the elder.
   - ◆ increase involvement with other people in a social context, family, friends. (RN, LPN, Family)

10. Instruct elder as to the complexities of pain and the many factors that precipitate and intensify pain.
    - ◆ precipitate—injuries, deterioration
    - ◆ intensify—focused attention, fatigue, increased emotional stress, anxiety. (RN, LPN)

11. Decrease tension, fear and anxiety by:
    - ◆ demonstrating resident's own control over pain
    - ◆ relaxation techniques
    - ◆ passive or active exercise program
    - ◆ appropriate application of hot and cold
    - ◆ use of massage
    - ◆ guided imagery
    - ◆ music
    - ◆ myotherapy
    - ◆ prayer and meditation.

12. If the perception of chronic pain is shown to be a learned response, a behavior modification approach should be used.
    - ◆ increase expectation of self-care and involvement in activity (begin gradually)
    - ◆ decrease talk of and complaining about pain by focusing conversation on other topics
    - ◆ reinforce positive non-pain behavior

- ◆ relaxation and deep breathing when pain occurs
- ◆ gradual reduction of pain medications
- ◆ increase rest if fatigue is a problem.

UNCOMPENSATED SHORT-TERM MEMORY DEFICIT

Definition: Impaired ability to recall recent or current events or activities.

Memory is a complex phenomena, which allows us to adapt to our environment. Through this process of recalling information, we are able to be responsive, interactional, and to independently care for ourselves. Memory is essential for functioning in our society and gives us our sense of identity. The use of memory is involved in everything we do.

There are three basic phases of memory: 1. acquiring information, 2. storing information, and 3. recalling or retrieving information. It is necessary for the individual to have an intact sensorium to perceive stimuli coming in. Also, the ability to recognize and associate input must be present. Physical, psychological, and social alterations can impact upon the memory process.

Memory is generally referred to as being short term or long term. Short-term memory includes the recall of those immediate or current events. Long-term memory is typically thought of as those events that have occurred in the distant past.

In addition to the time-referenced classifications of memory, there are two types that relate to the complexity of the memory process. *Episodic memory* refers to the recall of recent episodes or experiences. The individual remembers the event as it happened, the situation surrounding it, where it occurred, when, and with whom. Many of the particulars of episodic memory can be lost over time. The other type of memory is *semantic.* This refers to a more complex process whereby an event is evaluated and synthesized by relating stimuli to past experiences and making some sense out of it. This process requires language skills and a sense of logic.

Recall of memory may be almost *automatic* in nature, such as recalling how to drive a car or play an instrument. Giving another person directions in how to drive a car may be referred to as *effortful* recall.

The function of short-term memory is complex and includes maintaining memory of current events long enough so that the necessary actions or behaviors can be executed. Also, the short-term memory must recognize what factors have been identified that must be placed in long-term memory for later retrieval.

◆ Short-Term Memory Deficit

Most problems with memory lapse reflect short-term memory loss. The non-pathological causes for memory lapse are common to all age groups.

Factors such as: 1) inattention, which interferes with the intake of stimuli, 2) anxiety, which can also interfere with stimuli intake and retrieval of information, 3) depression, which can impair the retrieval of current episodic data, and 4) societal pressures including living alone, stress of a complex living environment, finances, and losing a close relative can all lead to impairment of memory.

The overall result of an increasingly ineffective memory is a withdrawal from interaction and decreased contact with other people, which leads to a diminished sense of self-awareness and self-esteem. Losing one's ability to remember can be frustrating, anxiety producing, and frightening.

AGE-RELATED PHENOMENA

Forgetfulness and aging are often seen as natural companions. The stereotypical image of the elderly person in our society automatically projects the individual who has a difficult time recalling recent events, names, and places. There is some evidence indicating that the short-term or active recall of the elderly person is not as good as that of the younger population. The possible cause of these memory lapses must be examined to determine if age-related factors are responsible for this decline in the ability to remember.

As was noted earlier, several factors which are not age-specific can cause memory lapse. These are more situational or temporary in nature. The etiology of memory lapse in the elderly person seems to be more permanent in nature. Often the elderly view the advent of memory lapse as the beginning of their decline and the possible loss of control or the ability to remain independent.

Perhaps the most common etiology for memory deficit is the detrimental effects resulting when too little oxygen is made available to the brain. This phenomena can occur with a variety of pathophysiological conditions such as atherosclerosis, chronic obstructive lung disease, myocardial infarct, low cardiac output, pulmonary embolus, and anemia. Other disease processes that can also contribute to the lapse of memory include cerebral vascular accidents, cerebral tumors, cerebral edema, diabetes mellitus, thyroid and adrenal insufficiency. The central nervous system depressant effects of some drugs, as well as the side effects, are also responsible for a number of memory problems in the elderly. These drugs include the sedative-hypnotics, anti-anxiety agents, narcotics, and barbiturates.

Although situational factors are not specific to the elderly, there seem to be a number of these factors that affect the elderly consistently and appear to be related to memory lapse. Stressful life styles, caused by poor economy, inadequate housing, lack of support systems, regimented or repetitive patterns of activities, or complex living situations can all contribute to a lapse of memory because of the associated anxiety.

If the elderly person is lacking in actual sensory input or intake necessary for acquiring information or triggering clues for retrieval, memory may be impaired. Due to the prevalence of depression among the elderly, this particular cause of memory lapse must not be over-looked. Even when other physiological evidence is noted to be the causative agent, depression, which usually involves social isolation and decreased sensory input, must be considered as a major etiological factor in elderly memory deficit.

ASSESSMENT

To accurately assess memory loss in the elderly, it may be necessary to observe them over the period of several days or weeks. This type of in-depth investigation is essential for planning the care of the elderly, including education, self-care focus, and family involvement.

Initially, you can ask some very straightforward questions which will indicate whether the short-term, episodic memory is intact.

1. What is your phone number?
2. What is your address?
3. What is the month and year?
4. With whom did you eat your last meal?
5. What did you have for your last meal?
6. Give the person a simple pair of words or a phase, then ask him or her to repeat it later in the interview.
7. Simple recall can also be tested by having the person repeat a series of 4 or 5 numbers.

The use of semantic memory requires more abstract thought and can be tested with the following questions:

1. List all of the things you did this morning since waking up.
2. Describe the importance of taking your medication at the prescribed times.
3. Can you tell me how to drive a stick shift car? Knit? Use a camera? etc.

The accuracy of long-term memory can easily be assessed by asking some of the following questions: (Be sure you have access to the correct answers)

1. What is your date of birth?
2. Where were you born?
3. What is your mother's maiden name?
4. Could you tell me what you were doing during the Depression?
5. How many children do you have? What are their names? Where do they live? What are their occupations?

Other means of assessing for memory deficit include noting the response to subjective questions such as:

1. Do you have difficulty remembering to take your medication?
2. Do you have difficulty remembering *if* you have taken your medication?

3. Do you find that you often forget people's names or where they live?
4. Do you find yourself beginning a task and then forgetting to complete it?
5. Do you lose items such as keys and glasses because you have forgotten where you placed them?

Assessment of the elderly persons as they perform their daily activities can give you objective information about how they utilize memory. Noting that the person repeatedly asks the same questions of the same person in a short span of time may indicate a problem with short-term memory. Repetitious loss of items and demanding behavior can also signal the presence of a memory deficit. Confabulation, which is a clever means of covering up for one's loss of memory by making up responses to questions, is often used by those who are alert enough to know that they have a memory deficit, but who are unable to retrieve from memory the necessary information.

Because memory involves a number of phases, it is essential that we know the point at which the interruption is taking place. If for some reason there is perceptual impairment, such as with decreased vision or hearing, the person may not be able to integrate the stimuli because it is not fully perceived. Even if there is no sensory deficit, the lack of attention being given to stimuli may result in much the same situation. After the stimuli is perceived, it must be compared with "old" experiences and some sense made out of what is happening. This is commonly referred to as *encoding*. Once some sense has been made out of the experience and it holds significance, the event can be translated into a permanent record. This is called *consolidation*. Lastly, the use of information permanently placed in memory, is called *retrieval*. Unfortunately, there are factors that can block or interfere with the retrieval of information. Sometimes changing the context under which the information is recalled results in the lack of retrieval. One symptom of this type of retrieval problem might be when a person tells you that they learned something, or they know someone's name but just can't bring it to mind. Often when given a sufficient amount of time and enough clues, they will be able to recall the needed information.

ETIOLOGIES

INTERNAL

1. Depression due to loss of spouse or other close relative, loss of home, or other significant symbol of self-sufficiency
2. Anxiety due to stress of life situations, complex environment, or difficulty dealing with problem situations
3. Impaired sensory perception, such as poor vision, poor hearing, or poor tactile sensation.

EXTERNAL

1. Complexity of the environment. Congregate living situation with group dining or multiple generation family situation

2. Repetitious daily routine and surroundings, not allowing for differentiation of days and places

3. Lack of environmental cues to stimulate retrieval.

◆ Nursing Care Plan

NURSING DIAGNOSES WITH INTERNAL ETIOLOGIES

1. Impaired ability to recall recent or current events or activities related to depression and anxiety

2. Impaired ability to recall recent or current events or activities related to impaired sensory perception.

NURSING DIAGNOSES WITH EXTERNAL ETIOLOGIES

1. Impaired ability to recall recent or current events or activities related to complex living situation

2. Impaired ability to recall recent or current events or activities related to repetitious daily routine and sameness of the environment

3. Impaired ability to recall recent or current events or activities related to the lack of cues to stimulate retrieval.

DEFINING CHARACTERISTICS

The elderly individual will have difficulty being able to:

◆ Recall his or her address and phone number

◆ Recall the month and year

◆ Recall what was eaten in a previous meal, what activity was just completed, or what was just said in a previous conversation

◆ Repeat paired words or phases shortly after given

◆ Repeat a 4 or 5 digit number

◆ Recall the events of the day

◆ Understand directions and problem solve due to a deficit in short-term memory

◆ Recall a previously learned procedure or skill

◆ Recall names and places which are familiar.

When observing the elderly individual you note that:

◆ Items are often "lost" or "misplaced"

◆ The elder is found entering the "wrong" room or going down the "wrong" hall

◆ Repetition of phrases, questions or stories is common

◆ Some tasks are not completed due to memory deficit

◆ There is use of confabulation to cover up the inability to remember specific factors.

GOALS/OUTCOME CRITERIA

The short-term memory deficit of the elderly person will be compensated for as evidenced by the following:

1. The elderly person will be able to:
   ◆ recall names, places, and recent events
   ◆ recall instructions and procedures
   ◆ locate items commonly used such as glasses, keys
   ◆ use landmarks to locate destination
   ◆ complete tasks without interruption from memory deficit
   ◆ recognize when a question or story has been previously stated.

INTERVENTIONS AND ACCOUNTABILITY

INTERNAL

1. Provide an atmosphere of acceptance toward the individuals with memory lapse. (RN, LPN, NA)
2. Help to focus the elder's attention by addressing them by name. (RN, LPN, NA)
3. Develop a group experience which will address the issue of short-term memory deficit, why it occurs, what aggravates the memory lapses, attitudes and emotions that often accompany memory deficits, and how memory aids can be utilized. (RN)
4. Use reminiscence to stimulate long-term recall and enrich the self-esteem and self-worth of the individual. This will also increase his or her ability to recall. Reminiscence can be triggered by using old photographs, news clippings, souvenirs, or keepsakes. (RN, LPN, NA)
5. Utilize repetitive cues to remind people of the date, time, and year. Put calendars and clocks in places where they will be seen frequently. Make sure that the days are consistently checked off or a single-day calendar is used. (RN, LPN, NA)
6. When giving instructions, include some written notes or outline to which the elder can refer at a later time. (RN)
7. Utilize pictures when giving instruction or teaching. The visual stimulation gives an added dimension and will provide another clue in stimulating recall. (RN)
8. If memory lapse seems to occur in episodic memory (forgetting if pills have been taken), then provide aids such as pill counters or posted calendars to check off when medication has been taken. (RN, LPN)
9. If memory lapse is more semantic in nature (forgetting that a specific pill is to be taken at 10 PM), the approach should include a definite reminder at the appropriate time, such as an alarm clock that goes off at 10 PM. (RN, LPN)

10. Allow for the elderly person to devote undivided attention to the task at hand, thereby perceiving available stimuli, and not being stressed by distractions or a hurried situation. (All Staff)

11. Have the elder keep a brief notebook of current events in his or her life, including the names of people, directions, or instructions that have been given.

12. For those with marked loss of short-term memory, it is essential that their daily routine be consistent, that personal items be returned to the same place after use, and that repeated verbal and/or written reminders be given to foster independence. (RN, LPN, NA)

13. When expecting the elder to recall information, utilize the same or similar contextual reference as the one in place when the information was originally received. (Don't start questioning the elder about how to perform the Accucheck test while he or she is playing shuffleboard.) (RN, LPN)

14. Use association, especially when giving information that must be recalled accurately and frequently, i.e. when telling someone how to schedule a treatment or medication, associate it with some other activity already established, such as foot care could be done in the evening while watching the news. (RN, LPN)

UNCOMPENSATED SENSORY DEFICIT

Definition: Uncompensated loss of acuity or absence of vision, hearing, touch, smell, taste, or kinesthesia.

Use of our senses allows us to interpret and appreciate our environment. This environment includes persons as well as physical surroundings. It is only through the use of our senses that we can determine where we are and what is happening to us. With a significant loss or total absence of one or more senses, the ability to perceive one's environment is markedly decreased.

AGE-RELATED PHENOMENA

Decreased acuity of the senses, primarily vision and hearing, is a physical aspect of aging. Expected vision changes include:

◆ decreased speed and ability to adapt to the dark

◆ narrowing of the visual field

◆ yellowing of the lens with resulting difficulty in distinguishing between blues and greens

◆ presbyopia—accommodation defect making it more difficult to focus (result of weakened ciliary muscles)

◆ increased sensitivity to glare (result of opacity in lens causing scattered light rays)

◆ decreased sensitivity to light (result of decreased pupil size).

Expected hearing changes include:

◆ decreased ability to detect the volume of sound

◆ decreased ability to detect the pitch of sound, in particular high-frequency loss is noted. This is referred to as presbycusis.

Hearing loss in the elderly may be due to sensory neural or conductive problems. A decrease in the movement of the tympanic membrane or ossicles is referred to as a conductive hearing loss, whereas damage to the cochlea is referred to as a sensory-neural alteration.

Although some deterioration of the visual and auditory senses is expected with aging, these changes should not significantly interfere with the ability of the older person to carry out his or her daily activities.

Alterations expected in the areas of touch, smell, taste, and kinesthetics include:

◆ less discrete perception of tactile stimulation including light touch, hot and cold

◆ decreased sensation of body movement and position

◆ decreased sensitivity to taste, with an 80 percent loss in taste buds. The taste buds most likely to diminish first are those that are sensitive to sweet and salty tastes.

ASSESSMENT

With some background knowledge of the expected alterations in sensory perception of the elderly, we can now focus on the assessment of the significant sensory deficits.

FUNCTIONAL ASSESSMENT

Interviewing the patient as to his or her perception of sensory acuity is often very unreliable. To accurately assess sensory loss, it is necessary to collect objective data through physical examination and observation of the patient while he or she is functioning in daily activities.

To assess for *visual acuity* the nurse should:

◆ note peripheral vision. Does the elder person acknowledge movement to the side or is it necessary for the elder to turn his or her head to visualize something off to the side? When eating, is the food on one side of the plate ignored?

◆ check for double vision by covering one eye at a time and holding up fingers or pencils, ask the elder person to indicate how many are present.

◆ use an eye chart (Snellen) for determining acuity at a distance.

◆ note if the person is able to read the newspaper. Validate this by having them read a segment to you. Can the person read medication labels or syringe markings?

◆ inspect eyes for pupil size, reaction to light, and ability to focus on objects that are near and far (accommodation)

◆ Observe smoothness of ocular movements. Do the eyes move together?

◆ note if the individual has difficulty visualizing whiskers, needlework

◆ note if the elder avoids bright light or complains frequently of inadequate lighting.

◆ what, if any, compensation has been made for the visual deficit noted?

To assess for *auditory acuity* the nurse should note:

◆ if the elder person is able to hear a ticking watch one inch from his or her ear

◆ if the elder responds to distant noises, such as outside traffic, sirens, intercom messages

◆ if the elder person is able to distinguish high frequency sounds such as consonants? To test this, the nurse should use words like *bed, cash, duck, fish,* and *juice,* while the person is NOT looking at the nurse's mouth

◆ if this elder person has difficulty understanding speech while in a group situation with background noise (dining room)

◆ if the individual has significantly more difficulty understanding when you speak when he or she is not able to see your face

◆ frequent blank expressions or lack of response when questioning the elderly person

◆ how is this person coping with or compensating for the loss of hearing? Use of the "Hearing Handicap Inventory for the Elderly" may be helpful.

To assess for *olfactory acuity* the nurse should note whether the person can:

◆ detect the various odors of food, smoke, chemicals, or perfume

◆ distinguish the smell of spices—cinnamon, cloves, peppermint, or vanilla.

Be certain that the nasal passages are clear when you test for olfactory sensation.

To assess for *taste acuity* the nurse should note if the elderly person:

◆ puts excessive amounts of seasoning on his or her food

◆ complains of the blandness of the food, or that all the food tastes the same

◆ has difficulty distinguishing between flavors of gelatin, jelly, or juices.

To assess for *tactile acuity* the nurse should observe the elderly person for:

◆ response to hot and cold temperatures on various parts of the body

◆ response to sharp pricking stimuli, light touch, and dull pressure. Can the elder distinguish between these? At what intensity are these perceived? Where on the body are these sensations perceived?

◆ the ability to distinguish between smooth and rough textures, ability to identify a coin, paper clip, or key by touch and not sight.

To assess for *kinesthetic awareness* the nurse should note whether the elderly person can:

◆ perceive movement of the body, change in direction or position while keeping eyes closed

◆ maintain self erect in one position while standing with eyes closed and not touching anyone or anything.

As was noted before, the loss of acuity in any of the senses may be related to a generalized deterioration; however, there may be a loss due to abnormal growth or injury to either the neurological structures (brain, neural transmission, and receptors) or the organ responsible for receiving the stimuli (eyes, ears, nose).

Alterations in sensory function may result from:

◆ *infections,* such as encephalitis, glossitis, sinusitis, neuritis, or otitis

◆ *circulatory impairment,* such as CVA and peripheral vascular insufficiency

◆ *traumatic injury,* such as subdural hematoma, enucleation, blow to side of head

◆ *drug side effects,* such as decreased taste sensation, increasing instability and loss of kinesthesia, decreasing peripheral circulation

◆ *lesions,* such as neoplasms and skin changes

◆ other *disease entities,* such as diabetes, Parkinson's, or multiple sclerosis

◆ *obstruction to the receptors* of sensory input, such as cerumen in the ear canal, nasal congestion, coating of the tongue.

ETIOLOGIES

INTERNAL

1. Lack of understanding or acceptance that a deficit exists
2. Lack of knowledge about the cause of the sensory deficit
3. Lack of knowledge about available resources and devices to compensate for and adapt to sensory deficit
4. Lack of motivation to seek resources to help compensate for the sensory deficit.

EXTERNAL

1. Lack of resources (finances, accessibility, and availability) to make it possible to obtain corrective devices thereby compensating for the sensory deficit.

◆ Nursing Care Plan

NURSING DIAGNOSES WITH INTERNAL ETIOLOGIES

1. Uncompensated sensory deficit related to a lack of knowledge regarding the existence of the deficit, its cause, and the possible resources available to compensate for the deficit.
2. Uncompensated sensory deficit related to the lack of motivation necessary to seek out the resources available.

DEFINING CHARACTERISTICS

VISION

◆ Decreased ability to read small print (newspapers, telephone books, medication bottles, syringes)

◆ Decreased ability to see fine needlework (crocheting, knitting)

◆ Poor color combinations especially with blues and greens

◆ Decreasing ability to read room numbers

◆ Lack of recognition of persons from a distance

◆ Lack of interest in reading or previously enjoyed art work.

HEARING

◆ Avoidance of large group gatherings. Complaints of others not speaking distinctly

◆ Frequently asking to have things repeated

◆ Having the TV or radio volume up very loud

◆ Giving no response or one indicating that the message given was not heard correctly.

SMELL

◆ Failing to correctly identify odors in the room (burned food, soured milk, flowers)

◆ Difficulty differentiating between odors of various foods. Loss of appetite

◆ Applying excessive amounts of perfume or cologne

◆ Ignoring obvious, offensive body odor.

TASTE

◆ Using large amounts of salt and sugar with food

◆ Ignoring foods with mild flavors, preferring foods with spicy or vinegar tastes

◆ Complaints of bland food

◆ Lack of interest in eating.

TOUCH

◆ Clumsiness in handling small objects (needles, thread, buttons, small coins)

◆ Denial of pain or discomfort with significant pressure and prick of finger. Multiple unexplained bruises with no note of associated pain

◆ Use of very hot or very cold water without any note of the extreme temperature

◆ Difficulty distinguishing between various textures

◆ Complaints of numbness in fingers and toes.

KINESTHETICS

◆ Unable to maintain balance with eyes closed

◆ Difficulty identifying the extent, direction, or weight of movement of body or body part.

GOALS/OUTCOME CRITERIA

The sensory deficits of the elderly will be compensated for to the extent that optimal functioning is made possible. This will be evidenced when the elder is able to:

GENERAL

1. Understand the extent of the deficit and how it affects his or her ability to function effectively and safely

2. Seek out and utilize aids and alternate approaches in daily activities, which will compensate for sensory losses.

VISION

1. Read, without difficulty, printed material routinely used in daily activities

2. Recognize familiar faces at 20–30 feet

3. Read signs while driving/riding in a car or signs in buildings

4. Accurately carry out needlework activities or other hobbies requiring detail work

5. Maneuver about residence without accidents, which result from poor vision.

HEARING

1. Accurately hear conversations in a group setting

2. Hear telephone conversation without difficulty

3. Hear various pitches of voice spoken in moderate volume

4. Listen to TV or radio with "normal" volume.

SMELL

1. Ask for verification of suspected odors
2. Utilize another person's sense of smell to assist in identifying the presence of odors
3. Recognize other factors that may signal the presence of unpleasant odors such as discoloration and mold.

TASTE

1. Maintain a nutritional intake with perceived variety in flavor without excessive use of salt, sugar, or spices.

TOUCH

1. Recognize the existing tactile loss and ask for verification from individuals with unimpaired sensory perception
2. Avoid harmful pressure, extreme temperature, and skin insults, which might result in injury.

KINESTHETICS

1. Recognize the lack of kinesthetic perception and purposely utilize measures to compensate for deficit. Use of grab bars in bathroom, shower, and stairs.

INTERVENTIONS AND ACCOUNTABILITY

GENERAL

1. After a complete assessment of the elder's sensory deficits, discuss these deficits with the elder, noting possible causes and means of compensating for deficits. (RN)

VISION

1. Assess for possible drug side effects, which may be causing visual problems such as blurring or inability to accommodate. (RN, LPN, or MD)
2. Have resident's eyes examined to determine need for corrective lens. Obtain if necessary. (RN, LPN) Maintain lens in good repair, keep clean and remind elderly person to use lens if prescribed. (RN, LPN, Family and NA)
3. Use sunglasses and/or visor when in bright light or outside in the sun. (RN, LPN, NA)
4. Utilize magnifying device to aid in detail work and some types of reading. (NA, Family)
5. Provide adequate lighting without glare and shadows. Non-glare floor wax, muted window light. (Administration, Maintenance)
6. Utilize reds, yellows, and highly contrasting colors in decor to assist with visual orientation. (Admin, Maintenance)

7. Place frequently used articles in obvious, easily accessible location. (NA, Family)

8. When conversing with elderly, sit facing them. (All)

9. Allow additional time for elder to adapt to light when coming from a dark area. (All)

10. Provide large print books, magazines, or "talking books" for those unable to use regular print. (RN, LPN, Soc. Services)

11. Place large numbers on phone, room door, etc. to facilitate ease of recognition.

12. Use bold block lettering, white on dark background for signage in buildings.

13. Assist elders with selection of clothing to coordinate colors. (NA)

14. Remove all articles that may be difficult to see, i.e. wrinkled rugs, shoes, cords, stools, etc. (NA, Family)

15. Provide sufficient constant night lighting to allow for identification of objects, doors, etc. (Maintenance)

HEARING

1. Discuss the hearing deficit with the elder and determine the person's awareness of the problem and need for compensation. (RN)

2. Discuss how hearing deficit may be negatively affecting socialization and interaction with others.

3. Direct speech to the ear with the greatest acuity. (All)

4. Avoid shouting. Speak in moderately loud, low-pitched voice with clear enunciation of consonants. (All)

5. Allow elders with severe, uncompensated hearing loss to wear a stethoscope while listening to others speak. This is especially helpful when giving instructions or interviewing. (All)

6. Verify patency of external ear canals. (RN)

7. Increase volume of doorbells, telephone ringer, and receiver. (Family)

8. Encourage use of hearing aide prescribed by audiologist. Check for proper fit, functioning batteries, and amplifier. (RN, LPN, NA and Family)

9. Decrease extraneous noise when speaking with the elder who has a hearing deficit. Close door to hall, turn TV/radio off or down, temporarily remove elder from group setting. (All)

10. Use facial expressions and gestures with speech to further reflect the message being conveyed. Use touch to draw attention. (All)

11. Have person with hearing deficit sit in the middle of a group, near the source of sound. (NA, Family)

12. Write out messages of importance, which may be misunderstood due to hearing deficit. (All)

SMELL

1. Discuss olfactory sensory loss and its impact on appetite and safety.
2. Establish routine hygiene schedule, preventing undetected body odors. (Elder, Family, NA)
3. Stimulate sense of smell with colognes, potpourri, spices, etc. (NA, Family)
4. Insure installation of smoke detector. (Admin., Family)
5. Inform family and associates of sensory deficits and ways in which they can facilitate compensation for the loss.
6. Enhance appeal of eating by making mealtime a pleasant experience, visually, socially, etc. to offset the deficit in smell. (RD, RN, LPN)

TASTE

1. Discuss gustatory sensory loss with the elder and point out the impact that this may have on nutritional intake.
2. Present food in an attractive manner. (RD, Family)
3. Comment on type of food and flavor when serving. (RD, NA, Family)
4. Separate various foods to keep flavors distinct. (NA, Family)
5. Provide regular oral hygiene before eating. (Aide, Family)
6. Encourage elder to eat favorite foods with flavor he or she can easily recall. (RD, Family)
7. Continue to stimulate the taste buds with new and varied flavors. (RD, Family)

TOUCH

1. Discuss loss of tactile sensory perception and the effects this may have on function and safety.
2. Use increasing touch stimulation—hair brushing, body rubs, and hugs. (NA, Family, All)
3. Warn elder of potential dangers regarding touch deficit—i.e. temperature extremes in water or food, sharp or abrasive surfaces, etc.
4. When giving the elder an object, make sure he or she has a firm grasp of it before releasing it. (All)
5. Inspect desensitized areas of body for possible injury frequently. (RN, LPN, NA)
6. Use velcro instead of buttons or laces to facilitate ease of fastening. (Family, RN, LPN)
7. Give elder rubber thimble to aid in turning pages. (NA)

KINESTHETICS

1. Discuss the loss of kinesthetic sensory perception and the safety implications.

2. Change position of the elder person slowly, giving prior warning about the direction of movement and limb placement. Instruct elder to keep eyes open throughout the procedure. (RN, LPN, NA, Family)

3. Allow the elder to hold onto something stationary while being moved. (RN, LPN, NA, Family)

NURSING DIAGNOSES WITH EXTERNAL ETIOLOGY

1. Uncompensated sensory deficit related to a lack of resources (financial or supportive) necessary to establish adaptive methods of dealing with sensory loss.

DEFINING CHARACTERISTICS

◆ Individual notes lack of funds, transportation, and supportive services.

◆ Availability of family or other supportive persons to assist with household repairs and management is not evident.

GOALS/OUTCOME CRITERIA

Compensation of sensory deficits will occur through physical means as evidenced by securing, installing, and utilizing adaptive equipment, such as:

◆ corrective lens
◆ hearing aids
◆ hand rails
◆ smoke detectors
◆ enlarged numbers on phone
◆ magnifying devices
◆ amplified phone receiver
◆ modified clothing fasteners
◆ increased lighting
◆ control glare window covering
◆ "talking books"
◆ large print books and magazines.

INTERVENTIONS AND ACCOUNTABILITY

1. Through assessment of financial status, determine the need for referral to Social Services. Will insurance cover any of these expenses? (RN)

2. Contact philanthropic groups, which assist in serving those with sensory loss, i.e., Lions Clubs, Deaf Society. (RN, Social Services)

3. Contact Senior Citizens groups which provide home repair services and transportation for the elderly. (RN, Social Services)

4. Contact elder's church, synagogue, or other support groups interested in increasing the quality of life for the elderly through:
   ◆ visitation
   ◆ home repairs
   ◆ transportation
   ◆ securing supplies
   ◆ financially supporting (RN, Social Services).
5. Contact family if available to assist in securing necessary equipment and making adjustments in the home. (RN, Social Services)

IMPAIRED THOUGHT PROCESSES

Definition: Discrepancy between manifested cognitive operations and expected cognitive operations for chronological age. (Included in these cognitive operations are memory recall, attention, perception of external stimuli, ability to grasp ideas, judgment, and decision-making. Multiple factors can affect these processes.)

ASSESSMENT

Assessment of the cognitive functioning of the elderly requires a systematic and conscientious collection and analysis of data. Attention must be focused not only on the physiological data but also on the environmental, developmental, social, and perceptual factors.

In an effort to determine the cause(s) of the impaired thought processes, it is necessary to view the individual wholistically. Historical data should be obtained from the elderly person, friends, neighbors, or relatives. Those living in closest proximity to the elder would most likely have seen him or her function on a daily basis. While interviewing the elder, it is essential that the elderly person feel at ease and not be threatened by the many questions. Heightened anxiety may give a false impression of impaired thought processes when none exists. Provide a quiet, comfortable environment with few distractions for the interview setting.

After fully introducing yourself and explaining the intent of the interview, factual questions may be asked to establish rapport and determine recent and distant memory recall.

◆ What is your full name?
◆ What is your age? Date of birth?
◆ How long have you lived here? Where did you live prior to this?
◆ What is the highest level of education you have achieved?
◆ What has been your past occupation(s)?
◆ What types of activities, hobbies interest you now?

These types of questions are non-threatening but will allow you to discover more about the elders' background and determine something about their remote and recent memory recall status. Relatives, neighbors, health care providers, and friends can comment on problems the individuals may have in locating personal articles, locating rooms within a facility, or losing their way back from the grocery store. Have the persons become disoriented to the extent that they believe themselves to be in some other location? One point at which confusion seems to develop is when an elder is relocated. This can mean a move within a facility, down the street, or to another state. All relocations carry with them a great deal of new stimuli and require extensive coping.

Questions which will explore the elder's response to a move include:

◆ How do you like this "new" apartment (room, facility, home)?
◆ Is it what you had expected?
◆ Is it similar to your previous residence?
◆ How does it differ (size, furnishings, neighbors, pets, plants)?
◆ Are there things which concern you about this place?
◆ What would you like to see changed?

As you observe and listen to the elderly person, note if his or her perceptions are reality based or may reflect some distortion in perception. Ask specific questions about the adequacy of the lighting, etc.

◆ Is there too much noise? Enough light?
◆ Are all of the sounds recognizable?
◆ Do you understand the function of the different staff who work here?
◆ Do you have any concerns about what people are doing for you and to you?
◆ Is the pace of activities acceptable?
◆ Are you bored? Or do you feel too busy?

CONCENTRATION

To determine the individual's ability to concentrate, take note of how often the elder "changes the subject," or has difficulty focusing on your questions.

◆ Is this person easily distracted by noise or other activities?
◆ Is this person able to follow through on a series of commands?

ABSTRACT THINKING

Evidence of the ability to think abstractly can be demonstrated by appropriately describing the meaning of the following idioms:

◆ "Don't count your chickens before they're hatched."
◆ "The grass is always greener on the other side of the fence."

CONCEPTUALIZATION

If you are concerned over the person's ability to conceptualize, you might ask the elder to tell you why certain items are similar: pears and apples (fruit), a boat and a plane (transportation), a knife and a gun (weapons).

PSYCHOMOTOR ABILITIES

Possible problems in carrying out psychomotor skills may be determined by asking the person to complete a series of instructions, i.e.

◆ touch your nose with your right hand, then turn your head to the left, and close your eyes

◆ ask the person to write their name, address, and date of birth

◆ ask the person to read a short poem or verse.

JUDGMENT

◆ Does this person demonstrate through action and communication sound judgment regarding safety, use of resources (money), and expectations about their own ability?

◆ Is there evidence within their dwelling of carelessness with fire or heating elements? Use of medication? Preparation of food?

◆ Is the person's choice of clothing appropriate for the weather? Occasion?

◆ Are the interactions of this person with others in the facility or neighborhood appropriate? Does the interaction demonstrate an accurate perception of what is really taking place?

◆ Does the quality of judgment seem to be better at certain times of the day?

DECISION-MAKING

◆ When given the opportunity to make a simple decision about something, such as which activity to become involved in, which dress/pants to wear, or with whom to sit at mealtime, does this person have difficulty?

◆ Is there adequate time allowed for making decisions? Are the options limited?

◆ Is the data which is needed to make the decision available to the elder?

◆ Is there always someone there to make the decision if the person is unable or unwilling to do so?

DEVELOPMENTAL LAG/DEFICITS

Establishing a clear picture of the developmental level of the elderly individual will assist the nurse in determining the positive coping skills which might be available to her or him. An interruption or lag in the developmental process may be a cause for impaired cognitive abilities.

◆ Is this elderly person controlled by her or his experiences and situations, or does the elder master them?

◆ Has this person experienced a number of losses recently? Car, home, finances, personal possessions, or home furnishings? How has this person reacted to these losses?

◆ Is this person mentally flexible or rigid?

◆ Is this person preoccupied with her or his own health or illness? Does the elder focus on the decline of her or his physical condition, pain, impending death, or does the elder focus on those around her or him?

If the elderly person has not learned the necessary coping skills and achieved the developmental level appropriate to her or his age, the elder may experience impairment in thought processes as evidenced by poor judgment, lack of decision-making abilities, and unrealistic perception of external stimuli.

The assessment for impaired thought processes and possible etiologies must include findings from a medical and psychiatric examination. Be alert to such factors as:

◆ electrolyte imbalance

◆ congestive heart failure

◆ organic brain syndrome (Alzheimer's)

◆ cerebral arteriosclerosis

◆ anemia

◆ neoplasm

◆ infection

◆ metabolic imbalance

◆ head trauma

◆ drug side effects

◆ sensory impairment

◆ depression

◆ excessive anxiety.

AGE-RELATED PHENOMENON

Intellectually, the elderly are generally as capable of cognitive functioning as their younger counterparts; however, the speed with which this process occurs is slower, especially within the realm of perceptual-motor activities.

In the majority of the elderly, recall of early events is much easier than recall of recent events. More obvious problems of memory in the elderly are often associated with depression or lack of environmental stimulation, or both.

Cerebral changes in the elderly include a progressive loss of neurons, increase in senile plaque, and increase in neurofibrillary tangles. It is not clear at this time just what the relationship is between the physical and the behavioral changes in the elderly.

Reaction time is extended in the elderly and performance time increased. The elderly fatigue more easily and are more quickly distracted by irrelevant stimuli. They tend to have more difficulty in organizing information and problem-solving. Generally the elderly are more concrete in their thinking and their creativity is somewhat diminished.

The variance in cognitive abilities in the elderly is contingent upon multiple factors including physiological alterations, developmental deficits, psychological impairment, and social and environmental complexities.

Most of the elderly whose thought processes have been severely impaired suffer from some type of cerebral injury or deterioration. Although milder forms of impaired thought processes may indicate the advent of such deterioration, it is often the case that altered cognition is temporary and has a nonphysiological etiology.

Many elderly seen in long-term care facilities or retirement centers are noted to display some impairment in their thought processes at the time of relocation. The familiar surroundings of the elders former "home" have been taken away, and they are now subject to a barrage of strange people, sounds, lighting, funiture arrangements, odors, textures, routines, and messages. Just the sheer volume of unfamiliar stimuli with which the elderly must deal is overwhelming (Refer to Nursing Diagnoses: Sensory-Perceptual Alterations).

ETIOLOGIES

EXTERNAL

SENSORY OVERLOAD

◆ change in living environment
◆ added responsibilities with loss

SENSORY DEPRIVATION

◆ limited stimuli associated with restricted living space, lack of variety in routine, activities, interactions, food, and surroundings

INTERNAL

SENSORY OVERLOAD

◆ heightened sensitivity to stimuli due to increased anxiety
◆ physical impairment causing heightened sensitivity to certain stimuli, i.e. pain

SENSORY DEPRIVATION

◆ impaired physical operation of senses (vision, hearing, taste, smell, or touch)
◆ blocking of stimuli due to preoccupation with self

DEVELOPMENTAL LAG/DEFICIT

◆ has inadequate coping skills for chronological age

◆ Nursing Care Plan

NURSING DIAGNOSIS

1. Impaired thought processes related to sensory overload or sensory deprivation.

DEFINING CHARACTERISTICS

1. Demonstrates impaired attention span
   - ◆ is easily distracted while talking to someone
   - ◆ has difficulty carrying out activities of daily living without repeated direction and encouragement.
2. Impaired recall ability
   - ◆ difficulty locating personal items
   - ◆ difficulty remembering names of people, places, etc.
   - ◆ difficulty remembering sequence of events, instructions.
3. Impaired ability to grasp ideas (conceptualize) or order ideas (reason and reflection)
   - ◆ thoughts are very concrete, triggered by visual or experiential events
   - ◆ difficulty seeing relationships between various situations or ideas
   - ◆ does not see how one event or action may lead to subsequent factors.
4. Impaired perception, judgment, decision making
   - ◆ lack of response or inappropriate response to stimuli
   - ◆ actions are unsafe
   - ◆ difficulty making decisions, relies on others for directions.

NURSING DIAGNOSES

2. Impaired thought processes related to developmental lag.

DEFINING CHARACTERISTICS

1. Inappropriate behavior; non-reality based thinking
   - ◆ social interaction is inappropriate, may be suspicious, paranoid, or insecure due to misinterpreted cues. Unrealistic expectation of self and others.
2. Increased self-concern (egocentricity)
   - ◆ pre-occupation with own body
   - ◆ little if any focus beyond self to others and more global interests.
3. Hypo- or hypervigilance
   - ◆ excessive concern or neglect regarding own body, events, surroundings.

GOALS/OUTCOME CRITERIA

RELATIVE TO NURSING DIAGNOSIS 1: Cognitive operation will be appropriate for chronological age. This will be evidenced when the elder:

1. Will not be easily distracted by internal or external stimuli
2. Will be able to concentrate on tasks necessary for daily independent functioning
3. Recall of recent events, actions, names, etc. will allow for efficiency in independent living and optimal social interaction
4. Will be able to reflectively examine ideas, events, feelings, and reactions to situations
5. Will be able to correctly identify stimuli and their significance
6. Will demonstrate caution and good judgment regarding potentially harmful situations
7. Will demonstrate appropriate decision-making ability.

RELATIVE TO NURSING DIAGNOSIS 2: Cognitive operation will be appropriate for chronological age. This will be evidenced when the elder:

1. Will demonstrate behavior and social interactions that reflect reality-based perception, interpretation, and management of environment
2. Will focus interest and concern beyond self to others
3. Will demonstrate appropriate sensitivity to incoming stimuli.

INTERVENTIONS AND ACCOUNTABILITY

1. Attitude and approach of staff must be calm, unhurried; interacting with elderly as adults. Recognizing their individual worth, strengths, and capabilities. (RN, LPN, NA)
2. Decrease irrelevant external stimuli, noise, interruptions. Clutter should be kept to a minimum. (RN, LPN, NA)
3. Allow elders to perform some activities with others who are doing similar tasks, taking cues from them. (RN, LPN, NA)
4. Give praise and encouragement when elder demonstrates ability to overcome distractions and adequately handle external stimuli. (RN, LPN, NA)
5. Orientation cues should be made available in environment.
   - ◆ Day, month, and year should be posted in a frequently noted location.
   - ◆ Post a personal calendar in the client's room indicating special days (birthdays, anniversaries, outings, and appointments). Keep updated. Family should participate in this.
   - ◆ Use seasonal decorations to remind elder of time of year. (Activities Director, RN, LPN, NA)

- ◆ Clocks, watches which are easily read should be readily available. (RN, LPN, NA)
- ◆ Post notice of activities in bold print with attractive contrasting colors, situated at appropriate height for easy reading. (Activities Director)
- ◆ Identify all staff with easily read name tags. (All staff)
- ◆ Place name of resident or easily identifiable object on or beside door of room or apartment. (RN, LPN)
- ◆ Post names of communally used rooms on or beside the doors. (Maintenance)
- ◆ Post elder's name on closet, dresser, etc. (RN, LPN, NA)
- ◆ When giving directions to a specific location, use landmarks which are not likely to change, i.e. "third door on the right, across from water fountain." (RN, LPN, NA)
- ◆ Seek out newly relocated persons and escort them to activities to insure proper destination. (LPN, NA)

6. Establish auditory and visual cues to remind elders of safety factors, i.e. (RN, LPN)
   - ◆ Note on the door about locking and taking key
   - ◆ Setting timers when stove or oven is being used.

7. Offer group sessions for memory retention skills.
   - ◆ Approach should include:
   - **a.** Reassurance (lessen anxiety and embarrassment)
   - **b.** Using association, improving concentration
   - **c.** Use motivation and repetition as learning tools
   - **d.** Discuss attitudes toward memory lapses; how do you cope?
   - **e.** Use of humor.

8. Allow for reminiscence individually and in groups. Focus on accomplishments, self-worth, and evidence of cognitive abilities. Trigger reminiscence with old photographs, articles of interest, or just historical questions about background. (RN)

9. Through reminiscence have elder point out own strengths, and begin to identify own needs, prioritize these. (RN)

10. Have elder involved as much as possible in planning and carrying out a plan of care. (Recognize limited attention span, ability to concentrate, and ability to cope with increasing stimuli. Elder may not be able to focus on more than one simple item.) (RN, LPN)

11. Encourage decision-making by having elder:
    - ◆ Select what to wear, eat, etc.
    - ◆ Determine which optional activities the elder would like to do. (RN, LPN, NA)

12. Discuss with elder information needed to make decision but avoid making decision for her or him. (RN, LPN)

13. To avoid sensory overload and reduce perceptual problems the following measures should be employed (RN, Admin.)

    ◆ maintain adequate direct lighting for daily activities, soft night light for safety at night

    ◆ prevent glare on polished floors, severe shadows, or excessive light/dark contrasts in floor coverings

    ◆ avoid bright lighting for elders with glaucoma, cataracts

    ◆ avoid use of pattern fabric on furniture

    ◆ limit use of intercoms

    ◆ arrange furniture and personal articles in organized manner

    ◆ limit noise and interruptions with individual.

14. Systematically review "new" environment with the elder to determine if perceptions are correct. (RN, LPN)

15. Maintain many of elders' own personal belongings and furnishings in their room or apartment

    ◆ bed, dresser, chairs

    ◆ pictures, needlecraft, chiming clocks, plants, mirrors, picture albums.

16. If sensory deprivation is a concern, variation in stimuli can be provided through: (RN, LPN)

    ◆ change in menu—include ethnic foods, use different seasoning

    ◆ posting colorful pictures on walls

    ◆ use of scented sachets, occasional use of real flowers

    ◆ avoiding continual use of strong institutional deodorizers

    ◆ using a fuzzy soft pillow

    ◆ viewing "new" radio or TV stations which provide a variety

    ◆ providing alternate types of music with tapes, performers, or sing alongs

    ◆ providing exposure to live animals (pet therapy) for visual and tactile stimulation

    ◆ participating with a new group of people, doing a new activity (gardening, working with clay, painting)

    ◆ participating in an exercise program, taking regular walks outside or in a mall. (Again, this should be jointly planned and implemented with the elder and possibly his family.)

17. Recognize and encourage creativity in the elderly (begin gradually, use concrete activities at first) (RN, LPN, NA)

18. Encourage the elder to become involved in helping other persons in the following ways: (RN, LPN)

◆ physical assistance if the elder is able

◆ volunteer telephoning for service organization (Blood Bank, Heart Association)

◆ calling to check on shut-ins

◆ writing letters for those not able

◆ making small gifts for special occasions, sending cards

◆ recording audio or written account of elder's history for family members

◆ visiting others

◆ entertaining others with musical instruments, poetry, etc.

19. Allow for formal or informal group discussion of concerns common to the elderly (For those who can conceptualize and think abstractly) (RN)

◆ retirement

◆ relocation

◆ loss of control (finances, home, occupation, decisions)

◆ fears: illness, mental discipline, dependency, being attacked, robbed, being alone.

◆ effective methods of coping with above items.

References: *Knowledge Deficit*

Corkadel, Linda and McGlashan, ReNel. A practical approach to patient teaching. In *Journal of Continuing Education in Nursing*. 1983; 14:9–15.
  The authors develop a general approach to patient teaching while defining some basic concepts. Barriers to teaching/learning are described and methods of minimizing these barriers are outlined. Focus is placed on learner readiness and actual learning needs assessment.

Pease, Ruth A. Praise Elders to Help Them Learn. In *Journal of Gerontological Nursing*. March 1985; 11:16–18, 20.
  This article is based on a study of emotionally dependent elderly persons. The degree of learning is examined in light of the variable of giving praise to the elder while they are being taught. Evidence indicates that when elderly persons who are emotionally dependent study a programmed lesson they learn more when praise is given than when praise is withheld.

Picariello, Gloria. A Guide for Teaching Elders. In *Geriatric Nursing*. January–February 1986; 38–39.
  A concise but very helpful guide to assessing and teaching the elderly. Practical techniques are delineated with reference to some specific situations.

Whitbourne, Susan Kraus and Sperbeck, David J. Health Care Maintenance for the Elderly. In *Aging and Health Promotion*. Edited by Thelma Wells, Rockville, Maryland: Aspen Pub., 1982; 111–126.
  An excellent overview of the elderly person's ability to learn. Multiple variables that may affect learning are examined, including environmental, physiologic, and psychosocial factors. Techniques and approaches that help to compensate for age-related problems in learning are explored.

Yurick, Ann Gera, et al. *The Aged Person and the Nursing Process.* New York: Appleton-Century-Crofts; 1980; 255–273.
Specific attention is given to the ability of the elderly person to learn and
process new information. Cognitive and sensory alterations and the effects on
learning are considered.

References: Sensory Overload/Deprivation

Bernardini, Losi. Effective communication as an intervention for sensory deprivation in the elderly client. In *Topics in Clinical Nursing.* January 1985; 72–81.
An excellent look at the causative factors leading to sensory deprivation and
the use of specific communication techniques to reduce that deprivation.
Assessment and the normal aging process and its effects on the sensory perception of the elderly is explored.

Fitzsimons, Virginia M. Maintaining a positive environment for the older adult. In
Orthopaedic Nursing. May–June 1985; 4:48–51.
Concise yet well-written article on both sensory overload and sensory deprivation. Focus is also given to the developmental levels of the elderly and how
certain behaviors can indicate potential problems. Some nursing interventions are outlined.

Gates, Sharon J. Helping your patient on bedrest cope with perceptual/sensory
deprivation. In *Orthopaedic Nursing.* March–April 1984; 3:35–38.
Implications of sensory/perceptual deprivation are examined. A case study of
a 40-year-old is developed with an accompanying care plan including nursing
diagnoses and interventions.

Kopac, Catherine A. Sensory loss in the aged: The role of the nurse and the family.
In *Nursing Clinics of North America.* June 1983; 18:373–383.
General sensory loss is explored in detail. The general effects of sensory deprivation due to institutionalization are highlighted and nursing and family
interventions described.

Yurick, Ann Gera, et al. *The Aged Person and the Nursing Process.* New York: Appleton-Century-Crofts; 1980; 278–284.
Brief attention is given to the nurse's role in providing adequate stimulation
within the elderly person's environment. Avoidance of overload and its effect
on teaching are noted.

Zachow, Kathleen M. Helen, can you hear me? In *Journal of Gerontological Nursing.*
1984; 10:18–22.
A personal account of an encounter with a disoriented elderly woman. Specific techniques were used to reestablish contact with an elderly woman and
provide much needed sensory stimulation. A vivid picture is portrayed and
helpful hints given.

References: Pain, Chronic Pain

DeCrosta, Tony. Relieving Pain: Four noninvasive ways you should know more
about. In *Nursing Life.* March–April 1984; 29–33.
A concise and practical guide to non-invasive techniques which can be used
to manage pain including TENS, ice massage, myotherapy, and distraction.

Fordyce, Wilbert. An operant conditioning method for managing chronic pain. In *Post Graduate Medicine*. May 1973; 53:123–128.
   A realistic look at chronic pain and the possibility that sufferers may become conditioned in their response. Insight is given into how one should care for this type of individual and hopefully decrease the disabling effects of chronic pain.

Fordyce, Wilbert. Evaluating and managing chronic pain. In *Geriatrics*. January 1978; 59–62.
   Detailed description of the theory of operant conditioning as it relates to chronic pain management. Environmental and iatrogenic factors affecting conditioning examined. Management techniques explored.

Kulich, Ronald J. and Warfield, Carol A. Relaxation in the management of pain. In *Hospital Practice*. December 15, 1985; 117–121.
   This article explores the rationale and physiologic basis for using relaxation techniques. Specific procedures are described with notation about possible contraindications and problems.

Melzack, Ronald and Wall, Patrick. Pain mechanisms: A new theory. In *Science*. November 19, 1965; 971–978.
   Original publication on the Gate-Control theory. Includes specifics of theory, physiology, anatomy, and practical implications.

Witt, Jimmie Ruth. Relieving Chronic Pain. In *The Nurse Practitioner*. January 1984; 9:36–38, 78.
   Focus of this article is on the independent techniques nursing can use in managing chronic pain. Therapeutic touch, myotherapy, guided imagery, and relaxation are briefly discussed.

References: **Short-Term Memory Deficit**

Baas, Linda S. and Allen, Gordon A. Memory error. In *Nursing Clinics of North America*. December 1985; 20:731–742.
   An informative look at how memory functions and the utilization of memory in complying with medication schedules. Two types of memory error are identified in association with medication compliance. Further in-depth study reveals the need for nursing to adequately assess the memory functioning of clients who are to be responsible for their own medication administration.

Church, Mike. Forgotten something? In *Nursing Times*. July 24, 1985; 23–24.
   A careful look at the possible etiologies of memory deficit including the neuropsychological aspects. Focus on complete assessment and its importance in evaluating memory loss are brought out.

Clites, Joan. Maximizing memory retention in the aged. In *Journal of Gerontological Nursing*. October 1984; 10:12–15.
   A helpful description of the use of group interaction and discussion sessions as designed by Garfunkel and Landau to enhance memory retention. The basic focus of each of six sessions is discussed.

Garfunkel, Florence and Landau, Gertrude. In *A Memory Retention Course for the Aged*. Washington DC: National Council on Aging; December 1981.
   A well-written guide for group leaders dealing with memory retention. A six-session format is outlined and appendix contain valuable strategies for the aged to utilize.

O'Hara-Devereaux, Mary, Andrus, Len Hughes, and Scott, Cynthia D. In *Eldercare: A Practical Guide to Clinical Geriatrics.* New York: Grune and Stratton Inc. 1981; 51–53.
A multi-disciplinary look at the cognitive and psychomotor functioning of the elderly and the many age-related factors that can impact on that functioning. The effect of memory on learning is briefly discussed.

Ozuna, Judy. Alterations in mentation: Nursing assessment and interventions. In *Journal of Neurosurgical Nursing.* February 1985; 17:66–70.
Addresses specifically the assessment and nursing interventions associated with memory deficit. Suggestions are made as to how the nurse can alter the patient's environment and enhance memory retention.

Tariot, Pierre, Sunderland, Frey, Murphy, Dennis, Cohen, Robert, Weingartener, Herbert, and Makhohon, Rennie. How memory fails: A theoretical model. In *Geriatric Nursing.* May–June 1985; 144–147.
An excellent article, which gives a descriptive outline of the various components of memory, its function, and causative disorders. Assessment of the type of memory loss being experienced is clearly discussed and implications for intervention and approach are described.

Yurick, Ann Gera, Robb, Susanne S, Spier, Barbara Elliot, and Ebert, Nancy J. In *The Aged Person and the Nursing Process.* New York: Appleton-Century-Crofts; 1980; 260–278.
A systematic approach to assessment of the cognitive functioning of the elderly. Questions to ask and content to cover is outlined. Specific nursing interventions are noted.

References: Sensory Deficits

Bernardini, Lois. Effective communication as an intervention for sensory deprivation in the elderly client. In *Topics in Clinical Nursing.* January 1985; 72–81.
An excellent look at the changes in visual and auditory perception in the elderly. Focus is placed on how these changes and more exaggerated loss can interfere with communication. Specific interventions are identified.

Bozian, Marguerite W. and Clark, Helen M. Counteracting sensory changes in the aging. In *American Journal of Nursing.* March 1980; 80:473–476.
The author has given a brief description of the sensory problems, which may exist in the elderly. A concise outline of how to assess the various senses is also included for quick reference.

Calvani, Dorothy. How well do your clients cope with hearing loss? In *Journal of Gerontological Nursing.* July 1985; 11:16–20.
An interesting study dealing with the way in which elderly people cope with hearing loss. *The Hearing Handicap Inventory for the Elderly* is used as a tool for measurement. A copy of the tool is included in the article.

Cohen, Stephen. Sensory changes in the elderly. In *American Journal of Nursing.* October 1981; 1850–1880.
A programmed instruction unit dealing with the pathophysiology, assessment, and interventions necessary in dealing with sensory changes. Terminology is defined and scenarios are given to help clarify.

Eliopoulos, Charlotte. *Gerontological Nursing,* New York: Harper and Row Publishers; 1979; Chapter 19.
Extensive description of common vision and hearing problems in the elderly.

Pictorial diagrams of the eye and ear help to clarify the location of pathology. Practical application of nursing interventions is given.

Hollinger, Linda M. Perception of touch in the elderly. In *Journal of Gerontological Nursing.* December 1980; 6:741–746.

The author carefully looks at the meaning of touch, referring to various theorists and examining the use of touch throughout the life cycle. Assessment is made of the need for, and use of, touch with the elderly. A sensitive piece which shows the multi-dimensional use of touch.

Kopac, Catharine. Sensory loss in the aged: The role of the nurse and the family. In *Nursing Clinics of North America.* June 1983; 18:373–383.

A detailed discussion of all of the senses with age-related considerations is developed. The role of the nurse, her or his interventions, and those of the family are also clearly stated.

Sullivan, Nancy. Vision in the elderly. In *Journal of Gerontological Nursing.* April 1983; 9:228–235.

A two-part comprehensive investigation of the visual functioning of the elderly and their ability to cope with a visual deficit. Nursing interventions are spelled out.

Thronbury, Julia M. and Mistretta, Charlotte M. Tactile sensitivity as a function of age. In *Journal of Gerontology.* January 1981; 36:34–39.

A controlled research study investigating the tactile acuity of individuals of various ages. Changes in the skin and touch receptors of the elderly are correlated with increasing tactile threshold.

Yurick, Ann Gera. *The Aged Person and the Nursing Process.* New York: Appleton-Century-Crofts; 1980.

A solid clinical reference aimed at the practicing nurse. It applies the nursing process to fifteen separate concepts including sensory changes.

References: Thought Impairment

Bartol, Mary Anne. Reaching the patient. In *Geriatric Nursing.* May–June 1983; 234–236.

The author carefully delineates the nursing process that should be carried out when caring for a confused elderly person. Assessment, goal development, establishing a relationship with the elderly, and definite steps to take in modifying the environment to meet the needs of the confused elder.

Clites, Joan. Maximizing memory loss in the aged. In *Journal of Gerontological Nursing.* August 1984; 34, 39.

An excellent description of the effects of memory loss on the elder's daily functions, self-concept, and level of anxiety. Specific approaches are outlined for group sessions, which should help to lessen the memory lapses and increase the functioning level of the elder.

Hamner, Mildred. Insight, reminiscence, denial, projection. In *Journal of Gerontological Nursing.* February 1984, 16–19.

Coping or defense behaviors of the elderly are discussed, including insight, reminiscence, denial, displacement, and projection. Effective and destructive use of these is explored.

Hayter, Jean. Modifying the environment to help older persons. May 1983; 265–269.

Age-related changes in the sensory capabilities of the elderly are discussed. Effects of the diminished sensorium on the elder and nursing interventions suggested are very helpful.

Huber, Kay and Miller, Pat. Reminiscence with the elderly—DO IT! In *Geriatric Nursing,* March–April 1984; 84–87.
The effects of group reminiscence on the memory and cognitive abilities of the elderly are discussed. Recommendations for implementation are given.

Lederer, Ann. Confusion: Recognition and remedy. In *Geriatric Nursing.* July–August 1983; 224–227.
Several vignettes about different confused elderly people paint vivid pictures of the individuality of each. An effective tool used in sensitizing those new employees who will be working with the cognitively impaired elder.

Nowakowski, Loretta. Accent capabilities in disorientation. In *Journal of Gerontological Nursing.* September 1985; 15–20.
The author identifies the strengths of the elderly, even though they may be experiencing some disorientation. The nursing tendency of making patients dependent and discouraging decision-making is skillfully brought out with solutions to correcting that approach.

O'Hara-Devereaux, Mary, et al. *Eldercare—A Practical Guide to Clinical Geriatrics.* New York: Grune and Stratton; 1981; 49–57, 333–335.
A multidisciplinary view of health problems common to the elderly. Although focus is primarily on physical problems, there are sections on the psychological, social, and ethical considerations of care. Community resources are cited.

Ozuna, Judy. Alterations in mentation: Nursing assessment and intervention. In *Journal of Neurosurgical Nursing.* February 1985; 66–70.
Specific methods of evaluating mentation, including communication, memory, and psychomotor skills is discussed. Nursing implications and interventions are spelled out in a very practical way.

Schafer, Susan C. Modifying the environment. In *Geriatric Nursing,* May-June 1985; 157–159.
A simple yet practical look at the methods used to decrease environmental confusion for the elderly. Examples of what may overstimulate the senses or distort the senses are given.

Schrock, Miriam M. *Holistic Assessment of the Healthy Aged.* New York: Wiley Medical Publications; 1980; 88–113.
A truly holistic look at the elderly and their physical, social, financial, and psychological needs. In depth review of theories relating to developmental and cultural perspectives make this a valuable book.

Tolbert, Bennie Mae. Reality orientation and remotivation in a long-term care facility. In *Nursing and Health Care.* January 1984; 40–44.

Yurick, Ann Gera, et al. *The Aged Person and the Nursing Process.* New York: Appleton-Century-Crofts; 1980; 221–253.

10

Self-Perception/ Self-Conflict Pattern

Elaine Jensen Amella

◆

BODY IMAGE DISTURBANCE

Definition: Negative feelings about characteristics, functions, or limits of the body or a body part. The belief by elder persons that changes related to the aging process or changes related to functional losses diminish sense of worth.

AGE-RELATED PHENOMENON

As an individual ages, various physiological changes take place; these changes vary among individuals for a number of reasons, e.g. genetics, diet, exercise, stress. The body image of the elderly is often linked to a form of prejudice called ageism. The physical appearance of older persons does have similarities: wrinkling of the skin, decreased muscle tone, change in hair color, change in distribution of fat stores. Unfortunately, these physical changes cause many individuals to stereotype older persons as undesirable.

Body image of the elderly is also at higher risks because of fear of permanent loss or dependency related to changes. Chronic illness, stroke, loss of a limb, paralysis, all threaten an individual's mobility and consequently his or her independence. Most older people assume that they will not recover as quickly from serious changes in their physical functioning. In fact, those persons who feared aging had a strong inverse relationship with current subjective well-being.

Abrupt change is usually traumatic. However, as we age we gradually shift our perception of our body. Disturbance of that image is most likely to precipitate when a stigmatizing event occurs such as loss of a body part, especially if that loss causes disfiguration, loss of ability to control bowel and/or bladder, obesity, or physical limitation.

The defining characteristics of this category can all be embodied in the older person's reaction to aging whether it be normal age-related changes or unexpected or traumatic changes.

219

ASSESSMENT

The adequate assessment of older people's disturbance in body image varies. The numerous threats to the elders' bodies can change both their conscious and unconscious view of themselves. Some older people subjectively report feeling different in their bodies because of changes related to normal aging. Those changes brought about by illness, immobility, and loss of function can drastically disturb an individual.

Three tests commonly administered to individuals to determine body image disturbances in older women have been compared. It was found that the Body-Perception Interview in which residents were asked open-ended questions about their body image was fairly accurate in disclosing disturbances. Questions could be "How do you see yourself now?" "How do others see you?" "Have you ever known anyone that had a stroke?" "How did that affect you?" The Body-Cathexis Scale had only minimal use in capturing the subtleties of aging body changes. The Draw-A-Person assessment whereby the individuals draw a picture of themselves or others is by far the clearest demonstrator of areas of need. The indicators are area—self-assessment in relation to environment, height—feelings of relative significance, and centeredness—general security and orientation to reality. When young and older women's drawings were compared, the older women's showed self-devaluation. When non-institutionalized and institutionalized elders drawings were compared, those in the community showed elevated status through larger, taller, and more centered drawings.

For those individuals undergoing amputation of a body part, the nurse is certainly obligated to assess the individual's knowledge regarding the phantom limb syndrome. The very real sensation that the body part is still in place occurs in almost all persons. Some however, may be reluctant to acknowledge this, believing staff will consider them "crazy." Pre-operative teaching and post-operative assessment of this phenomenon should not be avoided.

ETIOLOGY

EXTERNAL

- Non-integration of change
- Inability to acknowledge motor, sensory changes
- Sudden, traumatic change
- Loss of body function
- Loss of body part
- Societal devaluation of aging versus youth
- Inability to remain well-groomed
- Inability to find attractive, well-fitting clothing.

INTERNAL

- Perceived developmental imperfections
- Inability to acknowledge changed energy levels

◆ Former negative feelings for individuals who had similar changes
◆ Inability to cope with normal aging process
◆ Life-long view of older individuals as less desirable
◆ Chronic illness.

◆ Nursing Diagnosis

Body image disturbance related to nonintegration of change.

DEFINING CHARACTERISTICS

Verbalized actual or perceived change in structure and/or function of body or body part.

GOALS/OUTCOME CRITERIA

Verbalized acceptance of actual or perceived change.

INTERVENTIONS

◆ Assess resident's perception of self through Draw-A-Person testing or open-ended questioning. (MD, RN, SW, LPN)
◆ Assess resident's perception of self through grooming, if this is resident's responsibility. (MD, RN, LPN, SW)
◆ Work with resident one-on-one to work through or explore possible grief at changes. (MD, RN, LPN, SW)
◆ Use grief counseling skills so that changes might be assimilated into resident's perceptions. (MD, RN, LPN, SW)
◆ Include in peer group of those experiencing similar changes or losses for supporting, e.g. Reach to Recovery. (RN, LPN, SW)

◆ Nursing Diagnosis

Body image disturbance related to lifestyle change.

DEFINING CHARACTERISTICS

◆ Verbalized change in life style because of negative feelings or perceptions of body.
◆ Change in social involvement or social relationships.

GOALS/OUTCOME CRITERIA

Life style will be independent of perception of body image.

INTERVENTIONS

◆ Assess resident's interaction with peers or staff through observation. (RN, LPN, SW, NA)
◆ Assess resident's interaction with family or significant others through observation. (RN, LPN, SW, NA)

◆ Note any active refusals to interact with others and rationale for same being negative image. (RN, LPN, NA, SW)

◆ Note any passive refusals especially if they seem to be in conflict with previous life patterns, e.g. resident who enjoyed shopping refuses to go because he or she states "nothing fits." (RN, LPN, NA, SW)

◆ Involve in support group of peers who might have had similar experiences. (RN, LPN, SW)

◆ If resident refuses to leave home or room, visit resident regularly on a scheduled basis. (RN, LPN, NA, SW)

◆ Assist family members to adjust to resident's changed perception and change in lifestyle.

◆ Discourage family from further devaluing resident by criticizing life style.

◆ Encourage interaction on resident's terms until resident feels more comfortable with self and family's acceptance. (RN, LPN, NA, SW)

◆ Reinforce all attempts at socialization no matter how minimal. (RN, LPN, SW, NA)

◆ Assess former interests and leisure life style. (RN, SW, RT)

◆ Develop plan to reintegrate into areas of strength that do not depend upon losses. (RT, LPN, SW)

◆ Engage in activities that develop cognitive, social, and emotional strengths.

◆ In areas of sexuality, acknowledge implications of loss to feelings of self-identity.

   ◆ counsel resident as to need to integrate change into sexual patterns

   ◆ acknowledge person's right to sexual identity

   ◆ include in support groups of persons who have had similar experiences

   ◆ offer resident alternatives to sexual expression through education to alternatives. (RN, LPN, SW)

◆ Nursing Diagnosis

Body image disturbance related to verbalized fear of rejection by others.

GOALS/OUTCOME CRITERIA

Verbalization of decreased fear and increased acceptance.

INTERVENTIONS

◆ Assess fear and resident's perception of others reaction. (RN, LPN, NA, SW)

- Assess any similar experiences resident may have had in past when they acted either positively or negatively.
- Focus on resident's reactions that may have been based on lack of knowledge. (RN, LPN, SW)
- Attempt to counsel others in resident's family or peer group as to resident's needs, fears, or limitations, with resident's permission. (RN, LPN, SW)
- Educate resident as to realistic expectations of others. (SW, RN, LPN)
- Include in support group of peers who may have had similar experiences. (SW, RN, LPN)
- Gradually reintroduce to social situations as resident's level of fear decreases.
  - Do not have unrealistic expectations
  - Offer encouragement and support
  - Have staff member accompany to such situations until resident is more comfortable with independent participation
  - Support any friendships that may develop by assisting resident to visit friends through transportation, placing telephone calls, arranging for meeting places. (SW, RN, LPN, RT)

◆ Nursing Diagnosis

Body image disturbance related to repeated verbalizations focusing on past strength, function, or appearance.

GOALS/OUTCOME CRITERIA

Verbalizations are more focused on here and now.

INTERVENTIONS

- Assess premorbid condition by interviewing resident. (RN, LPN, SW)
- Whenever possible, validate any claims to strengths that seem exaggerated.
- Speak with resident and spouse, family, significant others. (RN, LPN, SW)
- Assist resident to chose simple, short-term goals that capture elements of past strengths.
- Be creative in involving resident in decisions. (SW, RN, LPN, RT)
- Give specific feedback focusing on present strengths. (RN, LPN, NA)
- Do not allow entire social climate to focus on those with similar losses.
- Include in mixed groups whenever possible with those having a variety of needs. (RT, SW, RN, LPN)

◆ Do not negate resident's feelings of loss but offer realistic support and acceptance. (SW, RN, LPN, NA)

DEFINING CHARACTERISTICS

Verbalized feelings of helplessness, powerlessness in relation to body.

GOALS/OUTCOME CRITERIA

Verbalizes feelings of increased control.

INTERVENTIONS

◆ Assess resident's perception and areas affected by change in body. (RN, LPN, SW)

◆ Whenever possible, give resident feedback as to areas of deficit and areas of control. (RN, LPN, SW)

◆ Assess areas of limitation and any forces or causal factors that tend to exaggerate feelings of loss. (RN, LPN, SW)

◆ Families or significant others may dwell on changes and limitations of resident.

◆ If area of loss held great significance for resident, attempt to find out in what way.

◆ Assess support systems available to resident and counsel them on allowing resident control over areas of perceived loss. (RN, LPN, SW)

◆ Counsel family members to relate to the resident and to their strengths and areas of control. (RN, LPN, SW)

◆ Allow resident empathetic support while grieving over losses of control. (RN, LPN, NA, SW)

◆ Assess any knowledge deficits resident may have in relation to loss of power/hope, e.g. diabetic resident may feel so overwhelmed by diagnosis and lack of knowledge that they may feel they will never be able to control their life again. (RN, SW, LPN)

◆ Perform resident teaching with significant others included so that all may realize resident's needs and strengths. (RN, LPN)

◆ Nursing Diagnosis

Altered body image related to perceived developmental imperfections.

DEFINING CHARACTERISTICS

Verbalized negative feelings about body (unsightly, wrinkled). Guilt and shame.

GOALS/OUTCOME CRITERIA

Integration of body or loss of part into a more positive perspective.

INTERVENTIONS

◆ Assess resident's perspective of normal aging. (RN, LPN, SW)

◆ Assess what meaning has held for the resident in the past, i.e. questions such as "How did you view older people when you were younger?" "Did you see any value in old age?" "What types of older persons did you know when you were younger, especially any significant others?" (RN, LPN, SW)

◆ Assess resident's physical appearance especially areas of deficits or excesses, e.g. poor grooming, body odors, meticulous dress, over-use of makeup, matted beard. (RN, LPN, NA)

◆ Assist resident with grooming and, if needed, teach skills necessary to perform grooming. (RN, LPN, NA)

◆ Whenever possible, allow resident to make decisions about self-care and grooming. (RN, LPN, NA)

◆ Reinforce all positive attempts at proper grooming or statements that reveal a more realistic view of self. (RN, LPN, NA)

◆ Counsel family or significant others to be patient with resident while they are adjusting to changes.

◆ Positive feedback from these persons is a strong motivator (SW, RN, LPN)

DEFINING CHARACTERISTICS

Preoccupation with, or refusal to verify, actual change in body or body part.

GOALS/OUTCOME CRITERIA

Realistic verbalizations and actions regarding body changes.

INTERVENTIONS

◆ Assess resident's perception of body changes.

◆ Utilize the Draw-A-Person assessment tool to ascertain areas of preoccupation or lack of acknowledgement. (RN, SW)

◆ Set limits for resident if lack of acceptance or acknowledgement or preoccupation might pose a threat to the resident's well-being. (RN, LPN, NA)

◆ In dealing with resident convey recognition that resident is accepted as a total person. (RN, LPN, NA)

◆ Counsel family or significant others to acknowledge resident's need to dwell on loss or refuse to accept it.

◆ Family should not negate resident's feelings but give positive feedback whenever resident is acting or speaking realistically of self. (SW, RN, LPN)

DEFINING CHARACTERISTICS

Missing body part.

◆ not looking at
◆ not touching
◆ hiding or overexposing

GOALS/OUTCOME CRITERIA

Demonstrate an appropriate attitude to missing body part.

INTERVENTIONS

◆ Assess resident's perception of body change or loss through questioning or Draw-A-Person. (RN, LPN, SW)
◆ If resident has received no teaching on phantom limb syndrome, acquaint him or her with this phenomenon (occurs in almost all amputees).
◆ Consider using alternative treatment modalities for these residents: hypnosis, guided imagery, voluntary muscle relaxation. (SW, RN, LPN)
◆ If resident's behavior is hindering his or her socialization, set limits on exposing behavior.
    ◆ consider behavioral modification—rewarding appropriate behavior.
    ◆ be sure to convey the goals to all members of team and family. (RN, LPN, SW, NA)
◆ In dealing with resident, convey attitude of acceptance as a total person. (RN, LPN, NA)

POWERLESSNESS (SEVERE, MODERATE, LOW)

Definition: Perceived lack of control over a situation. Resident relinquishes control of self to others and assumes a passive role in life situations.

AGE-RELATED PHENOMENON

Powerlessness for the older person has components that are associated with this phenomenon in all age groups. However, for the elderly loss of control, learned helplessness, and attribution are key components. These ideas are also commonly associated with depression and a link has been established among the factors. This does not imply that depressed persons have an inaccurate perception of their control. As discussed by McClure, depressed persons had a surprisingly accurate perception of their personal control in situations where they did and did not control outcomes, while the nondepressed had an inflated sense of control. If dependency is associated with powerlessness, as it often is by both professionals and lay people, it would also be surprising to note that in many ways elderly people are less dependent than the younger people who depend upon status, position, work, recognition, and physical prowess to gain a sense of self. It is those attributes we bring to old age that we consider most important that give us a sense of control. Attribution theorists focus on the need to relearn and redefine our significant attributes as life situations dictate. If during our lifetime, we have learned to be helpless, we will exercise very little power over our attributes.

If during the individual's lifetime, he or she learns that unpleasant events are uncontrollable it will be difficult for him or her to make adjustments during old age. Contributors to a feeling of helplessness in old age are isolation and loneliness. The clinician can often lessen these environmental causes through a therapeutic relationship where formerly unallowable feelings of pessimism and despair, so inconsistent with previous feelings of self-esteem and confidence, can be expressed.

Control for the elderly is of primary importance; without it they lose self-sufficiency. However, several factors undermine the older person's control. Lack of financial security diminishes an individual's choices in many areas of life from housing to health care. Chronic illness and exacerbations of illnesses may limit an individual's options for life styles from always monitoring grams of food, to carrying an oxygen pack about. Dependence in self-care skills change an individual's requirements for outside support. Change in cognition has perhaps the greatest number of restrictions for choice.

The vicious cycle of loneliness—powerlessness—social isolation—decreased self-esteem occurs all too frequently for the institutionalized elderly. Isolation is iatrogenic in institutions and fosters the following scenario: The individual is unable to function alone yet does not recognize the cause; relationships are disrupted as significant others may be out of reach of institution; the feeling of loneliness is feared and defended against; the individual is left feeling impotent and segregates himself or herself; isolation sets in along with decreasing self-esteem. Actions do not effect outcomes at this point.

Nurses and other health care providers must guard against fostering helplessness and powerlessness out of a self-directed need to help and rescue. Restorative nursing should clearly remain in focus for all older residents.

ASSESSMENT

A pattern of powerlessness and a belief in the inability to control events can probably be easily demonstrated through the OARS Multidimensional Functional Assessment (available from Duke University, Durham, North Carolina). Focusing on social resources, economic resources, mental health, physical health, and activities of daily living, it gives the clinician an excellent baseline of information on factors that could contribute to powerlessness. The Geriatric Hopelessness Scale was developed to assess subclinically depressed elderly and gives an index of hopelessness.

The nurse should try to determine which attributes had the most significance for the resident and which losses are most devastating. This type of interview is best accomplished when an environment of trust has been established. Assessment should include questions regarding social isolation and the ability to form new support systems or networks. Perceived social support is significant to a sense of well-being. The resident's unfamiliarity with expectations and routines, whether they involve medications, how to obtain a physician appointment, or how to summon help, all lead to a sense of powerlessness. Finally, establishing the degree of social isolation as an indicator of loneliness and low self-esteem should be explored.

Questioning family members or significant others as to the degree of dependence or feelings of powerlessness is a legitimate alternative for validation. Observation of the resident in decision-making situations reveals a significant amount about their perceptions. The resident's ability to negotiate the health care system will give a good indicator of perceived control.

ETIOLOGIES

ACTUAL

EXTERNAL

◆ Health-care environment: Forced dependency by care-givers, isolation of institution, loss of decision-making

◆ Illness-related regime: dependence on medication, diet, machinery for life maintenance, loss of livelihood or money for expenses, inability to negotiate health care system.

INTERNAL

◆ Interpersonal interaction

◆ Lifestyle of helplessness: Lifelong inability to affect change, desire by others to rescue resident from situation, religious, cultural beliefs.

POTENTIAL

EXTERNAL

◆ Health-care environment: Lack of knowledge of health care system, inability to make decisions regarding care/placement

◆ Illness-related regime: Dependence on others for maintenance of life style, change in life style.

INTERNAL

◆ Interpersonal interactions: Submissive life style, feeling that control is held by others, idealization of care-givers, especially professionals, lack of knowledge.

◆ Nursing Diagnosis

Altered perception of powerlessness related to illness-related regime.

DEFINING CHARACTERISTICS

Depression over physical deterioration (occurring despite compliance with regimes).

GOALS/OUTCOME CRITERIA

Decrease depressed behavior or verbalizations.

INTERVENTIONS

- ◆ Assess resident's depressive behavior (see previous care plan) and integrate plan. (RN, LPN, SW)
- ◆ Assess resident's attempts at compliance with health care regimes:
  - ◆ note any areas of deficit especially in knowledge of supportive actions and rationale. (RN, LPN, SW)
- ◆ Assess resident's knowledge of disease process:
  - ◆ do not overwhelm resident with information; however, do not hide information from resident as this will decrease trust in relationship. (RN, LPN, SW)
- ◆ Assess family's or significant other's knowledge of disease process and resident's care needs:
  - ◆ others should not be placing unrealistic expectations on resident. (RN, LPN, SW)
- ◆ Counsel resident on a therapeutic relationship:
  - ◆ do not negate resident's feelings
  - ◆ assist resident to focus on accomplishments and successes
  - ◆ help resident to develop a "legacy", if that is their desire, through tape recording life experiences to share with others. (RN, LPN, SW, RT)
- ◆ Include resident in support of group of person's with similar problems. (RN, SW)
- ◆ Counsel significant others who may be called upon to give ever-increasing support:
  - ◆ include in family support groups where ventilation, sharing, and successful caring strategies are discussed. (RN, SW)

DEFINING CHARACTERISTICS

Does not monitor progress, seek information regarding care, or defend self-care practices when challenged.

GOALS/OUTCOME CRITERIA

Adopt a more active role in relation to illness/need.

INTERVENTIONS

◆ Assess value of attributes resident disregards through interview.

  ◆ have resident re-tell history of problem and note any areas of denial

  ◆ attempt to determine resident's exposure to these problems/needs in the past, especially if they were present in significant others, e.g. grandfather also had diabetes and died of complications. This may distort resident's perceived ability to control diet and life style.

  ◆ assess any particular significance area of problem may have held, e.g. may feel that removal of cancerous testicle so decreases his sense of masculinity that he will not knowledge need for chemotherapy. (RN, LPN, SW)

◆ Assess resident's knowledge of problem/need—his or her reaction may originate from lack of knowledge, misconceptions, or "old wives tales."

  ◆ may be associated with mistaken belief that illness, discomfort, and dependency are to be expected in old age. (RN, LPN, SW)

◆ Give resident realistic feedback regarding effects of lack of acknowledgement of problem/need. (RN, LPN, NA)

◆ Perform resident teaching to make him or her aware of his or her role in the control of problem/need. (RN, LPN)

◆ Involve in support group of others who might be coping with similar problems/needs. (RN, LPN, SW)

◆ Consider use of behavior modification—positive reward system—when resident is resistant to acknowledgement and situation is deteriorating, e.g. very obese resident with cardiac disease who continues to overeat. (RN, LPN, SW)

◆ Whenever possible, return control of situation to resident. Do not foster increased dependency on care givers to monitor progress or cares. (RN, LPN, NA)

◆ Nursing Diagnosis

Altered perception of powerlessness related to health care environment.

DEFINING CHARACTERISTICS

Dependence on others that may result in irritability, resentment, anger, and guilt.

GOALS/OUTCOME CRITERIA

Acceptance of need to depend upon others when appropriate with some measure of life control.

INTERVENTIONS

◆ Assess present level of dependence and those areas of life affected:
◆ perform "OARS" test of functional abilities (RN, LPN)
◆ Interview resident to determine his or her perception of the dependence:
◆ which areas of life do they perceive affected?
◆ what significance did those areas have in the past for this person?
◆ what has been his or her experience with these problems, especially if occurred in person close to resident?
◆ Do not try to focus on area of dependency, if possible, and acknowledge strengths whenever possible. (RN, LPN, A)
◆ Whenever possible attempt to integrate restorative nursing techniques to lessen degree of dependence:
◆ provide adaptive equipment and make certain it is available and used by resident (RN, LPN, NA)
◆ Do not fall into the "pity-sympathy-rescue triad" (Ebersole).
◆ Support residents whenever they acknowledge their negative feelings regarding dependency:
◆ do not negate feelings
◆ give realistic feedback and support (RN, LPN, NA)
◆ Assist resident to relearn decision-making skills in areas of independence whenever possible:
◆ allow resident to chose times of care, clothing, food, activities
◆ give positive feedback so that resident realizes continued progress he or she is making
◆ counsel family to allow resident this right in their care of resident
◆ assist resident to negotiate social systems, e.g. food stamps, senior housing, social security, and health care system (making clinic appointments, obtaining needed therapy, obtaining special permits) so that they might feel more in control. (RN, LPN, NA)

DEFINING CHARACTERISTICS

Reluctance to express true feelings fearing alienation from caregivers

GOALS/OUTCOME CRITERIA

Will confide and trust care-givers.

INTERVENTIONS

◆ Assess resident's verbalizations for absences, denial, or minimizing affect of problem/need. (RN, LPN, NA)

◆ Investigate value of problem/need for resident before development of same. (RN, LPN, SW)

◆ Assess resident's need to control negative emotions:

    ◆ Are any negative statements made?

    ◆ Has resident always been emotionally reserved? (RN, LPN, SW)

◆ Do not express any judgmental statement regarding residents contribution to current situation. (RN, LPN, NA)

◆ Plan consistency in care givers so that resident may develop trust. (RN, LPN)

◆ Involve in support group where others may be expressing their feelings in an open, nonjudgmental, supportive environment. (RN, LPN, SW)

◆ Nursing Diagnosis

Altered sense of power related to interpersonal interaction.

DEFINING CHARACTERISTICS

Apathy, passivity

GOALS/OUTCOME CRITERIA

Active interest in life situation.

INTERVENTIONS

◆ Assess history of present situation, especially resident's ability to control any factors. (RN, LPN, NA)

◆ Assess role of family or significant others in development of this attitude. (RN, LPN, SW)

◆ Counsel family or significant others to allow resident some measure of decision-making. (RN, LPN, SW)

◆ Educate resident in decision-making beginning with familiar tasks and working from the concrete to the more abstract, e.g. choosing clothes to wear, washing clothing, purchasing clothing (RN, LPN, SW)

◆ Respect individual's territory and right to privacy as this will increase sense of control. (RN, LPN, NA)

◆ Focus on any area of interest and attempt to rekindle interest through therapeutic activity. (RN, LPN, REC. THERAPY)

◆ Do not socially isolate, but accept into groups even as passive observer. (RN, LPN, REC. THERAPY)

DEFINING CHARACTERISTICS

Expressed doubt regarding role performance.

GOALS/OUTCOME CRITERIA

Acceptance of role.

INTERVENTIONS

◆ Assess resident's perception of role expectations. (RN, LPN, SW)

◆ Focus on other areas of contribution to situation. (RN, LPN, NA)

◆ Counsel family or spouse if alteration has caused changes for resident. (RN, LPN, SW)

◆ Support all attempts to re-establish role or compensating strengths. (RN, LPN, SW)

◆ Nursing Diagnosis

Altered power related to a life style of helplessness.

DEFINING CHARACTERISTICS

Verbalization of having no control.

GOALS/OUTCOME CRITERIA

Increased control.

INTERVENTIONS

◆ Assess resident's perception of control:
  ◆ Does it lie outside himself or herself, e.g. luck, controlled by others?
  ◆ Does it lie within himself or herself?
  ◆ What types of situations has resident controlled in past, and what changed to cause a loss of control? (RN, LPN, SW)

◆ Respect any cultural or religious beliefs surrounding control of actions and environment. (RN, LPN, NA)

◆ Assess present functional status using "OARS" assessment tool or "Geriatric Hopelessness Scale." (RN, LPN, SW)

◆ Whenever possible give resident control over situations; do not foster climate of excessive dependency.

◆ Counsel family and others as to need to have resident's involvement in decision-making and care. (RN, LPN, NA, SW)

◆ Give positive feedback and reinforcement for all attempts at establishing control.(RN, LPN, NA)

◆ Include in skills-building group so that resident might relearn skills in a supportive environment. (RN, LPN, NA)

DEFINING CHARACTERISTICS

Nonparticipation in care or decision-making when opportunities provided.

GOALS/OUTCOME CRITERIA

Appropriate participation.

INTERVENTIONS

- ◆ Assess resident's life-long pattern of decision-making to ascertain a pattern of learned helplessness. (RN, LPN, SW)
- ◆ Assess resident's perception of self in relation to others:
  - ◆ Do they see themselves as effective?
  - ◆ Do they feel they make contributions to their or other's welfare? (RN, LPN, SW)
- ◆ Involve in reminiscence to draw upon past strengths and effective relationships. (RN, LPN, SW)
- ◆ Do not negate resident's feelings. (RN, LPN, NA)
- ◆ Develop a consistent, therapeutic relationship with resident that fosters an environment of inclusion, control, and affection. (RN, LPN, NA, RT)
- ◆ Give positive feedback whenever attempts at decision-making/control are attempted. (RN, LPN, NA)

DEPRESSION, REACTIVE (SITUATIONAL)

Definition: Acute decrease in self-esteem/worth related to a threat to self-competency. Although sadness is usually associated with depression, a sense of hopelessness in response to a situation is implied. Often depression is accompanied by physical symptoms but might not be identified in the elderly if passivity is mistaken for dementia.

AGE-RELATED PHENOMENON

Depression in the elderly is a frequently occurring phenomenon. Studies cite a range of statistics, but there is general agreement that depression is greater among older adults, from 5 percent to 50 percent. Successful suicidal attempts are also highest among the elderly. Predisposing factors for depression in the elderly include: over 80 percent have chronic health problems; one out of five persons over 65 has limited mobility; multiple personal losses—ten percent of men 65 and older are widowed, and in those 75 and older, 25 percent are, 50 percent of women over 65 and 70 percent of women over 75 are widows; isolation—one out of seven men and one out of three women over 65 lives alone; and poverty. It has long been recognized that loss and depression are closely linked.

Often is is the cataclysmic nature of losses that overwhelm the older person, leading to a reactional depression. Deaths of younger relatives or siblings often have a more profound effect than the death of of a peer. Professionals will often need to work closely with residents after such a loss, but often grief is delayed and depression is not realized for many months. Nurses and others might neglect signs of depression at this time, as they seem unrelated to a specific event.

Suicide is greater in older persons who are single, widowed, or divorced, or who experienced a recent loss. Elderly widowers have the highest rate of suicide. Those persons suffering from terminal illnesses, have a history of alcoholism, or acute or chronic brain dysfunctions are also at high risk. Statistics clearly point to the high correlation between attempts at suicide and success in the elderly. Seventy-five percent of elderly persons committing suicide spoke with a physician or clergyman before their attempt. It cannot, therefore, be too strongly emphasized that all verbalizations by older persons should be taken seriously.

One of the most tragic phenomenon related to depression in the elderly is misdiagnosis (see Assessment Section). Because of assumptions on the part of health professionals and family members, persons suffering from depression are labeled as demented. Pseudomentia is a type of depression that closely mimics dementia, as its onset is gradual and the individual's loss of interest in life is displayed in memory impairments, vague to inappropriate answers to questions, defective orientation, delusions, and mental retardation. The professional falsely assumes a dementia to be in progress and the underlying depression is not treated. These residents will rapidly deteriorate as their prophecy of diminshed self-concept is fulfilled.

Older persons are also more prone to depression from electrolyte disturbances and various chronic or acute illnesses. Often medications, especially anti-hypertensive agents, have produced side-effects of depression. Hormones, anti-Parkinsonian agents, corticosteroids, antituberculosis and anticancer medications have been associated with depression.

ASSESSMENT

Assessment of depression in older persons can pose a major challenge for the nurse. Unlike younger people who might be more able to express their inner feelings, especially the loss of self-worth or self-competency, elders were raised in a time when such discussion was considered inappropriate. Most elders will not use the same terminology to express dysphoria or sadness. Instead somatic problems, apathy, or difficulty concentrating often are the presenting chief complaint.

The vegetative symptoms reported in younger individuals are also present in the elderly. These symptoms include loss of appetite and weight, sleep disturbances, changes in psychomotor activity from feeling jittery to retarded movement and speech, and constipation. Other reported symptoms include anxiety, loss of pleasure in things that were once important, fatigue, difficulty concentrating, low self-esteem, and feelings of helplessness. For these individuals, the mistaken diagnosis of dementia might be assigned, especially if symptoms are focused on the mental sphere. However, in the demented there is a true loss of cognitive abilities and the individual should be evaluated using valid, standardized examinations. With careful questioning, individuals will be able to recall and focus on questions especially if the resident has some degree of trust in the examiner. The demented elderly or those who are nonverbal may have difficulty completing the standard mental status assessment instruments. Nurses may wish to use the Haycox Dementia Behavior Scale.

A mental health examination is central to assessing the resident. There are five areas of suggested questioning: overt behavior ranging from psychomotor retardation to agitation; mood status—a depressed affect will be sustained with less fluxuation; process of thinking—responses are generally negative, such as "I just can't do anything" or "I don't remember"; distorted perceptions—false perception of movement, body sensations, sounds, smell, task, touch; and cognitive impairment—15 percent of elderly show signs of cognitive losses or dementias.

It cannot be too strongly emphasized that the nurse also should investigate medications that may have depression as a side effect and poor nutrition as a precursor to confusional states. Hearing and vision losses must also be examined.

Tylor points out several valid areas for assessment to determine if despair exists or if a sense of well-being can be established. Physical health—those individuals who have maintained good physical health respond better to stressors. Also, it is appropriate for an older person to experience a period of dependency until his or her physical health returns. Autonomy—if the individual is able to make choices regarding issues that are important to them, i.e. housing, he or she maintains better mental health. Availability of a confidante—this eases adaptation to changes. The ability to maintain stability in the face of change—the known and familiar should be preserved as much as possible. Control over the speed of change—preplanning is important, it gives the individual a chance to mentally rehearse the change.

ETIOLOGIES

ACTUAL

EXTERNAL

◆ Loss of significant other—younger

◆ Loss of significant other—contemporary

◆ Loss of role in family

◆ Loss of health or worsening of chronic illness

◆ Loss of home

◆ Loss of income

◆ Loss of job

◆ Isolation

◆ Relocation trauma

◆ Loss of control over body and functions

INTERNAL

◆ Perceived powerlessness
◆ Loss of sensory awareness through vision and hearing
◆ Loss of self-esteem

POTENTIAL

EXTERNAL

◆ Inability to find meaningful replacements for roles and activities
◆ Fewer and less significant relationships
◆ Accessibility to other people and places
◆ Inability to maintain culture, customs, or religious practices
◆ Loss of privacy

INTERNAL

◆ Perceived powerlessness
◆ Reaction to disease states:
  ◆ Parkinson's disease
  ◆ brain tumor
  ◆ vascular compromise
  ◆ endocrine disturbances
  ◆ cancer
  ◆ nutritional deficiency, especially B_{12} or folate.
◆ Reaction to medication:
  ◆ antihypertensives
  ◆ reserpine
  ◆ propranolol
  ◆ methyldopa
  ◆ L-dopa
  ◆ digitalis toxicity
  ◆ steroids
  ◆ chemotherapy.
◆ Loss of sexual partner
◆ Loss of libido

◆ Nursing Diagnosis

Altered self-perception related to reactive depression.

DEFINING CHARACTERISTICS

Expressions of hopelessness, despair.

GOALS/OUTCOME CRITERIA

Decreased expressions of hopelessness, despair.

INTERVENTIONS

- ◆ Assess resident for perception of event precipitating feelings. (RN, LPN, NA, SW)
- ◆ Assess for recent or past losses (see Etiology). (RN, LPN, NA, SW)
- ◆ Be alert to complaints of physical problems, apathy, sleep disturbances, constipation, weight loss as presenting symptoms of depression. (RN, LPN, NA, SW)
- ◆ Perform physical examination with diagnostic work-up if illness, medication usage, or nutritional deficiency is suspected as exacerbating cause. (MD, RN, RD)
- ◆ Whenever possible, allow resident control over variables of situation, especially change. (MD, RN, LPN, NA, SW)
- ◆ Keep resident informed of all changes pending. (SW, RN, LPN, MD)
- ◆ Allow resident time to assimilate changes and do not rush decisions. (MD, SW, RN, LPN, NA)
- ◆ Involve resident in therapeutic relationship by primary care givers built on control, inclusion, and affection. (MD, RN, SW, LPN, NA, RD)
- ◆ Minimize isolation whether in community or institution by fostering relationship with peers and staff.
- ◆ Encourage involvement in meaningful leisure activities.
- ◆ Assist in developing replacements for lost roles/identity through activities, volunteering, new life skills. (RT, RN, SW, LPN, NA)
- ◆ Involve in group therapy with focus on resocialization, learning problem-solving techniques.
  - ◆ encourages communication
  - ◆ encourages independence
  - ◆ develops feeling of self-worth
  - ◆ encourages use of problem-solving skills (simple, economical, easy to implement) (SW, RN, RT)
- ◆ Increase social support systems through involvement in community centers, family counseling, visits by volunteer agencies or inclusion in same (Widow-to-Widow Program), part-time or full-time work in same or related field. (SW, RN, MD, REC. THERAPIST)
- ◆ Assess resident's level of depression using standardized examinations:
  - ◆ Zung Self-Rating
  - ◆ Beck Depression Inventory

- ◆ Minnesota Multiphasic Personality Inventory
- ◆ Geriatric Depression Scale (MD, RN, SW)
- ◆ Consider the use of anti-depressant medication but be especially alert for anticholenergic and sedative potential. Tricyclic antidepressants should be used with great caution in residents with heart disease. Begin medication allowed, allow divided doses, and gradually adjust. Administer dosage at bedtime, once stabilized, to reduce injury and confusion. (MD, RN, LPN)
- ◆ Consider use of one of the psychotherapeutic modalities:
  - ◆ supportive—geared to limited goals
  - ◆ behavioral—present behavior is target for change, emphasizes self-change and self-reliance
  - ◆ cognitive—(only type of therapy designed for depression and works well with elderly) time-limited, problem-solving orientation with emphasis on present problems and coping skills. (MD, RN, SW)
- ◆ Consider inclusion in reminiscence group—focus on retelling life experiences chronologically from childhood onward with focus on past resolutions of problems/losses as aid to dealing with present situation, improving self-esteem and integrity. Social skills and cohort effect are also improved. (RN, SW, RT)

DEFINING CHARACTERISTICS

Inability to concentrate.

GOALS/OUTCOME CRITERIA

Improved thought processes.

INTERVENTIONS

- ◆ Assess thought process—can be anxiety provoking in elderly and good rapport needs to be established.
- ◆ Assess possibility of pseudodementia existing (dementia is mimicked by functional psychiatric illness, usually depression). Be alert for the following:
  - ◆ more recent onset of symptoms
  - ◆ rapid progression after onset
  - ◆ recognition and emphasis on disability
  - ◆ more pervasive affect change
  - ◆ more frequent "I don't know" answers to mental status exams.
- ◆ Assess for loss of sensory input: hearing, vision, touch, taste, smell through diagnostic testing. (MD, RN, LPN, AUDIOLOGIST, OT)
- ◆ Assess for pain as overwhelming stimulus to resident's system. (MD, RN, LPN)

◆ For residents who have been socially isolated, introduce new phenomenon and staff persons slowly.

   ◆ respect right of privacy

   ◆ do not rush resident in decisions or dealings with others. (RN, SW, LPN, NA)

◆ Keep environment familiar:

   ◆ encourage personal possessions be brought into hospital or long-term care setting

   ◆ refer to these items from the past and/or familiar when conversing with resident. (SW, RN, LPN, NA)

◆ In evaluating thought process, focus on familiar or past. (SW, RN, LPN)

◆ Allow periods of rest interspersed with nonstrenuous activities of daily living. (RN, LPN, NA)

◆ Structure daily life so residents can feel they have control over situations and can predict outcomes. (RN, LPN, NA)

◆ Continuity in care givers. (SW, RN, LPN, NA, REC. THERAPIST)

DEFINING CHARACTERISTICS

Change in physical activity, eating, sleeping, sexual activity.

GOALS/OUTCOME CRITERIA

Establish homeostasis in life patterns.

INTERVENTIONS

◆ Assessor should be aware of relationship of somatic symptoms and depression and evaluate accordingly, focusing on stressors, crisis, losses. (MD, RN, LPN, SW)

◆ Attempt to assist resident in defining relationship of physical changes to possible provocative events. (MD, RN, LPN)

◆ Be sensitive to resident's inability to link somatic problems with depression—not socially or culturally acceptable to some elders. (RN, LPN, NA)

◆ Provide support for resident in areas of activities of daily living, discouraging total dependence while allowing resident to feel supported. (RN, LPN, NA)

◆ Effect on physical health can soon become profound if condition allowed to exist. Consider use of antidepressant medication in cases of anorexia or insomnia. (MD, RN, LPN, RD)

◆ If possible, allow resident to have control over environment, including sleeping and eating schedules, rather than intervening in a manner that would further increase a loss of self-esteem, e.g. insertion of naso-gastric tube, sedation. (RN, LPN, NA, RD, MD)

◆ Plan time for daily activity especially physical exercise to increase functioning—allow rest periods, as needed. (RN, LPN, NA, RT)

◆ Include in pet therapy programs and groups. When possible, allow resident to be responsible for care of pet.

  ◆ establishes trusting relationship

  ◆ increases self-esteem through responsibility

  ◆ gives some purpose to living

  ◆ gives resident another focus outside of self

  ◆ can provide replacement for other lost relationships. (RN, LPN, NA, RT)

◆ Include in inter-generational programs with younger children:

  ◆ provides caring and nonjudgmental relationship

  ◆ provides replacement for other lost relationships

  ◆ fulfills need to feel useful and important to others, especially future generations. (RN, SW, RT)

◆ For residents whose physical health is rapidly declining, consider referral for electroconvulsive therapy (ECT). Now considered a safe and effective alternative for residents (contraindicated in cases of recent coronary thrombosis, decompensated heart failure). (MD, RN, SW)

◆ Consider family counseling for care givers: children, spouse, sibling.

  ◆ support groups available for family members to discuss issues, air feelings, discuss plans for action

  ◆ if possible, include older resident so that resolution of latent problems may be achieved

  ◆ encourage family not to neglect personal needs to make drastic sacrifices of time or well-being. (MD, RN, SW)

DEFINING CHARACTERISTICS

Threats or attempts to commit suicide.

GOALS/OUTCOME CRITERIA

Elimination of desire to commit suicide.

INTERVENTIONS

◆ Assess disguised life-threatening actions as possible suicidal attempts: overdose of drugs, failure to take life-sustaining medication, anorexia. (MD, RN, LPN, RD, SW)

◆ Assess for precursors of suicide: serious physical illness, history of depression, alcoholism, drug dependency, chronic insomnia, prolonged grief, multiple major losses, loss of social support network, economic difficulties. (MD, RN, LPN, SW, PSYCH.)

◆ Consider all verbalizations about desire to commit suicide as legitimate (elderly have highest successful suicide rate) and be alert for other disguised attempts to communicate desire: reuniting with friends and family, putting estate in order, sudden interest in church, religion, funerals. (MD, RN, LPN, SW)

◆ Directly question resident as to plans, means available, reasons for self-injury. (RN, MD, SW)

◆ Prompt hospitalization, including one-to-one supervision, removal of all dangerous items. (RN, LPN, NA)

◆ After crisis subsides can return home or to long-term care facility with definite plans to supervise resident. (RN, LPN, NA)

◆ Consider use of antidepressant medication or electroconvulsive therapy (see previous plan). (MD, RN, SW, PSYCH.)

◆ Establish therapeutic relationship with therapist establishing control of process communicating empathy, perspective, control, and hope. (MD, RN, SW)

DEFINING CHARACTERISTIC

Extreme dependency on others with related feelings of helplessness and anger.

GOALS/OUTCOME CRITERIA

Resume control over issues in question, express autonomy.

INTERVENTION

◆ When resident has become extremely dependent, assess areas of dependency and any gains achieved by same. (MD, RN, SW, LPN, NA)

◆ Foster autonomy whenever possible in all therapeutic relationships; do not allow resident to elevate care givers to parental role.

   ◆ offer positive reinforcement for all decisions made

   ◆ set limits in resident's ability to rely on care givers for decisions. (RN, LPN, NA, SW)

◆ Counsel children, spouse as to methods of dealing with resident's dependency:

   ◆ include in support groups—provides emotional support and ability to deal with role reversal

   ◆ depressed spouse may communicate need for constant help to spouse then reject same—spouse might then pull away increasing dependency and depression in partner.

◆ Assess areas of depression. (see previous plans)

◆ Focus on areas of achievement:

   ◆ build on these areas in choosing therapeutic activities

   ◆ praise all attempts at control or mastery

◆ include in skills building group. (RN, LPN, NA, OT, REC. THERAPIST)

◆ Include in support group to receive perspective and feedback from peers. (RN, SW, RT)

◆ Give feedback when resident's perception of level of functioning is not appropriate, focusing on positive accomplishments. (RN, LPN, NA, SW, RT, OT)

ANXIETY: MILD, MODERATE, SEVERE

Definition: Increased level of arousal associated with expectations of a threat (unfocused) to self or significant relationship. A feeling of helplessness or powerlessness with an impending sense of dread. The numerous changes and losses associated with aging, especially the shattering of the sense of invulnerability, promote an unsettled and insecure perception of self. May be manifested in a continuum from mild to severe.

ASSESSMENT

Anxiety may be revealed when obtaining a detailed psycho-social history with emphasis on recent losses, changes in life style, or bereavements. The nurse will need to differentiate between other physical conditions that may have anxiety as a symptom (hyperthroidism, cancer, cardiac failure) and psychological factors that originated and now maintain anxiety. Depression, which is often accompanied by agitation and restlessness in the elderly, may be mistaken for anxiety. However, in anxiety the vegetative symptoms (sleep and eating disorders, constipation) are often absent. Those persons who are experiencing a loss of mental capacities, will often be aware of this decline and a general increase in anxiety may be observed.

The DSM-III lists four classes of anxiety disorders. Phobic disorders are seen as a persistent avoidance behavior secondary to irrational fears of a specific object. Panic disorders are noted by recurrent attacks of intense anxiety involving feelings of extreme apprehension or terror. With generalized anxiety there is a chronic, however less severe, manifestation of the panic disorder. Usually the resident will demonstrate autonomic hyperactivity and an attitude of apprehensive expectation with increased perceptual vigilance. In the obsessive-compulsive disorder, ideas and behaviors are outside of voluntary control. Generalized anxiety and panic disorders are most often found in the elderly.

Assessment of physical care needs may reveal a pattern of anxiety. Lengthy rituals may prevent adequate intake of food or adequate sleep. The resident may experience regular periods of vomiting or extensive diaphoresis. Inability to carry out activities of daily living (ADL), when anxiety is severe, is found. Physical assessments should be performed on the resident during periods of noncomplaining so that more accurate reporting is obtained.

AGE-RELATED PHENOMENON

Anxiety is not a new phenomenon for many elders who are symptomatic. A history of anxiety in earlier life is often found. This state becomes reactivated as the older person is faced with new and increased stresses brought about by aging. Whether the individual is facing increased social isolation, a decline in the number of relationships, or a loss of status or role, anxiety can be rekindled. Upon interview the family may characterize the resident as always having "bad nerves" or some other similar statement.

When extreme forms of anxiety are experienced by the elderly, dependent behaviors and helplessness are reinforced. The older person lives in dread that the panic attack may occur again. Often the family will attempt to intervene and in their attempts to make the older relative's world less anxiety-provoking, they foster increased dependency, especially for those individuals suffering from some mild to moderate memory or cognitive loss. Loss of independence in the elderly can be manifested through serious illness, injury, sudden deterioration in a once well-managed chronic illness, or by loss of a friend or neighbor that assisted with errands, spouse, sibling, or significant other.

ETIOLOGIES

ACTUAL

EXTERNAL

◆ Separation from those roles, status, and life styles that gave definition to self

◆ Loss of significant others, either through death or inability to sustain relationships

INTERNAL

◆ Physical illness

◆ Life-long history of anxiety; anxiety as coping mechanism

◆ Serious illness, surgery that may alter level of independence

◆ Change in severity of chronic illness

POTENTIAL

EXTERNAL

◆ Change in life style

◆ Loss of significant others

◆ Need to depend upon others for ADL assistance, shopping, cooking, handling finances

INTERNAL

◆ Declining cognitive/memory powers

◆ Reduced feeling of mastery over life

◆ Development of chronic illness

◆ Change in severity of chronic illness

◆ Use of psychotropic medications
◆ Incontinence
◆ Perceptual changes: loss of vision and hearing

◆ Nursing Diagnosis

Altered anxiety related to future events perceived as threatening to self or others *(anticipatory)*.

DEFINING CHARACTERISTICS

Increased level of arousal.

GOALS/OUTCOME CRITERIA

Reduce aroused state.

INTERVENTIONS

◆ Assess resident perception of threatening event:
  ◆ use reality testing, when possible, to compare event to others resident has dealt with in past
  ◆ assess coping skills
  ◆ interview family or significant others to determine past experiences and coping strategies. (RN, LPN, MD, SW)
◆ Consider resident for inclusion in support group of peers.
◆ Builds cohort effect. (RN, SW)
◆ Encourage financial planning so that assets are allocated to proper areas. (SW)

◆ Nursing Diagnosis

Altered anxiety level *(mild)* related to threat to self or significant relationships.

DEFINING CHARACTERISTICS

Expressed feelings of increased arousal and concern.

GOALS/OUTCOME CRITERIA

Decrease in feelings to level appropriate to situation.

INTERVENTIONS

◆ Assess residents perception of threat:
  ◆ use reality testing with feedback
  ◆ encourage resident to focus on event rather than peripheral issues/concerns
  ◆ allow resident to ventilate "worst case" fears regarding events. (RN, SW, LPN, MD)

- Assess resident's previous coping mechanisms:
  - interview resident
  - interview family. (RN, SW, LPN)
- Evaluate if anxiety is appropriate for situation or if result of secondary problem:
  - disease-related
  - medication side effect
  - nutrition deficiency related. (MD, RN, RD)
- Obtain needed diagnostic tests to verify or rule out physical origin. (MD, NP, CNS)
- Encourage resident to join support group of peers:
  - builds cohort effect
  - gives feedback
  - gives emotional support
  - validates feelings. (RN, SW)
- Establish priorities and routines for daily needs:
  - block-time day with reminders of special events
  - encourage independence in grooming and other ADL skills
  - encourage proper diet.
- Teach effective use of leisure time
  - assess previous interests and hobbies
  - encourage participation in developing new interests, skills, or areas of socialization
  - encourage mastery of skills to reduce feelings of being out of control, increase feelings of self-worth. (OT, RT, RN, LPN, NA)
- Teach relaxation techniques to decrease anxious feelings:
  - deep-muscle relaxation
  - self-hypnosis. (RN, SW)
- Teach/use guided imagery
  - guide resident through imagined visit to peaceful place where he or she can then return. (RN, SW, RT)

DEFINING CHARACTERISTICS

Increased restlessness.

GOALS/OUTCOME CRITERIA

Reduce restlessness.

INTERVENTION

◆ Assess if sleep/wake cycle is disturbed
  ◆ periods of insomnia
  ◆ encourage to follow own sleep routines
  ◆ periods of fatigue from loss of sleep. (MD, RN, LPN, NA)
◆ Teach resident to establish habitation patterns to reduce stress of needlessly redoing previously accomplished tasks
  ◆ use check-off sheet with events listed. (RN, LPN, NA)
◆ Evaluate medication, especially antipsychotic and antidepressant drugs, for side-effects of restlessness
  ◆ attempt to reduce dosage. (MD, RN)
◆ Consider involvement in activity therapy group, focusing on immediate gains
  ◆ dance/movement
  ◆ drama
  ◆ music
  ◆ exercise. (RN, SW, RT, PT, OT)
◆ Assess for hyperkalemia, hyperventilation, chronic liver disease, hyperthyroidism, infectious process displaying atypical symptomatology. (MD, RN)
◆ Assess for intermittent incontinence, UTI, inability to use toilet
  ◆ check voiding and defecation pattern
  ◆ establish toileting routine
  ◆ assess for abnormal UTI or other GU problems such as prostatitis
  ◆ clearly mark toilet room, especially at night. (MD, RN, LPN, NA, FAMILY)

DEFINING CHARACTERISTICS

Increased questioning, awareness.

GOALS/OUTCOME CRITERIA

Appropriate level of awareness, questioning.

INTERVENTIONS

◆ Communicate an understanding of residents emotional state:
  ◆ clarify ideas
  ◆ use feedback
  ◆ validate need for concern, if appropriate
  ◆ focus on the "here and now." (MD, RN, LPN, NA, SW)

◆ Explain all procedures, problems, or concerns to resident in a matter-of-fact manner. (RN, LPN, NA, SW)

◆ Focus on control of items that he or she can manage; assist in delegating items that resident does not need or want to manage.

◆ Nursing Diagnosis

Altered anxiety level *(moderate)* related to expectations of an unfocused threat to self or significant others.

DEFINING CHARACTERISTICS

Expressed feelings of unfocused apprehension, nervousness, or concern.

GOALS/OUTCOME CRITERIA

Reduced feelings of apprehension, nervousness, concern.

INTERVENTION

◆ Assess resident's appraisal of threatening situation to validate realistic from unrealistic concerns. (MD, RN, SW, LPN)

◆ Whenever possible, reduce environmental influences that may be increasing anxiety
  ◆ delegate responsibilities for complex tasks to others, if possible
  ◆ explore alternative ways of dealing with situation
  ◆ involve family members that may be able to assist resident or may be provoking increasing anxiety. (MD, RN, SW, LPN)

◆ Involve resident in support group if anxiety related to discernible cause:
  ◆ chronic illness
  ◆ change in life style
  ◆ change in living arrangements
  ◆ loss of role
  ◆ loss of others. (MD, RN, SW)

◆ Refer to psychologist or psychiatrist for therapy emphasizing a supportive relationship. (MD, RN, SW)

◆ Consider use of behavioral treatments: systematic desensitization, progressive muscle relaxation, hypnosis, biofeedback, group training in relaxation. (MD, RN, SW)

◆ Assist with ADL when anxiety increased. (RN, LPN, NA)

◆ Retain consistency in care givers to increase feeling of security.

◆ Allow resident to make simple decisions and gradually increase quality of decisions.

◆ Nursing Diagnosis

Altered anxiety level *(severe)* related to expectations of a threat to self or to significant relationships.

DEFINING CHARACTERISTICS

Expressed feelings of unfocused severe dread, apprehension, nervousness, or concern.

GOALS/OUTCOME CRITERIA

Reduction in feelings to appropriate levels.

INTERVENTIONS

- ◆ Establish strong therapeutic relationship
  - ◆ visit resident regularly to convey sense of security and closeness.
- ◆ If anxiolytic drugs not effective, consider use of major tranquilizers— trifluroperazine or thioridazine or one of the tricyclic antidepressants.
- ◆ All have significant side effects in the elderly, including sedation, anticholinergic, cardiovascular effects.
- ◆ Consider administering at bedtime when symptoms are controlled to reduce experiencing side-effects. (MD, RN)

DEFINING CHARACTERISTICS

Increased heart rate, hyperventilation, diaphoresis, increased muscle tension, dilated pupils, pallor.

GOALS/OUTCOME CRITERIA

Decreased cholingeric symptoms.

INTERVENTIONS

- ◆ Assess physiological response to anxiety attack
  - ◆ monitor vital signs
  - ◆ encourage rest whenever possible
  - ◆ assess affect of stressors on major systems especially, if resident has chronic or acute illness. (MD, RN, LPN, NA)
- ◆ Consider use of major tranquilizers to quickly reduce symptoms. (MD, RN)
- ◆ Provide nonthreatening, nonstimulating environment. (RN, LPN, NA)
- ◆ Communicate an understanding of resident's feelings without comment on behavior or symptoms.

DEFINING CHARACTERISTICS

Altered verbalizations, activity, change in perception of reality.

GOALS/OUTCOME CRITERIA

Increased perception of reality and control.

INTERVENTION

◆ Focus communication on "here and now" when dealing with resident. (RN, SW, LPN, NA)

◆ Set limits on behavior that is exhausting resident, i.e. pacing. (RN, SW, LPN)

◆ Provide quiet place where resident can rest without feelings of being threatened or judged. (RN, SW, LPN)

◆ Have staff members that the resident knows well remain with resident to increase security. (RN)

◆ Have continuity in care givers. (RN)

◆ Assist with ADL. (RN, LPN, NA)

◆ Praise all attempts to regain control over environment from less complicated decisions—choice of slacks or skirt—to more complex—choice of programs to attend. (ALL)

◆ When attack has subsided, do not deny resident's experience but attempt to communicate (ALL)

FEAR OF FALLING

Definition: Apprehension brought about by a history of falls and often anxiety, which leads to a higher mortality and further falls. Resulting behavior is manifested in the inability to move one's self secondary to belief that one will fall again from either standing or walking.

ASSESSMENT

Assessment of the nonambulatory resident should include muscle strength, integrity of weight-bearing joints, coordination of movement and balance. Medication should be reviewed for side-effects that would influence balance. Experience of syncope and vertigo that might be related to either cardiac or vestibular changes should be explored further.

A careful history should include information regarding serious falls or serial falls over a specified period of time. The nurse should explore the circumstances surrounding the falls, such as amount of time elapsed before the resident was found/assisted, mental functioning, balance, anxiety, whether the resident was home bound (or room bound if institutionalized) prior to the fall. A syndrome will develop for those individuals who display a higher frequency of these factors. Suspicion of an increased morbidity and mortality among these residents is great.

AGE-RELATED PHENOMENON

Older persons have great justification for a fear of falling; as one ages the normal decalcification of bones predisposes them to more extensive injury from trauma. Often the elderly are taking medication that produces orthostatic hypertension as a side-effect. Vascular changes also incline many individuals toward this condition. Atrophy of the musculature can cause difficulty in righting oneself and remaining upright. However, despite these and other obvious conditions that might lead to a normal cautious approach to ambulation, a syndrome has been noted in the literature that has been labeled the "post-fall syndrome." These residents expressed great fear of falling when they stood erect, tending to grab and clutch at objects within their view. They showed great hesitancy and irregularity in their walking attempts. This condition was not apparent prior to recent fall and/or falls, and therefore a syndrome is suspected.

After developing this syndrome, a general immobility develops, which predisposes the individual to further complications. Morbidity and mortality is high among this group. When factors are controlled for, it appears that those living alone in the community are at higher risk. Fifty percent of the fallers lived alone and 40 percent of the remainder lived with an aged spouse only.

It has been hypothesized that the interconnectedness of dementia and depression to falling, lack of attention to gait, or obstacles would predispose the resident to falling; but one's preoccupation with self associated with depression leads to unusual inattention to gait and therefore falling. Especially in subcortical dementia associated with movement disturbances, e.g. Parkinson's disease, the incidence of depression is high and the potential for fear of falling syndrome is greater.

The nurse must attempt to identfy individuals at risk with an increased number of factors for post-fall syndrome: anxiety, increased time on floor, depression, isolated, increase in number of falls. By working with the resident in collaboration with other health professionals, the possibility of mobilizing the resident increases.

ETIOLOGY

ACTUAL

ENVIRONMENTAL

◆ Living alone or with aged spouse

◆ Increased time alone before receiving assistance

◆ Hazardous environment (obstacles, stairs, poorly maintained living quarters)

SOMATIC

◆ Expressed anxiety or fear

◆ Decreased sensory status (poor sight, hearing)

◆ Decreased functioning of proprioceptors

- Vestibular disease
- Vascular disease
- Medication causing hypotension (especially tricyclic antidepressants)
- Depression
- Subcortical dementia

POTENTIAL

- Sense of isolation from resources

◆ Nursing Diagnosis

Fear of falling related to perceived inability to control event.

DEFINING CHARACTERISTICS

Hesitant and irregular gait, clutching and grabbing, immobility.

GOALS/OUTCOME CRITERIA

Regular gait.

INTERVENTIONS

- Assess resident for integrity of joints and musculature to insure strength and endurance required for ambulation. (RN, PT)
- Assess resident for fear of falling syndrome: verbalization of fear, immobility without supporting cause, sense of isolation, history of serious or serial falls, depression/dementia. (RN, SW)
- Attempt desensitization through development of regular treatment regime. (RN, LPN, PT)
- Design plan with resident's input as to time and place. (RN)
- Promote hazard-free environment. (RN, LPN, NA)
- Beginning with movement from sitting to standing, progress at a pace within resident's tolerance. (RN, LPN, NA, PT)
- Insure that plan will be carried out from three to four times daily. (RN, PT)
- Instruct all level of staff as to resident's regime so there is continuity. (NA, RN, LPN, PT)
- For home-bound individuals, consider use of tape recorder with instructions so that plan may be supported by other caregivers/family. (RN)
- Discourage family or significant others from supporting dependent behavior. (RN, LPN, PT)
- Focus on positive strides made in mobility and appropriate ventilation of concerns. (RN, PT)

FEAR OF ABUSE/CRIME

Definition: Fear can be directed toward family, caregivers, or community environment. Rather than supporting the elderly, these persons or factors place the older person in a position of extreme vulnerability.

ASSESSMENT

Assessment of victims of abuse would include observations for unusual bruising; contractures and pressure ulcers, which seem unreasonable in light of overall presentation; dehydration with supporting laboratory data to indicate it occurred over time; diarrhea or impactions. Assess for malnutrition, especially with serum protein and albumin levels and eating patterns.

The nurse should attempt to study the family dynamic for patterns of multiple dependency, which pose a burden for care givers. History of abusive relationships between spouses, siblings, and parent-child are revealed on interview, especially if this family system used domestic violence as a pattern of conflict resolution.

Aside from physical abuse, the elderly can be victimized by those who would take money or property either directly or covertly be means of various schemes. This type of abuse should be suspected when funds or property are disproportionately depleted when the elderly person may be existing within a moderate life style. Elderly women, who have not managed their property as this responsibility was assumed by their husbands, are more easily victimized when they are widowed.

AGE-RELATED PHENOMENON

Elder abuse is a very unfortunate phenomenon in our society. This abuse can take the form of physical violence against the person, either in the form of assault by care givers or strangers, neglect or failure to provide goods or services, or exploitation such as improper use of resources. Psychological abuse and abandonment are also practiced.

Elder abuse is reportable by health professionals in all but seven states, and failure to report has various penalties attached, depending on the state. It is projected that annually 500,000 to 1,500,000 cases of abuse toward the elderly are reported. The elderly are also more at risk for violence in the community at large; robberies make up about 90 percent of crimes against the elderly and 8 percent are assaults. As the criminal takes advantage of the older person's sensory deprivation, difficulty with ambulation, possible confusion, or difficulty with decision-making, the elderly become easy victims. Thus, many elderly isolate themselves behind locked doors refusing available services and becoming more detached from society.

In developing a theoretical framework of the explanation of abusive family relationships, several factors have been identified; in particular, using past experiences to develop a composite identity of the elder, the present behavior is seen by the caregiver only as it relates to the past. In abusive patterns the present image is lower than the past, e.g. there is a "dignified" past image and "normal" present image or a "normal" past image and a "stigmatized" present image. The elder is viewed as "spoiled" by the care giver. The care giver customarily uses control to resolve conflicts, with such negative strategies as tripping and slapping. The role then becomes one of prison guard for the care giver, "constantly" observing for inappropriate behavior that requires corrective action. These individuals will often reveal, in an interview, strong, unyielding opinions about how elders should and should not behave, close-mindedness, personal projection of right and justice in action and thoughts. Care giver stress is a major component in elder abuse. The average care giver is a middle-aged female "sandwiched" between care of her family and the added responsibility of a parent or relative. The personal and financial stress can be overwhelming.

Nurses employed in long-term care facilities and hospitals have an obligation to report all cases of suspected abuse, mistreatment, or neglect. Whether required by state statute or not, the role of nurse as advocate has long existed as a professional ethic. Disciplinary proceedings must be followed through on all staff suspected of abusing a resident in their care.

Protective Service Agencies should be notified for all persons who have been victims of abuse who return to the community. If the elderly person does not wish to leave an unsafe environment, consider placing a home health aide in the home with follow up by a community service agency.

ETIOLOGY

ACTUAL

EXTERNAL

Inability to control event:

- living in high-crime neighborhood due to either poverty or reluctance to leave familiar surroundings
- abusive relationship with care givers.

INTERNAL

Inability to control

- inability to make decisions
- dependent, demanding personality
- history of domestic violence.

POTENTIAL

EXTERNAL

- Care giver is involved in multiple dependency relationship
- Elderly person lives alone or with minimal contact with persons outside the home
- Care giver has difficulty dealing with role-reversal, eg. assuming a caregiving role for a parent

◆ Care giver has rigid standards and expectations for elder
◆ Financial affairs not clearly managed by reputable financial advisor

INTERNAL

◆ Multiple needs that cannot be met by resident
◆ Sensory deprivation
◆ Confusion
◆ Unrealistic expectations of care giver
◆ Recently assumed responsibility for property after death of spouse

◆ Nursing Diagnosis

Fear of abuse related to dependency on abusive care givers.

DEFINING CHARACTERISTICS

Physical examination reveals lack of care or mistreatment.

GOALS/OUTCOME CRITERIA

Free of injury, well-nourished.

INTERVENTIONS

◆ Assess for signs of neglect or mistreatment: unexplained injury, mal-nourished, pressure ulcers/contractures, diarrhea/impactions, unclean. (RN, MD, RD)
◆ Interview family/care givers for unusual dynamics or expectations of resident. (RN, SW)
◆ Note especially:
   ◆ "prison-guard" mentality, close-minded, rigid expectations
   ◆ lowered status of resident in view of care giver
   ◆ descriptions of resident as "spoiled"
   ◆ history of abusive behavior, domestic violence
   ◆ care giver/companion refuses to allow resident to be interviewed alone
◆ Report all cases of suspected or actual abuse to proper authorities for further investigation. (RN)
◆ Encourage alternate living arrangements with other family members or institutionalization, if dependencies are numerous. (RN, SW)
◆ Within institution, change care givers and unit, if possible. (RN, SW)

◆ Nursing Diagnosis

Fear of exploitation, of personal safety, of property.

DEFINING CHARACTERISTICS

Refusal to leave dwelling, depletion of funds.

GOALS/OUTCOME CRITERIA

Property will be managed appropriately; state that they are at ease with leaving dwelling.

INTERVENTION

◆ Assess for possible exploitation not related to hoarding of funds. (RN, SW)

  ◆ living in deprived surroundings despite statements regarding pensions, annuities, etc.

  ◆ sudden depletion of funds

  ◆ use of unorthodox persons for financial management.

◆ Refer resident to social service agencies in community. (RN)

◆ Refer case to proper authorities for legal action. (RN)

◆ Encourage resident to have property managed by reputable bank or attorney. (RN, SW)

◆ Assess resident for reluctance to leave home

  ◆ lack of food, goods needed to sustain self

  ◆ statements regarding reluctance to leave dwelling.

◆ Assess community for crime rate, support systems for elderly. (RN)

◆ Refer resident to community-based support systems. (RN, SW)

◆ Arrange for paraprofessional to assist with obtaining food/goods. (RN, LPN)

◆ Encourage resident to consider move to a more protected environment—senior housing. (RN, LPN)

SELF-ESTEEM DISTURBANCE

Definition: Negative feelings regarding conception of self, social-self, or self-capabilities. Perceived loss of worth, competence, or productivity.

AGE-RELATED PHENOMENON

Martha Rogers, an eminent nurse theorist, views life on a space-time continuum growing ever more complex and negentropic. Evolution is always occurring for the individual and behavior is synergistic. This perspective allows the clinician to see disruptions in self-esteem as part of a continuum rather than as a positive/negative dynamic. Interventions are then based on growth and increasing change. In Rogers' model, regression is not possible—only change.

Perhaps the change in roles and expectations are the most profound factors affecting self-esteem. The role of provider is challenged as the resident reaches retirement. Even with adequate financial support, which all too few persons have the luxury of amassing, much of an individual's identity is linked to their occupation. Forced retirement, even at age 70, is still difficult to accept for the viable worker. Relocation may become necessary as cost of living prohibits fixed-income support. Loss of spouse is the most significant life stress. Redefinition of roles at this time becomes even more difficult as options for finding a new love are limited. Sexual roles for those remaining unmarried may be distorted by societal pressures to negate this human need. For the husband whose wife becomes impaired so that he must assume nurturing tasks, or the wife who must assume management of the household affairs as a husband declines, these expectations can be both overwhelming and a potential for growth.

The individual's ability to cope with the changing roles and expectations of later life strongly depends upon his or her former coping skills and perceived social support. For one individual, self-esteem may be profoundly disturbed, while another may feel free to explore new roles. Other issues such as ability to contract chronic illness, previous dependence on alcohol or other substances, control over decisions, influence in families or with significant others, ability to remain functional both mentally and physically all contribute to the self-worth perception.

Reminiscence group work has been particularly helpful with older residents experiencing diminished self-esteem. Respect of territoriality, privacy, and ability to have personal possessions all contribute to self-worth. For most individuals, these are hallmarks of respect and reminders of a rich heritage.

ASSESSMENT

The nurse assessing self-esteem in the older resident should be alert for negativistic self-statements, e.g. "I'm no good." Expression of uselessness are often encountered, sometimes including a wish to die. Depression and self-esteem are highly correlated, therefore assessment and interventions for one often entail inclusion of the other dynamic. A loss of motivation to perform any task, whether pleasurable or functional, would indicate a possible loss of self-esteem as the feeling of competency is devalued. Therefore a functional assessment tool such as OARS might reveal a loss of self-esteem.

Affect will change with a change in this dynamic. Residents often appear depressed, hostile, negativistic, or demanding. Nothing satisfies them. They are not personally satisfied. Masochistic or self-sabotaging behavior may appear, ranging from non-compliance with therapeutic regimes to anorexia or self-mutilation.

An objective assessment tool that can be easily used was introduced by Rosenberg, Silbers, and Tippett in 1965. It has since been validated with elderly, disabled, and elderly-disabled residents. The scale consists of ten declarative statements regarding a persons self-conception. Each statement is then scored on a scale from one to four; level is computed by summing cross items.

◆ Nursing Diagnosis

Self-esteem disturbances related to loss of significant roles.

DEFINING CHARACTERISTICS

Lack of eye contact, head flexion, shoulder flexion.

GOALS/OUTCOME CRITERIA

More positive nonverbal communication.

INTERVENTIONS

◆ Assess resident's perception of life situation through observation of nonverbal communication, placement in room, verbal interaction. (RN, LPN, NA)

◆ Convey to resident an environment of trust and acceptance through active listening and touch (if resident is comfortable with touch). (RN, LPN, NA)

◆ Develop therapeutic relationship with resident attempting to use principles of inclusion, control, and affection. (RN, LPN, NA)

◆ Reinforce every attempt at positive nonverbal communication with recognition. (RN, LPN, NA)

◆ Interact with residents on their terms until they can extend themselves into a more appropriate situation. (RN, LPN, NA)

◆ Counsel family and others not to negate resident's feelings and encourage continued interaction even if feedback is minimal.

◆ Consider inclusion in pet therapy program (has been very effective with the resident who is interacting minimally or regular visits to institution's pet. (RN, LPN, NA, SW, RT)

DEFINING CHARACTERISTICS

Self-negating verbalizations. Expressions of shame or guilt.

GOALS/OUTCOME CRITERIA

More positive self-statements.

INTERVENTIONS

◆ Assess previous coping mechanisms with change, respect any religious or cultural norms. (RN, LPN, SW)

◆ Assess any significant losses, whether in the recent past or unresolved losses from the more remote past. (RN, LPN, SW)

◆ Consider assessing using Rosenberg Self-Esteem Scale (see References) or Depression Scales (see Diagnosis Section). (RN, LPN, SW)

◆ Note any loss of functional abilities or mental activity.
  ◆ Use OARS tool
  ◆ Use standardized Mental Acuity Questionnaire

◆ Include in care regime mastery over small tasks, breaking them into simplest tasks so that resident may feel satisfaction with successes and be motivated to continue. (RN, LPN, NA)

- ◆ continuity in care givers
- ◆ communicate to all shifts.
- ◆ Include in skills-building group that focuses on success in areas of former strengths. (RN, LPN, OT, RT)
- ◆ Encourage participation in activities that focus on mastery. (RT, RN, LPN)
  - ◆ build on skills that resident has intact, then move into areas of deficits, e.g. cognitive, emotional, social.
  - ◆ Include in reminiscence therapy groups or individual discussions if resident unable to tolerate groups.
- ◆ Include in pet therapy groups or have resident responsible for their own pet.
- ◆ Keep personal possessions and heirlooms in positions where resident can easily see them. Encourage staff to reminisce with resident using possessions as props, as springboards for discussion.
- ◆ Respect resident's right to privacy and territory. Encourage ancillary staff, e.g. housekeeping, not to move or change resident's possessions. (RN, LPN, NA)

DEFINING CHARACTERISTICS

Evaluates self as unable to deal with situations, events.

GOALS/OUTCOME CRITERIA

States they perceive mastery over life situations.

INTERVENTIONS

(see Powerlessness Section)

- ◆ Assess areas of perceived inability to control. (RN, LPN)
- ◆ Administer Rosenberg Self-Esteem Scale and OARS Scale to determine perception of self-esteem and areas of mastery/deficit. (RN, SW)
- ◆ Interview family or significant others to determine resident's ability to handle affairs in community—validate with resident. (RN, SW)
- ◆ Determine if this has been a life pattern or is the result of a single or series of traumatic events, e.g. forced retirement, loss of spouse. (RN, LPN)
- ◆ Assist residents to structure daily routine so they have some predictability in their life. (RN, LPN, NA)
  - ◆ if needed, post schedule
  - ◆ keep reality cues such as clock and calendar available.

◆ Encourage mastery over simple tasks. (RN, LPN, NA)
  ◆ break complex tasks into fundamental areas
  ◆ have resident focus on one area of task at a time
  ◆ give constant feedback and recognition.
◆ Include in support or reminiscence group to receive cohort effect and sense of total life accomplishment. (RN, LPN, NA)
◆ Give realistic feedback to resident. (RN, LPN, NA)
◆ If resident has functional deficit, refer to Rehabilitation Nurse clinical for evaluation. (RN)
◆ Assess any environmental or community forces that may be exerting additional pressure on resident. (RN, SW)
  ◆ living in walk-up building
  ◆ having difficulty obtaining health care for self or significant other
  ◆ unable to obtain economic support as planned
  ◆ unable to visit family or friends
  ◆ consider involvement in intergenerational program, e.g. Foster Grandparents or volunteer programs, such as Retired Senior Volunteer Program (RSVP), as avenue to develop social support and increased feeling of worth.

References

Anderson, A. and Sivesand, B. Assessment and intervention with depressed elderly. In Roger, C. and Lanen, J. *Nursing Interventions in Depression.* Orlando: Grune and Stratton, Inc.; 1985; 195–216.
Clearly stated guidelines for assessing the elderly resident, focusing on developing a therapeutic relationship. Various treatment modalities outlined.

Bauer, Barbara B. and Hill, Signe S. *Essentials of Mental Health Care-Planning and Intervention.* Philadelphia: W.B. Saunders; 1986.
A useful reference in planning the care of the client with a mental illness. Focusing on the nursing process throughout, it details care giving for a variety of client needs.

Bhala, Ram P. O'Donnell, John and Thoppil, Ephrem. Ptophobia: Phobic fear of falling and its clinical management. In *Physical Therapy.* February 1982; 62:187–190.
Case study and management format of six patients who developed an intense fear of falling. Differentiates agoraphobia (fear of open spaces/crowds) and ptophobia.

Blau, David. Depression and the elderly: A psychoanalytic perspective. In Breslau, Lawrence and Haug, Marie. *Depression and Aging.* New York: Springer Publishing Co.; 1983; 75–94.
General theories of depression are explored in light of psychoanalytic theory. Case studies included.

Butler, Robert. The life review: An interpretation of reminiscence in the aged. In *Psychiatry.* 1963; 26:65–76.

The classic article defining life review as a valuable intervention and model in working with the elderly, especially the depressed and those with low self-esteem.

Butler, Robert N. and Lewis, Myrna I. *Aging and Mental Health.* 3rd edition. St. Louis: C.V. Mosby Company; 1982.
A classic work outlining the psychosocial needs and changes associated with aging. Authors advocate against ageism and all the stereotypes that foster dependency for the elderly. Includes an excellent appendix section with referral agencies and literature.

Cadoret, RJ and Widmer, RB. The development of depressive symptoms in elderly following onset of severe physical illness. In *Journal of Family Practice.* January 1988; 27:71–76.
Predictors of depression among a group of elderly institutionalized patients was determined. Original research focussing on illness and stressful life events.

Chenitz, WC, Stone, JT, and Salisbury, SA. *Clinical Gerontological Nursing: A Guide to Advanced Practice.* Philadelphia: W.B. Saunders, 1991.
Excellent guide for the GNP or CNS for management of major clinical problems including depression, alcoholism, dementia/delirium, medication, and behavioral problems.

Costen, Joseph J. *Abuse of the Elderly: A Guide to Resources and Services.* Lexington, Mass.: Lexington Books; 1984.
An excellent resource citing demographics, legalities, and trends. Analysis of several state's approaches to the problem of abuse. There is a lengthy appendix including state by state referral agencies and resources.

Cusack, Odean and Smith, Elaine. *Pets and the Elderly: The Therapeutic Bond.* New York: Haworth Press; 1984.
Worthwhile book devoted to the use of pets in developing therapeutic programs with elderly persons both in institutions and in the community.

de la Cruz, Lourdes. On loneliness and the elderly. In *Journal of Gerontological Nursing.* November 1986; 12:22–27.
A humanistic approach to the problem of loneliness and its contribution to powerlessness in the long-term care setting. Dynamic of factors explored.

Dernham, Pamela. Phantom limb pain. In *Geriatric Nursing.* January–February 1986; 34–37.
An interesting article explaining the phenomenon of phantom limb syndrome and pain. Nursing interventions for dealing with pain are outlined as well as those at risk.

Dreyfus, JK. Depression assessment and interventions in the medically frail elderly. *Journal of Gerontological Nursing.* September 1988; 14:27–36.
Article highlights the differential diagnosis of depression among the aged. Nursing assessment techniques are stressed.

Dye, Celeste. *Assessment and Intervention in Geropsychiatric Nursing.* Orlando, Florida: Grune and Stratton; 1985.
This excellent book guides the reader through normal aging, assessment of mental/emotional problems in the older client, and a superior section on interventions. The chapter on Drug Therapy is one of the most useful in the literature.

Ebersole, Priscilla and Hess, Patricia. *Toward Healthy Aging: Human Needs and Nursing Responses.* St. Louis: C.V. Mosby; 1990.

Classic text outlining gerontological nursing. Holistic approach to client's problems. Body image disturbance is viewed as a dynamic process.

Ehrlich, P and Anetzberger, G. Survey of state public health departments procedures for reporting elder abuse. *Public Health Reports—Hyattsville.* February 1991; 106:151–154.
Exploratory study of state health departments to determine current reporting laws concerning elder abuse.

Fry, PS. *Depression, Stress, and Adaptations in the Elderly: Psychological Assessment and Intervention.* Rockville, MD: Aspen Publishing; 1986.
A most comprehensive guide to depression in the elderly. The author combined an extensive review of research and theorists to produce an excellent reference text.

Fry, PS. Development of a geriatric scale of hopelessness: Implications for counseling and intervention with depressed elderly. In *Journal of Counseling Psychology.* July 1984; 322–331.
Research into development of scale to establish link between hopelessness and depression. Interventions for clinicians cited.

Fulmer, Terry T. Mistreatment of elders: Assessment, diagnosis, and intervention. *Nursing Clinics of North America.* March 1989; 24:707–716.
Offers the reader insight into the problem of elder abuse and a framework in which the nursing process can be integrated. Highlights the possible problems that may result with changing demographics.

Fulmer, Terry and Wetle, Terrie. Elder abuse screening and intervention. In *The Nurse Practitioner.* May 1986; 11:33–39.
Excellent form for assessment of elder abuse included in this article. Discusses situations seen in the community.

Harris, Marilyn. Helping the person with an altered self-image. In *Geriatric Nursing.* March–April 1986; 7:90–92.
An article focused on planning care for the resident with an altered self-image. Author focuses on interventions, acceptance, and rejection.

Haycox, James A. A simple, reliable clinical behavioral scale for assessing demented patients. *Journal of Clinical Psychiatry.* 1984; 45:23–24.
This scale can be used with nonverbal patients for whom other mental status tests may be inappropriate. Nurses observations correlated well with assessments by families.

Herman, Steve. Anxiety disorders. In *Mental Health Assessment and Therapeutic Interventions with Older Adults.* Whanger, Alan D. and Meyers, Alice C. (eds) Rockville MD: Aspen Publications; 1984; 75–87
A very clear description of anxiety disorders in the elderly including origin, assessment, approaches, and a case history.

Hinchcliffe, Ronald E. *Hearing and Balance in the Elderly.* Edinburgh: Churchill-Livingstone; 1983.
Explores psychological and sociological facets of balance disorders. Establishes link between balance disorders and psychosomatic factors.

Holzapfel, Sally Kennedy. The importance of personal possessions in the lives of the institutionalized elderly. In *Journal of Gerontological Nursing.* March 1982; 8:156–158.
Using Roger's theoretical framework, the author advocates that the elderly should maintain their personal possessions.

Janelli, Linda. The realities of body image. In *Journal of Gerontological Nursing.* October 1986; 12:23–27.
An excellent article outlining the effects of changing body image on the elderly. Author compared three assessment tools to determine the most appropriate for the older client.

Klermack, David and Roff, Lucinda Lee. Fear of personal aging and subjective well-being in later life. In *Journal of Gerontology.* November 1984; 39:756–758.
Original research to examine the relationship among situational factors, fear of personal aging, and subjective well-being.

Klerman, G. Problems in definition and diagnosis of depression in the elderly. In Breslau, Lawrence and Hang, Marie. *Depression and Aging.* New York: Springer Publishing Company; 1983; 3–20.
A fine introduction to the demographics of depression, background, and problems in diagnosis.

Lang, NM, Kraegel, JM, Rantz, MJ, and Krejci, JW. *Quality of Health Care for Older People in America: A Review of Nursing Studies.* Kansas City: American Nurses' Association; 1990.
A review of salient nursing research addressing the issues of underuse, overuse, technical issues, and interventions in gerontological nursing. A useful tool for nurse researchers seeking an outstanding bibliography.

LaRocco, Susan A. A case of patient abuse. In *American Journal of Nursing.* November 1985; 85:1233–1234.
A first-person account of a nursing administrator's battle to terminate an abusive staff member.

Lesser, Jay, et al. Reminiscence group therapy with psychotic geriatric inpatients. In *Gerontologist.* June 1981; 21:291–296.
Original research comparing traditional group therapy and reminiscence therapy with residents. Helpful to clinician establishing a group.

McClure, John. The social parameters of learned helplessness: Its recognition and implications. In *Journal of Personality and Social Psychology.* June 1985; 48:1534–1539.
Interesting article regarding history of learned helplessness and locus of control. Implications for working with depressed clients.

Marks, Issac, and Bebbington, Paul. Space phobia: syndrome or agoraphobic variant. In *British Medical Journal.* August 1976; 7:345–347.
Early article proposing a link between inability to ambulate and a phobic disorder. A syndrome is outlined that relates to agoraphobia.

Mossey, Jana. Social and psychological factors related to falls among elderly. In *Clinics in Geriatric Medicine.* August 1985; 1:541–553.
Author does a retrospective review of the literature on research surrounding falls. Common variants are explored as they appear throughout articles. Suggestions are made for future research, especially in the areas of dementia and depression.

Murphy, John and Issac, Bernard. The post-fall syndrome. In *Gerontology.* 1982; 28:265–270.
Careful examination of factors that led to increased morbidity and mortality among fall victims. Table with relationship between syndrome and factors establishes possible causal links.

Nelson, PB. Social support, self-esteem, and depression in the institutionalized elderly. *Issues in Mental Health Nursing.* January 1989; 10:55–68.

Research focussed on elderly living within institutions determined that social support correlated significantly with depression. Nurses used three scales to measure depression and support.

Phillips, Linda. Elder abuse—What is it? Who says so? In *Geriatric Nursing.* May-June 1983; 4:167–170.
A most helpful guide to defining the problem of abuse, assessment, and the role of nurse as advocate. Very sound introduction to this topic.

Phillips, Linda R. and Rempusheski, Veronica, F. Caring for the frail elderly at home: Toward a theoretical explanation of dynamics of poor quality family caregiving. In *Advances in Nursing Science.* July 1986; 8:62–76.
Authors develop a theoretical framework based on nursing research on various types of care-giving relationships. Appendix to article illustrates each category of care giver and behaviors.

Pillemer, K and Moore, DW. Abuse of patients in nursing homes: Findings from a survey of staff. *Gerontologist.* 1989; 29:314–320.
Survey research presented on abuse within nursing homes. Staff self-reports are presented as well as subgroups of staff who are more likely to engage in abusive behavior.

Roberts, Sharon L. *Behavioral Concepts and Nursing Throughout the Life Span.* Englewood Cliffs, NJ: Prentice-Hall, Inc.; 1978.
The author devotes an entire chapter of this text to body image. Use of the impact, retreat, acknowledgment, and reconstruction model is a worthwhile nursing-based paradigm.

Rogers, Martha. *Theoretical Basis of Nursing.* Philadelphia: F.A. Davis Company; 1970.
Development of a theoretical basis of nursing based on Dr. Rogers' principles of a unified man. Positive view of aging for the gerontological nurse.

Rosenberg, M., Silbers, E., and Tippett, J. Self-esteem: Clinical assessment and measurement validation. In *Psychological Reports* 1965; 16:1017–1071.
Validated test of self-esteem used with elderly, disabled, and elderly-disabled.

Sampson, Edward and Marthas, Mary. *Group Process for the Health Professions.* 2nd edition. New York: John Wiley and Sons; 1981.
Helpful introduction to group work for the inexperienced in this area. Group dynamics clearly outlined.

Site, Jeanne, Craven, Ruth, and Bruno, Pauline. Late life depression: A guide for assessment. In *Journal of Gerontological Nursing.* November 1986; 12:4–10.
The gerontological nurse's point of view as both assessor and provider of care to the depressed elderly is clearly outlined. A good overview to the definition, theories, and various nursing assessments. Cognitive impairment of elderly resident explored, especially in area of family support and guidance. Contained in a sensitive nursing test focusing on psychogeriatric needs.

Thorabee, Marshelle and Anderson, Linda. Reporting elder abuse—It's the law. In *American Journal of Nursing.* April 1985; 85:371–374.
Legal terminology defined in various states in regard to reporting abuse. Excellent state-by-state chart of coverage, reporting, and investigation.

Tylor, Joyce. Mental status and dependency of the elderly: Helping families understand. In Hall, Beverly. *Mental Health and the Elderly.* Orlando: Grune and Stratton, Inc.; 1984; 145–165.

Verwoerdt, A. Anxiety, dissociative and personality disorders in the elderly. In *Handbook of Geriatric Psychiatry.* Busse, E.W. and Blazer, D.G. (eds) New York: Van Nostrand Rheinhold; 1980; 368–380.
A very thorough clinical examination of anxiety disorders in the older resident. This text is an excellent source for the nurse practitioner wishing to have a broad clinical reference.

Waller, M. and Griffin, M. Group therapy for depressed elders. In *Geriatric Nursing* October 1984.
Research conducted on effect of group therapy on depressed elders. Authors used scientific method to assess residents' progress in group. Original research.

Wernick, Mark and Manaster, Guy. Age and the perception of age and attractiveness. In *The Gerontologist* August 1984; 24:408–414.
Original research. Authors present an excellent article for nurse clinicians interested in the link between aging and attractiveness. Research is very clearly detailed.

Whall, Ann. Identifying the characteristics of pseudodementia. In *Journal of Gerontological Nursing* October 1986; 12:34–35.
A short but very clear article on the all too frequent misdiagnosis of dementia for residents who are actually depressed.

Wild, D., Nayak, USL., and Isaac, B. How dangerous are falls in old people at home? In *British Medical Journal* 1981; 282:266–268.
Relationship of acute and chronic illnesses and functional impairments to be incidence of morbidity in the home-bound elderly. Demographic data identified places at higher risk for increased mortality.

Yalom, Irwin. The Theory and Practice of Group Psychotherapy. New York: Basic Books, Inc.; 1975.
Classic text for the clinician wishing to do more advanced group work, especially with clients having special needs.

Yesavage, Jerome A. Depression in the elderly: How to recognize masked symptoms and choose appropriate therapy. *Postgraduate Medicine.* January 1992; 91:255–261.
Explains how to differentiate depression from dementia and describes a shortened version of the Yesavage Geriatric Depression Scale. Offers pharmacological treatment of geriatic depression.

11

Role Relationship Pattern

Mary Frances Madigan

◆

SOCIAL ISOLATION/REJECTION

Definition: A selected state of physical, emotional, or social withdrawal from others in response to perceived personal alterations in health of social status.

ASSESSMENT

Isolation infers the ability or choice to separate or cease interaction with persons, objects, or activities that are involved in the daily routine of life. This exercise of withdrawal from others implies a negative perceptual state of relationship in the family or community, for as human beings, the need for social communion, self validation, and recognition depends on consistent interplay with others.

Isolation need not always be construed as a singularly antagonistic event. As a personally selected time given to disassociate oneself from the routine of everyday tasks, to reflect, to ponder change, and to plan a new life design, it takes the form of solitude.

Social isolation, a societal phenomenon whose continuity is fostered by the health/economic events of a particular time in the life of the individual, is not a preferred interaction pattern. Here mobility restrictions or limited social/community contact exist. The elderly person is especially prone to non-selected isolation because of economic and health vulnerability. (Friedman, 1980)

Decreased social activity, the result of chronic isolation, blunts significant communication. Developed by the perception that one's social needs are curtailed, the result is a fragmented interaction mode, gradual disinterest in appearance, apathy in the opinions or comments of others. Once in place the "rude behavior" is not easily dislodged when the elderly person is placed in the company of others. Over time, previous socialization patterns prior to forced isolation will emerge with support and interest of the professional caregiver.

Behavioral patterns (i.e., hostile response to predominant cultural mores) indicating an individual's need to minimize meaningful interaction with others preclude isolation over long periods of time and reinforce the perception of rejection.

Isolation and rejection are co-existent behavioral states, interweaving individual actions of withdrawal from the dominant society one inhabits, rejecting its socially acceptable forms of expression in inappropriate verbalizations or action, (i.e. not bathing, wearing filthy clothes to workplace).

Isolation/rejection is, for some, expressed in the workplace as doing one's job, co-existing with many persons but having an absence of personal or intimate involvement other than to do the job and return to one's habitat without significant interpersonal involvement. There is usually no evidence of mental illness.

This pattern can continue for a lifetime, its predictability upset by illness or other social/economic incapacity.

Elderly persons displaying isolate interaction style require individual nursing care assessments to determine their accessibility and ability to participate in unity activity without anxiety.

AGE-RELATED PHENOMENON

A lifetime of social interaction patterns whose chief feature is isolation or rejection is not altered in the later life span. Entrenched in a pattern or belief system that trust or concern for others inflicts pain, the potential of alteration or loss of certain factors (i.e. biological, psychological, environmental) in the elderly years is perceived as further instances of a need to maintain the isolate stance—minimal interaction with others.

Social Isolation/Rejection is the preferred social mode.

A serious illness or economic crisis usurps the carefully constructed world of the lifetime social isolate. Attempts will be made to continue the security of a contained environment. The inability to stave off outside social involvement (i.e. non-payment of rent, injury/hospitalization) increases the long-term isolate need to utilize earlier distancing coping mechanisms (i.e. verbal insult, withdrawal).

In the event of a short-term crisis, the elderly isolate may exhibit tangential signs of cooperation (i.e. bathing, sitting quietly) in care. Conversations limited to health/economic planning will be met with resistance (i.e. indifference) if they do not mesh with previous concepts of problem-solving skills. (Magilvy, 1988)

The pattern of resistance escalates if treatment is prolonged or nursing home care is indicated.

Self-containment, a lack of interest in the life of others, a sadness pattern of indifferent social exchanges are indications of social isolation/rejection having its roots in selected interaction modes over a lifetime. Social isolation behavior may be imposed on the elderly client as the result of illness, fear of the environment/reduced mobility, or decreased social sensitivity and often may be the result of long-term isolation. The latter two nursing diagnoses are the result of the elderly person's social health factors that have altered former interaction patterns. The social/rejection behavioral pattern—a life-long development style. (Morrison, 1990)

ETIOLOGIES

EXTERNAL

SITUATIONAL CRISIS: Environmental accident; economic loss; insufficient community resources in social/educational activity; crime in neighborhood.

MATURATIONAL CRISIS: Retirement lessened social contact; health impairs mobility; children unavailable.

PERSONAL VULNERABILITY: Inability to defend personal self/belongings; potential for rejection in new environment.

KNOWLEDGE DEFICIT: Cognitive structure prepares for rejection; isolation disturbs ability to differentiate real vs. imagined threat.

PERCEIVED LOSS OF CONTROL: Health/socio-economic vulnerability given "outsider" control over life events.

INTERNAL

SITUATIONAL CRISIS: Need to restructure familiar role preparation for outcast class; reaction (i.e. anger-guilt); evolution of dependency needs that won't be met (individual perception).

MATURATIONAL CRISIS: Age-related health problems—change in body image, fear of rejection, inhibition of new social contacts.

PERSONAL VULNERABILITY: Resurrection of fears of rejection.

KNOWLEDGE DEFICIT: Intellectual capability diminished—lack of stimuli, verbalization thwarted—temporary if no organicity.

PERCEIVED LOSS OF CONTROL: Interaction with others no longer controlled by client (i.e. time, place, duration).

◆ Nursing Diagnosis

Social Isolation or Social Rejection.

DEFINING CHARACTERISTICS

- ◆ Inadequate social interaction diminishes self-fulfillment criteria
- ◆ Decreased social sensitivity (i.e. lack of interst in maintaining accepted social amenities)
- ◆ Expresses feelings of aloneness imposed by others/rejection or feelings of difference from others
- ◆ Perceived inability to meet expectations of others or insecurity in public
- ◆ Perceived inadequacy of significant purpose in life or absence of purpose in life
- ◆ Observed or expressed interest/activities inappropriate to developmental age/stage

- Express values acceptable to subculture but unacceptable to dominant cultural group
- Shows behavior unaccepted by dominant cultural group
- Seeks to be alone or exist in subculture
- Sad, dull affect
- Uncommunicative, withdrawn—no eye contact
- Projects in voice, behavior
- Preoccupation with own thoughts, repetitive, meaningless actions
- Absence of supportive other(s)—family, friends, group
- Apathy
- Verbalization of isolation from others
- Low contact with peers
- Absence or limited contact with community
- Lack of contact in absence of significant others
- Seclusion.

GOALS

- Reduce anxiety of interaction process with others
- Identify permissible limits of isolation in health-care setting
- Establish initial, tentative patterns of interaction
- Discuss comfort level rules for interaction
- Maintain minimal comfort levels of interaction
- Devise plan to alert staff/others to breech of comfort index
- Evaluate ability to realistically increase social contact with others (i.e. mobility)
- Determine extent of comfortable interaction
- Work with family/staff to coordinate potential change/increase in social options
- Learn available options to seek out community help networks (i.e. church, telephone, visitors, Office of Aging)
- Select personal guidelines for individual group involvement (i.e. stress reduction, fear of rejection)
- Determine occurrence of specific behavioral changes
- Assess impact of behavior on social systems
- Identify physical/social inhibitors to social contacts
- Coordinate assessment review with potential community resources/ unit resources
- Initiate self-proposed beginning steps—plan for change.

INTERVENTIONS

◆ Observe present behavioral patterns that thwart elderly clients' unit adaptation (RN/LPN)

◆ Utilize community resources/unit resources to identify previous behavioral patterns (RN, LPN)

◆ Construct atmosphere of purposeful interest in daily routine in initial contacts; review boundaries of care (RN/LPN/NA)

◆ Increase amount of client-professional contact as client's comfort level indicates; evaluate territorial boundary for anxiety (i.e. restless-shifting) (RN/LPN/NA)

◆ Re-evaluate after one week: a. territorial comfort, b. verbal interaction, c. time-quality of social interaction, d. ability to relate to others (RN/LPN/NA)

◆ Reinstitute previous care plan if no change observed, or increased withdrawal, hostility (RN/LPN)

◆ Consult with psychogeriatric nurse clinician team for further guidelines (RN/LPN)

◆ If progress noted, continue interview times for maximum of 30 min/day

◆ Discuss with client interest in unit activities

◆ Utilize services of activity therapist to identify available/applicable individual interest in games, walk, etc.

◆ As client comfort signals indicate, discuss feasibility of increased involvement with others

◆ As client comfort signals indicate, discuss future plan of health care and ability to become involved in it (RN/LPN)

◆ Utilize present information system (i.e. family/staff/social services) to identify health/social factors relating to isolation (RN/LPN)

◆ Introduce client to new social contacts (if care residence) (RN/LPN/NA)

◆ Negotiate with client 20 minute interview—set time, place for daily one-to-one interview (RN/LPN/NA)

◆ Create interview climate of concern (i.e. active listening—observation, non-verbal cues) (RN/LPN/NA)

◆ Organize interview construct about client present concerns of ability to interact with others (i.e. evaluate current perceptions of real life activities and ability to participate) (RN/LPN/NA)

◆ Identify with client past success in social interactions and where and why change occurred (RN/LPN/NA)

◆ Reinforce concept of success—determine with client realistic potential to initiate minimal social change in environment/social interaction (RN/LPN)

♦ Encourage client recognition of potential resources to alleviate isolation (RN/LPN)

♦ Participate in initial client requests for social participation in activities (as time allows) (RN/LPN/NA)

♦ Review client social progress with client and staff in areas concerning health modification, environmental constrictions (RN/LPN/NA)

♦ Coordinate planning effort to reestablish social links with family/ community via available resources (RN/LPN).

DYSFUNCTIONAL GRIEVING

Definition: Inability to resolve emotional loss of a significant other/object beyond socially defined norms for grieving process.

ASSESSMENT

Grief as defined in western culture is a subjective feeling that finds expression in a sense of "deep and poignant distress." An individual's need to grieve over the loss or perceived loss of a valued companion and the termination of the pleasure and security insured in the relationship is acknowledged in all societies. In the United States, confirmation of grief as an expression of loss generally extends from the time of death to the day of the funeral service and burial. Most of the open grief work is accomplished at this time. This sorrow, which others are allowed to witness, is expected to be completed as quickly as possible so the survivors can get on with the task of living. Private expressions of grief after this time are expressed covertly in the home, perhaps among the companionship of intimate friends and relatives.

Most religious denominations that are part of the American society have prescribed traditional rituals recognizing the importance of the need to grieve. Essentially time, support of others, and individual reaction to loss comprise the grieving experience. Jewish tradition recognizes certain time frames and personal involvement in the grieving process. Christian time-frame rituals are less clearly defined. Eighteen to twenty-four months is theorized as a rough estimate for the completion of the grieving process but is not applicable to all persons.

The physical and emotional expressions of loss are as varied as the individual experiencing them. High on the list of life stress activators is the death of a spouse. The resultant physical and emotional manifestations of stress comprise a list of over one hundred signs and symptoms that have been observed by many nursing practitioners.

Prolonged or dysfunctional grieving patterns are the province of all age groups. The ability of the elderly person to adapt to the death of a loved one is no less stressful than for younger adults. This adaptation to grieving may be altered if past grieving patterns have been dysfunctional—also, if social support systems are not available to console and comfort and if there is the physical potential of increased cerebral degeneration coupled with minimal life stressors (i.e. new table assignment, new mailperson).

Dysfunctional grieving patterns in the elderly can be assessed through the knowledge of previous behavior in reaction to stress. Some altered grieving patterns begin shortly after a loved one's death. Refusing to eat, visiting the gravesite for long periods in inclement weather, refusing to alert family or authorities to death of loved one, refusing to leave gravesite at closing time or denying the death long after the event are key signals of dysfunctional grieving. Continued persistence in these or development of other patterns incongruent with normal cultural grieving patterns necessitates assessment and restructuring of the nursing care plan.

AGE-RELATED PHENOMENON

Persons over 65 satisfied with the life they have lived interweave the loss of a loved one into a revised pattern of life activity. Loss, or the anticipated loss, of a loved one does not diminish the intensity of the emotional experience. Past coping mechanisms obviate the re-learning of familiar grieving methods if present ones are no longer acceptable.

An elderly person whose self-belief system reflects a lack of fulfillment views the loss of a loved one as further proof of inability to exert life destiny. The impact of the aging process reinforces feelings of despair, hopelessness and helplessness in preventing or changing the state of loss.

The need to establish a sense of control over loss precipitates for some the use of the defense mechanism of denial (of the death), emotional escape via a delusional or psychotic state. (McFarland, 1986)

For others, the socially accepted period of grieving (18–24 months) extends in varying forms of intensity. The usual social patterns of family life are focused on edification of the deceased and maintenance of a lifestyle revolving about the deceased's memory.

Dysfunctional grieving occurs in all areas/stages of life. It is important to recognize the importance of cultural mores in the expression of grief. In the United States, culturally assigned grieving tasks may take precedence over general social expectations.

ETIOLOGIES

EXTERNAL

SITUATIONAL CRISIS: Inability to participate in funeral/burial service; inadequate social outlets for grief, i.e. crying in public; isolation from family/friends.

MATURATIONAL CRISIS: Physical incapabilities narrow ability to participate in funeral arrangements; social networks diminished due to illness; mobility.

PERSONAL VULNERABILITY: Cultural expectations may be inhibited due to illness, i.e. going to gravesite wearing black, armband.

KNOWLEDGE DEFICIT: See Anticipatory Grieving.

PERCEIVED LOSS OF CONTROL: See Anticipatory Grieving.

INTERNAL

SITUATIONAL CRISIS: Belief that feelings of anger, abandonment by loved one need to be contained, containing need to weep, wail, guilt over feelings of anger.

MATURATIONAL CRISIS: Recurrent sense of failure to direct life path.

PERSONAL VULNERABILITY: Loneliness of survivor, constant feelings of abandonment.

KNOWLEDGE DEFICIT: Intellectual functioning-ability stabilized but perception of ability to create new life role without loved one and need to recreate life in old way maintained.

PERCEIVED LOSS OF CONTROL: Perceive life as being manageable with edification of deceased.

◆ Nursing Diagnosis

Dysfunctional Grieving

DEFINING CHARACTERISTICS

- ◆ Verbal expression of distress at loss
- ◆ Denial of loss
- ◆ Expression of guilt
- ◆ Expression of unresolved issues
- ◆ Anger
- ◆ Sadness
- ◆ Crying
- ◆ Difficulty in expressing loss
- ◆ Alterations in eating habits
- ◆ Alterations in sleep or dream patterns
- ◆ Alterations in activity, work, or socialization
- ◆ Altered libido
- ◆ Idealization of lost object
- ◆ Reliving past experiences
- ◆ Interference with life
- ◆ Developmental regression
- ◆ Labile affect
- ◆ Alteration in concentration and in pursuits of tasks
- ◆ Continued indicators of grieving beyond expected time.

GOALS

- ◆ Reduction of symptoms causing social malfunction
- ◆ Reduction of potential life threatening grief behaviors, (i.e. anorexia)

◆ Recognize individual need to express grief in own manner
◆ Work with caregiver to establish ability to express fears, concerns, about life change
◆ Recognize ability to set up individual plan for daily activities, (i.e. social, on gradually accelerated scale)
◆ Confirm importance of lost loved one in life, renegotiate social input
◆ Research availability of other social supports to assist in solution of grief
◆ Identify with caregiver need for further professional care if denial/ extended grief patterns persist.

INTERVENTIONS

◆ Coordinate physical health regime with ancillary staff, to improve eating/sleeping patterns, identify potential for possible organic impairment (RN)
◆ Create specific time frame/place each day for discussion of client concerns, i.e. inability to eat/social isolation (RN/LPN/NA)
◆ Active listening/observation to discern client involvement with continued grieving pattern, nonverbal cries, i.e. sad, slumped body language, angry stare (RN/LPN/NA)
◆ Allow client time to discuss implications of loss in life role, ventilate emotions constructively (i.e. verbalize, exercise, beat pillow) (RN/ LPN/NA)
◆ Integrate concept of reality testing, use of "I" experience, empathize concern (RN/LPN)
◆ Utilize discussion time to formulate with client impact of role loss (potential methods of adaptation, select one area) (RN/LPN)
◆ Select with client possible resources in home/unit/community to assist in adaptation to loss resolution (RN/LPN)
◆ Increase level of activity/socialization as client indicates ability to tolerate (RN/LPN/NA)
◆ If delusional content: avoid direct confrontation of delusion, use of "I" reality (RN)
◆ Refer to psychogeriatric nurse clinician for further evaluation (RN).

ANTICIPATORY GRIEVING

Definition: Expectation of disruption in familiar pattern of significant relationships. Anticipated alteration in familiar life routine due to changes in health, economics of self or significant others. Initiates a pattern of loss preparedness, restructuring of self-concept in relation to societal expectations.

ASSESSMENT

Sudden loss of a loved one/object confronts the bereaved with the reality that a valued, comforting relationship has been terminated by death. The emotional content interlaced with the recognition of the finality of death initiates a life event known as the grieving process. (Kubler-Ross, 1975)

The components of this crisis involve preparation for the ceremony of burial; verbal and physical manifestations of grief (i.e. crying, wailing) as appropriate and encouraged in most cultures as a means of ameliorating the loss. (Eberle, 1976)

The support of family and friends during the initial stage of loss includes verbal expressions of sympathy, emotional and social companionship. The resultant loss of the familiar role of wife, mother, or friend survivor and the social accommodation to a new one is difficult for many but physical death is tangible, concrete, and irrevocable.

The expectation of loss places the individual on a less clearly defined path of resolution and support. It initiates a sense of foreboding precipitated by sudden or gradual change in one's own health, social or environmental state or in a spouse, family member, friend, or caretaker.

Whatever the cause, the perception of potential loss presents a threat to the self-concept nurtured by one's status in a role over most of a lifetime in a particular society. (McConnell, 1990)

Anticipatory grieving restrains over-expression of grief that is not yet an event but the individual interpretation of a possible happening. One's sense of security and love is threatened. Initially it takes the form of decreased interest in valued social activity, minor alteration of eating and sleeping patterns, or difficulties in concentration on complex tasks. Verbalizations of anger or frustration not related to the identified person or objects are expressed. Crying, regressive behavior may be sporadic or increase over time if the feeling engendered by the anticipated loss is not resolved.

Older persons reflect societal expectations set in another historical or economic context that taught the importance of a stoic mien in the face of personal loss (i.e. the Depression, World War II). They believe they will "survive about like they always did" or deny true feelings in an attempt to "act graciously" and obtain the approval that is otherwise denied them. The call for help for a non-event is believed to be unnecessary or leads to self-chastisement for inability to handle one's own affairs.

In the long-term care facility, care plans, extensive intake record, patient care coordination (i.e. family, staff), familiarity with the social system of each elderly client, observation of coping behaviors facilitate the process of identifying the process of behavioral change.

The following factors contain the essential components influencing human behavior per Roy's Adaptation Model, and are presented to assist and guide the formulation of nursing care plans designed to attend to the complex and individual needs of each elderly client. Roy's Model identifies four factors: biological, psychological, environmental, and metaphysical.

Each factor, important to personal growth and development at whatever life stage, is also unique to the individual construct of self and place in society. The factors described interact continually, consistently, and cooperatively assisting individual accommodation to a perceived life transit.

AGE-RELATED PHENOMENON

Elderly persons understand and accept "life's turning points" and the inevitable patterns of loss/change. The unanticipated time event can become a stressor, such as early retirement or recognition of need to live in a long-term care facility. Preparation for these events can become stressful for many even though they are recognized as a fortuitous solution to a current health or social problem.

The gaining of a new role, such as retiree or nursing home resident, does not eliminate the recognition that such a gain engenders certain losses and privileges that were part of the old role, i.e. economic means, autonomy. (McConnell, 1990)

The patterns of readiness come into play as they have so many times before, hopefully to augment the emotional pain. Age, present health status, social support systems, each factor influencing the ability of the elderly person to prepare for what is his or her individual perception of change.

The 65-year-old having fair health, mobility, and an active social network of support may resolve the anticipation of loss through verbal interactions with peers and family.

The older debilitated individual, whose social system network is minimal and whose mobility is impaired, will react to anticipated change according to past patterns of behavior that are not easily recognized as anticipatory grieving (i.e. gradual disinterest in food, unit activities, sadness). This behavior can be precipitated by anticipation of the loss of a favored staff member, change of roommate, change in environmental setting.

It is important for professional staff caring for the frail elderly client to recognize that cultural mores of past times promoted the concept of "keeping your problems to yourself." Elderly clients who have lived in those times often attempt to hide the emotional content of anticipated change behind the facade of acceptance. (Kasch, 1986)

ETIOLOGIES

EXTERNAL

SITUATIONAL CRISIS: Illness of spouse, family member, friend, staff member, caretaker, favorite pet; pending transfer of roommate, family member, staff member caretaker.

MATURATIONAL CRISIS: From 65–75, lessened economic autonomy, decreased control over children, health relationship to mobility, ability to create/continue to expand social network; from 75–85, health and economic autonomy continue to lessen, decreased mobility, decreased sociability if health/economic problems; 85+, continued decrease in ability to create/continue to expand social networks.

PERSONAL VULNERABILITY: Decreased social/family contacts.

KNOWLEDGE DEFICIT: Anxiety clouds ability to objectively assess current perception of anticipated loss.

PERCEIVED LOSS OF CONTROL: Enforced sense of loss of autonomy.

INTERNAL

SITUATIONAL CRISIS: Anticipated role change; loss of significant other/s; loss of individual status in relationship to others.

MATURATIONAL CRISIS: Pending loss affect on ability to control destiny declining with physical deterioration/lessened social contact; gradual increase in dependency needs; lessened control over personal habits.

PERSONAL VULNERABILITY: Ability to judge, make decision, learning impeded by individual anxiety level.

KNOWLEDGE DEFICIT: Intelligence affected emotional content, sensory decrease.

PERCEIVED LOSS OF CONTROL: Impending fears may be realized.

DEFINING CHARACTERISTICS

◆ Potential loss of significant object
◆ Verbal expression of distress at potential (anticipated loss)
◆ Anger
◆ Sadness, sorrow, crying
◆ Crying at frequent intervals
◆ Change in eating habits
◆ Alteration in sleep or dream patterns
◆ Alteration in activity
◆ Altered libido
◆ Idealization of anticipated loss
◆ Development regression
◆ Alteration of concentration in pursuit of tasks.

GOALS

◆ Identify concern about pending loss of significant other; discuss impact of a pending change; establish sense of control over loss perceived; implement plan of role resolution via family friend/staff support networks.

INTERVENTIONS

◆ Observe present behavioral changes (RN, LPN, NA)
◆ Review possibility of physical determinants (RN, LPN)
◆ Medication change, social change in home (RN/LPN)
◆ Increase time spent discussing recent life event (LPN/NA)

◆ Active listening to health care concern—change in personal health, change in unit assignment, family change (health, mobility), non-verbal clue—nodding, sitting, staring into space, reduced verbal interaction, reduced social involvement, all reflect patient concern over present pending changes (RN/LPN)

◆ Discuss with client perspective about eventual change event may have on life activities—has this type of situation ever happened before, explore methods of solving concerns about perceived potential of role—loss in past (RN/LPN)

◆ Plan methods of resolution that are realistic and within scope of family/staff participation (RN/LPN).

ALTERATION IN FAMILY PROCESS

Definition: Inability of family system (household members) to meet needs of members, carry out family functions, or maintain communications for mutual growth and maturation.

ASSESSMENT

Family life cycles begin with a couple's establishment of a home. As individuals, they come to the union with personally defined concepts about family process expectations (i.e. methods of communication, ability to resolve differences, child rearing, and individual responsibility). Within the family unit, the partners seek to establish a sense of mutuality, family enrichment, compatibility, and enjoyment that coalesce into a pattern of interaction that is unique to each family. (McConnell, 1988)

The communication patterns between parents and children during the child rearing years cultivate a complex set of rules about issues that are openly discussed and those that remain covert in nature. The boundaries governing the expression of thought and feelings are firmly implanted. Most members adhere to the rules, those who refuse will eventually leave to design a life style allowing for minimal interaction with other family members or their presence will continue to inject a sense of disharmony at family gatherings.

Problem-solving skills may involve one or more children as an ally with one or both partners. Usually one child, because of proximity, age, or ease of relationship with parents is selected as interpreter or co-implementer of family decisions.

The reason for the selection of certain family members to carry out selected tasks remains obscure. However, once chosen, the individual's status within the family remains unless the person rejects it by complicity, absence at family gatherings, or a move to a distant locale.

Death or divorce in the post-parental family often unites the family to assist either elderly parent in renegotiating a new life role. Adult children may help their parents as demonstrated through verbal expressions, family visits, and/or phone calls.

Disruption in the health of the parent, economic setback, or the need of the parent or child to relocate may initiate a crisis in each family structure. Availability of children to visit provides economic and health-related assistance and extends the independence of older parent. Again a selected child/adult, usually a daughter, often initiates the change process, enhances its continuity with verbal and economic support from other siblings.

Alterations in the family interaction patterns may emerge if the selected caretaker moves away or becomes ill. If the parent's health worsens, necessitating home health care or placement in a long-term care facility, the selected family member must take on additional responsibilities. These will include presenting the decision for home care/nursing home placement to the parent; selecting the eventual location; and researching availability of services and negotiating the placement.

Even in the family with clearly defined lines of communication, the task may become difficult. In a family whose decision-making process was guided by the now low-functioning or resistant parent, a search for resolution becomes bogged down in the avoidance of any one member taking responsibility for determining the parent's destiny. The problem is seen in community service institutions responsible for the care of its inhabitants. It is expressed through denial of a problem, a sense of being overwhelmed by its presence, anger at the parent or caregiver by one or more members of the family.

AGE-RELATED PHENOMENON

An elderly person progresses through the later stages of the family life development cycle (65 + years) accepting the role of parent, abiding by its expectations, until familial social or economic reversal or change.

The inferred role of parent remains, but the status begins to crumble as the parent because of deteriorating health is no longer able to care for himself or herself, but instead must seek care from significant others. (Baum, CM, 1991)

The child or children, long in the role status of child, now must confront the issue of role-reversal, assuming the role of parent while maintaining the title and status of adult child.

This switching of roles, during the later stages of the parent's life and the mid-adult years of the child, creates a blurred, diffuse, and confused sense of family member identity.

The parental role/status reversal engenders a sense of loss for both parent and child. Conflicting needs to maintain the pattern against the realities of parental dependency/welfare often have a ripple effect on the original family siblings, the child's adult spouse and children.

The need for long-term care in the home or in a residential setting involves decision-making skills and preparation via contact with community resources. (Hayes, A, 1988)

Resolution of each of these areas of need necessitates family member participation if the problem of placement/care is to be resolved.

Communication of need, one's role/status in the family, the parental ability to make decisions with or without the children will now test the boundaries of family problem-solving skills. (Davies, H, 1991)

Previous family interaction, mannerisms, involvement/distancing, selection/avoidance, and resolution/non-resolution methods will once again surface as members strive to cope with an unfamiliar family situation.

ETIOLOGIES

EXTERNAL

SITUATIONAL CRISIS: Disruption of home routine of parent/child; child caretaker unable to continue role—economic/emotional depletion; lack of safety devices for elderly persons.

MATURATIONAL CRISIS: Parent health vulnerability; adult child assigned to caretaker role; adult children unable to assume parental care.

PERSONAL VULNERABILITY: Economic; health needs increase with age; resources to cope diminish; helpless to change or reverse; dependency on family members.

KNOWLEDGE DEFICIT: Cognitive structure based on social system that encourages independence.

PERCEIVED LOSS OF CONTROL: Intrusion of significant others into personal, private aspects of life (i.e. money management, time allotment).

INTERNAL

SITUATIONAL CRISIS: Deprivation of routine of social system; role ambiguity, grief/anticipatory grief over loss of personal space/privacy; intrusion into personal lives of children, guilt/anger.

MATURATIONAL CRISIS: Perceived need to adapt from mother to grandmother, matriarch/patriarch to retiree/nursing home resident; adult child caught in squeeze of parenting own family and parental family.

PERSONAL VULNERABILITY: Loss of roles is perceived as end of usefulness, productivity, beginning of increased dependency; adult child experiences loss of autonomy to care for patient; negotiate family reaction to crisis to acceptable levels of assistance.

KNOWLEDGE DEFICIT: Ability (in absence of organicity) to integrate dimension of problem; anxiety; depression over loss of control deters competency to resolve.

PERCEIVED LOSS OF CONTROL: Parental role-status in jeopardy; life situation managed by adult child(ren).

DEFINING CHARACTERISTICS

◆ Inability of family members to relate to each other for natural growth and maturation

◆ Failure to send and receive clear messages

- ◆ Poorly communicated family rules, rituals, symbols, unexamined myths
- ◆ Unhealthy family decision-making processes
- ◆ Inability of family member to express and accept wide range of feelings
- ◆ Inability to accept and receive help
- ◆ Does not demonstrate respect for individuality and autonomy of members
- ◆ Rigidity in function and roles
- ◆ Failure to accomplish current (or past) family developmental tasks
- ◆ Inappropriate, non-productive boundary maintenance
- ◆ Inability to adapt to change
- ◆ Inability to deal with trauma or crisis experience constructively
- ◆ Parents do not demonstrate respect for each other's views on child-rearing practices
- ◆ Inappropriate, non-productive level and direction of energy
- ◆ Inability to meet member needs (i.e. physical, emotional, security, spiritual)
- ◆ Family not involved in community activities.

GOALS

- ◆ Identification of compatible family communication system
- ◆ Ascertaining availability of member willingness to assume responsibility for delegated tasks of parent care
- ◆ Coordinating family members with parent-responsible adult-child perception of needs/realistic response
- ◆ Assigned family member will initiate immediate care plan
- ◆ Family members will identify ability to assist in initial transition of parental care plan
- ◆ Family members willing to identify community resources available to assist in care plan process
- ◆ Decision for placement will involve all family members.

INTERVENTIONS

- ◆ Identify patterns of family problem solving skills, via family visit, observations of other professionals involved in care (RN/LPN)
- ◆ Assess client parent perception of family capabilities in regard to care (RN/LPN)
- ◆ Facilitate family understanding of health concern via counseling/interview time—focus on immediate problems (RN)
- ◆ Discuss family potential methods of resolution (i.e. focus on *one* concern) (RN)

- ◆ Assess family ability/inability to resolve assigned task to date (i.e. issue of nursing home selection) (RN)
- ◆ Work with family in identification of inter/intra communications that cause stress (RN)
- ◆ Discuss with client/family crisis coping skill of past (RN)
- ◆ Work with family to identify potential strategies to resolve present placement in other crisis strategies (RN)
- ◆ Identify with client/family, what they wish to resolve (care for parent), who are family members willing to take on task, how individual family members could assist in resolution, how effort to resolve issue will be coordinated (RN)
- ◆ Encourage positive family efforts at resolution (RN)
- ◆ Explore with family availability of social networks outside of family structure to aid in resolution (i.e. church, friends, social service) (RN)
- ◆ If inability to resolve family decision—family tension—refer to specially trained nurse clinician/social worker, etc. (RN)

IMPAIRED VERBAL COMMUNICATION

Definition: Reduced or absent ability to use language in human interaction.

ASSESSMENT

The means through which the human mind experiences the world, both outside and inside the body, is accomplished through the functioning of the five senses. Each sense organ is charged with the task of picking up information concerning the environment and passing it along to the brain, which channels, organizes, and interprets the input.

At each level of human development, individual perceptions of the world are influenced by the ability to discern between important and irrelevant data. Mental functioning, the ability to perform psychomotor tasks, relies on information channeled through the nervous system. The initial step to resolution of the simplest task begins with sensory awareness.

Sensory experience and its eventual interpretation is unique to the individual. Time, life experience, emotional and cognitive facility cooperate in assisting each person's interpretation of the world about them. The aging process affects the acuity.

Vision reaches high degrees of performance in the 20's, beginning its decline after the 40th year. By the sixth and seventh decade, few people have normal vision.

The hearing sense has been influenced by modern technology in the form of machines and radio/television. It is believed to assist in the loss of certain high-pitched sounds early in the second decade of life. In later life both low-pitched and high-pitched sounds are more difficult to hear. People who have worked in manufacturing trades may experience this earlier.

Other senses such as the ability to taste qualities (i.e. sweet, sour, bitter, and salt) diminish in acuity after the fifth decade. There is a paucity of research on changes in the sense of smell as an individual progresses through the life cycle. The sense of touch, the ability to feel pain, vibrations are highly receptive to change until mid-life. There is some diminution of pain threshold as an individual ages. The need for comforting touch is pertinent to the sense of security, acceptance, and other non-verbal forms of caring.

The ability to verbalize the interpreted data in a rational and coherent form is the dynamic link between the person and the society. The complex functioning of the human mind encompasses our ability to learn, memorize, problem solve, and define emotional content attached to the perceptual process. The partial or complete cessation of speaking creates a social void in the interaction process. Inability to communicate our thoughts and concerns interrupts the familiar and comforting routine of social communion, creating the potential for social withdrawal and eventual isolation.

Research statistics note that persons over 65 have a higher propensity for verbal incapacity due to dementia. (Shapira et al. 1986) The authors note that within the dementia syndrome, "two patterns of mental deterioration reflect disruption of two general areas of the brain."

In either diagnostic category, the ability to verbalize and communicate effectively at some stage of either condition becomes inhibited. The potential for withdrawal, depression predominates. Nursing intervention based on the ability to crystallize the predominating symptomatology will involve listening, observation, and coordination of the staff efforts to determine an accurate diagnosis.

AGE-RELATED PHENOMENON

Youth does not guarantee immunity to the development of verbal impairment and the ability to communicate with the world outside the self.

Aphasia, temporary speech disorder patterns due to organic brain syndrome (i.e. fever, chemical/drug toxicity) and functional psychiatric illness, impede the young adult's ability to communicate.

The physical alterations found in the aging process and their effect on the five senses incur some dysfunction in communication. Adaptation takes place over time via the use of hearing aids, glasses, or the use of spicy food. Verbal communication flow may be impeded by the elderly person's need to process sensory input at a slower pace, resulting in speech hesitance or groping for appropriate words. (Phillips, A, 1981)

The two most common forms of mental impairment with resultant distorted cognitive and speech impairment are multi-infarct and Alzheimer's disease, which occur primarily in persons over 65.

Breakdown in verbal communication varies in awareness of difficulty and presentation of acute symptoms.

The cortical vs subcortical dementias noted by Shapira et al. (1986) are aphasia and intellectual deterioration. The clinical signs manifested in subcortical dementia are ability to understand what is being said but having difficulty in speaking.

Inability to communicate verbally alters the interaction patterns of a lifetime. Compounded by the diminution of the sense and the need for treatment in a strange place, it can be anticipated that elderly persons will perceive this environment much differently than the staff caring for them. Deliberate attempts to analyze each client's verbal communication capacity will involve definition of type of dementia, age-related impairment of sense function and present ability to communicate in nonverbal actions. (Rempusheski, U.F. et al 1988)

ETIOLOGIES

EXTERNAL

SITUATIONAL CRISIS: Long term isolation; accident.

MATURATIONAL CRISIS: Diminished contact with family; diminished physical ability (i.e. 5 senses).

PERSONAL VULNERABILITY: Inability to correctly process information to sensorium; decreased cognitive function.

PERCEIVED LOSS OF CONTROL: Dependency needs increase.

INTERNAL

SITUATIONAL CRISIS: Cortical dementia—development of dementia syndrome, Alzheimer's disease, Pick's disease; infarct dementia; sub-cortical dementia—Parkinson's disease, Huntington's chorea.

MATURATIONAL CRISIS: Difficulty in coping with ordinary routine in home/unit; increased vulnerability to anxiety; fear as disease progresses; verbal deficit continues or is maintained to minimal degree of former ability.

KNOWLEDGE DEFICIT: All areas of cognitive structure affected; memory—unable to retain information—in need of cues from outside self; ability to interpret abstract material is impaired; judgment in socio/economic sphere impaired; judgment in psycho-motor abilities is disturbed (i.e. gait, manual tasks).

DEFINING CHARACTERISTICS

◆ Unable to speak dominant language
◆ Speaks or verbalizes with difficulty
◆ Does not or cannot speak
◆ Stuttering
◆ Slurring
◆ Difficulty forming words or sentences
◆ Difficulty expressing thoughts verbally
◆ Inappropriate verbalization
◆ Dyspnea
◆ Disorientation.

GOALS

◆ Accommodate to Care Unit

◆ Identify nonverbal communication cues to staff/other patients

◆ Communicate verbally as able using short or simple words/phrases

◆ Utilize unit resources facilitating identifiable communication modes

◆ Continue to work with staff/others in identifying comfort areas for verbal/nonverbal interaction.

INTERVENTIONS

◆ Coordinate effort of family/caregiver/staff to identify type of disorder, present capabilities for communication (RN)

◆ Increase availability of time initially to acquaint client with assigned personnel, unit structure (RN/LPN/NA)

◆ Maintain consistent time-interview limit each day to visit client, create climate of trust (RN/LPN/NA)

◆ Work with client to identify accessible means of communication (i.e. verbal/nonverbal) (RN/LPN/NA)

◆ Discuss with client (i.e. verbal/nonverbal) areas of comfort/potential for anxiety (i.e. observations—hand/eye cues by staff), ability to tolerate "support touch" (RN/LPN)

◆ Identify with client a sense of definition of safe environment (i.e. leave on small light at night, lock medications, eliminate hazardous utensils) (RN/LPN/NA)

◆ Determine with client (or observation) ability to tolerate noise, loud colors (i.e. voice range) (RN/LPN/NA)

◆ Continued monitoring of medication, physical hygiene, eating habits (RN/LPN)

◆ Identify body/facial movements indicating anxiety, irritability, to reduce tension behaviors, depression, sadness (RN/LPN/NA)

◆ Locate best stance/verbalization reception via sensory assessment (i.e. ability to hear in right ear only) (RN/LPN/NA)

◆ Monitor own verbal tone, pitch, and range for client comfort/stress level in daily interactions (RN/LPN/NA)

◆ Assess client ability to tolerate social activity on unit/home (i.e. interact via sitting-walking about unit) (RN/LPN)

◆ Integrate use of physical/occupational therapies as client condition allows (i.e. pasting forms on paper, simple dance routine) (RN/LPN)

◆ Continue to monitor client activity, change in verbal expression ability (RN/LPN/NA)

◆ Assist family as needed in locating community resources available to discuss feelings, client's condition (i.e. self-help groups) (RN/LPN)

◆ Refer client for counseling if depression or continued acting out behaviors (RN)

◆ Initiate socialization regime for client in coordination with staff/social service/rehabilitation therapy/medical personnel, educational regime to trigger memory function for short-time period (i.e. special flower to identify room), to alert staff to tension building situations (i.e. ear rubbing), to assist client in use of elementary survival utensils (i.e. picture of table set with knives, forks, spoon, dish), to alert client to need for personal hygiene (i.e. sign with client name or special color near toothbrush, comb) (RN).

POTENTIAL FOR VIOLENCE

Definition: Presence of risk factors for self-directed or other-directed physical trauma.

ASSESSMENT

Violent or potentially violent clients elicit fear and concern within the environment they inhabit. Family and staff are not immune to the stress encountered when the threat to personal safety erupts without warning. The potential for violence creates a crisis situation and alleviating its source takes precedence over routine unit tasks.

Often the best solution to the threat is understanding the clinical predictors that the client is exhibiting and defusing the presenting issue before it culminates in a violent episode. If the client is known to the institution or the caretaker, the past physical, psychological, and environmental factors that played a role in the development of aggressive coping patterns is incorporated in the evaluation of the presenting behavior. The task now is to evaluate the precipitating events observed in the client's present pre-assaultive state. (Feil, 1989)

An aggressive, hostile stance (i.e. arms crossed, shoulders back, hip thrust forward), angry eye contact, curled lip, threatening arm or leg gestures increasing in motion, clenched fists or clenched jaw, increased pacing behavior, verbal abuse, profanity, and threats to harm self or others are pre-eruptive signals often seen 30–60 minutes before the outbursts. The staff belief that if ignored the behavior will go away may be an invitation to harm. The recognition of behavioral change, increasing anger, provocative stance, and the persistence of threat requires immediate evaluation of client status for the protection of the client and the staff members.

Aggressive or threatening behavior to self and others often represents a defense against feelings of helplessness, or as Ellison (1979) states "a state of inner tension causing some discomfort to the individual and energizing him to take some action vis-a-vis the environment, very often but not always involving gross motor behavior."

Recent demographic trends noting violence to self and others among the elderly indicate high rates of aggressive behavior for those living in institutional settings (Donat 1986). Suicide rates, especially among white males over 70, continue to escalate (Seiden 1981). Non-institutionalized elderly prone to suicidal ideation are difficult to evaluate as they rarely seek help for such thoughts. A suicidal attempt or threat discovered by a family member or friend is the first indication of a problem and a call for help.

Suicidal indicators among institutionalized elderly may take the form of depression (i.e. declined activity, refusal to eat, deep, moaning sighs, verbalizations of "I want to die," or the voices of dead relatives telling them to kill themselves (or others).

AGE-RELATED PHENOMENON

During the development stages of childhood and adolescence, individual perception as to the limits of socially acceptable forms of aggressive behavior is channeled into constructive areas of release (i.e. games, exercise, ability to express anger in an appropriate manner).

In the United States, individual cultural expressions of aggression are not always accepted by the society. The influence of the at-large societal institutions (i.e. school, peers outside culture) assist the child in recognizing the social limits of aggressive or potentially harmful behavior.

For some, innate genetic make-up, cultural or personality traits, the need to perpetuate an aggressive stance toward others is continued through adult years, making its presence known when autonomy is threatened.

The aggressive patterns of early years are dormant in the older years until precipitated by a sudden, incomprehensible change that threatens the client's autonomy (i.e. economic/family). As the crisis continues with little moves toward resolution, the emotions of anger and rage begin to surface. If intervention via family or professional means takes place, the situation may be diffused temporarily or permanently.

If it is not, the condition escalates in uncooperative behavior, angry threats or isolated stance until it erupts in self or other destruct behavior.

The diagnosis of dementia and resultant deterioration of cognitive function decreases the ability to control impulsive or violent behavior. The individual diagnosed may not have had the pre-morbid destructive patterns.

Their present organic condition creates anxiety about their gradual inability to control their lives, fear of being harmed and placed in a new and unfamiliar environment among strangers.

They react adversely to sharp commands, over-stimulating color, and loud noise. Effort to protect themselves from an impaired perception of cause takes the form of uncontrolled psychomotor activity.

ETIOLOGIES

EXTERNAL

SITUATIONAL CRISIS: Sudden change in noise level, environment, location, caretaker availability.

MATURATIONAL CRISIS: If prone to violence in young adult life, re-emergence of violent behavior occurs if sudden change forfeits autonomy.

PERSONAL VULNERABILITY: Perceive others as controlling life.

KNOWLEDGE DEFICIT: Organic brain syndrome or psychiatric disorder (functional) impede ability to judge rational action.

PERCEIVED LOSS OF CONTROL: Illness or socio-economic conditions initiate inability to control events.

INTERNAL

SITUATIONAL CRISIS: Feelings of hopelessness, helplessness, anger, and rage.

MATURATIONAL CRISIS: Amelioration of anger impulses in elder years.

PERSONAL VULNERABILITY: Unable to control own destiny.

KNOWLEDGE DEFICIT: Anxiety over loss of control impedes ability to control impulsive behavior (in absence of organic brain syndrome).

◆ Nursing Diagnosis

Potential for violence (i.e. suicide, homicide, physical injury to self or others).

DEFINING CHARACTERISTICS

◆ Clenched fists

◆ Angry facial expression

◆ Rigid posture

◆ Tautness indicating intense effort for self-control

◆ Hostility

◆ Threatening verbalizations

◆ Boasting prior abuse to others

◆ Increased motor activity, pacing, excitement, irritability, agitation

◆ Overt and aggressive acts

◆ Goal directed destruction of objects in environment

◆ Possession of destructive means (gun, knives, weapon, etc.)

◆ Rage

◆ Self-destructive behavior (active, aggressive, or suicidal acts)

◆ Substance abuse or withdrawal

◆ Suspicion of others (paranoid ideation, delusions, hallucinations)

◆ Increasing anxiety level

◆ Fear of self or others

◆ Inability to verbalize feelings

◆ High situational stress factors

◆ Anti-social character disturbance

◆ Catatonic or manic excitement

◆ Organic brain syndrome

◆ Rage reactions, child abuse

◆ Temporal lobe epilepsy

◆ Anger

◆ Repeated complaints, requests, and demands

◆ Provocative acts (argumentative/hypersensitivity, overreaction, dissatisfaction)

◆ Depression (active, aggressive, suicidal acts).

GOALS

◆ Reduction of anxiety/threat of harm

◆ Find trustful humane institutional environment

◆ Understand (within diagnostic limits) implications of behavior

◆ Define with staff limits to preserve safe, healthful environment

◆ Negotiate verbal/nonverbal cues to alert staff to increase in tension/fear

◆ Understand limit setting behavior to be imposed by staff for acting out behavior (i.e. medication, restraints).

INTERVENTIONS

◆ Utilize staff and personal observations of client presenting behavior to determine interaction/self-care abilities (RN/LPN)

◆ Close observation of verbal/nonverbal clues, indicating escalation of aggressive behavior (RN/LPN/NA)

◆ Coordinate plan client care with staff to thwart/understand aggressive behavior or dynamics (i.e. approach method, voice tone, eye contact, engage in tension reducing conversation, escape plan or route for staff), medication, PRN restraints, establish inservice education format—theory, practical steps to prevent staff injury (RN)

◆ Create climate of firm but trustful assistance to assist client in self-control abilities

◆ Daily discussion session predictable time-place to discuss client present concerns, gradually build trust relationship on one to one basis/other staff, involve client in negotiating best possible methods to contain behavior, allow client to identify "button" words, drug, actions, environmental material that triggers aggressive behavior, identify with client potential for self- or other-destructive behavior/define concretely potential for either (are you suicidal?), define nursing care intervention if aggressive behavior apparent starting at level of talk—medication/restraints (RN/LPN/NA)

◆ Involve client in group activity applicable to stage of illness

◆ Coordinate family and social service agency personnel in identifying ability to contain client behavior

◆ Refer client to use of specially trained psychiatric clinician to evaluate emotional cognitive functioning if no improvement demonstrated

◆ Organically impaired client—review interventions supplement non-verbal communication clues (as client able to interpret) i.e. written clarification, picture clarification, use of touch signals, code (RN/LPN/NA).

UNRESOLVED INDEPENDENCE-DEPENDENCE CONFLICT

Definition: Lack of resolution of current needs and desires to be dependent/independent with expectation (therapeutic, matu-rational, or social) to be independent/dependent. Conflictual expectations based on cognitive structure of past dependence/independence pattterns and currently applied to present needs (therapeutic, maturational, and social) for which they are no longer relevant.

ASSESSMENT

Each life-development stage engages its participants in confrontation and temporary resolution of dependence and independence needs. From birth to death the struggle to disengage the bonds of dependency on others contrasts with the recognition for most of us that isolation and loneliness are uncomfortable states for extended periods of time. Self-actualization depends on the provision of security, comfort, belongingness, and self-esteem reinforced by the presence or support of significant other (Kaluger & Kaluger 1984).

In Erikson's description of the first developmental stage, Trust vs. Mistrust (1963), the infant is totally dependent on the significant other or caring person to fulfill all of life's needs. Progression through each stage of growth and development witnesses acquisition of motor and social skills and the lessened need for dependence on the parental family. In the child-hood years occasional returns to the dependent state are indicated when health, economic, or social downturns deplete available resources.

The thrust for independence, to carve one's own destiny, to be responsible for a selected life course utilizing individual defined resources reflects the social ideal in American society and most of adult life is spent on the attainment of this ambition. Independence becomes the goal in life's interactions for some, while others perceived a predominantly dependent behavioral style as a mainstay in their interactions with others. The poten-tial for total dependence or total independence is unlikely for most persons in every factor of human growth and development (i.e. biological, psycho-logical, environmental, and metaphysical).

In the adult years a predominant mode of dependent/independent behavior in human relationships stabilizes. Recognition of the "need for affiliation" with others causing temporary change in dependent/indepen-dent patterns (i.e. illness, loss of business) implies that the individual's pri-mary method of interaction will have to be adjusted to adapt to a life crisis.

Interdependence, a comfortable balance between dependence and independence with others, is defined by McIntier (1976) as recognizing the "need for affiliation." These needs are usually temporary in nature (i.e. illness, loss of business). Reestablishment of the former independent/dependent patterns are assumed.

If return to the former health, social, or economic circumstance is not feasible, then new ones will surface in many areas of the individual's life as the struggle for adaptation continues. The desire for the old patterns confronts reality of the new situation creating conflict, evidenced in behavior as the individual confronts the past issues of dependence/independence in the adaptation process (i.e. effect of divorce on dependent partner/debilitating illness in life of independent executive).

AGE-RELATED PHENOMENON

Resolution of the dependence/independence conflict is attained for most adults through the various social contact/interactions that are part of the life-development stages (Maddi 1972).

The constant change that is part of each stage is influenced by biological, psychological, environmental, and metaphysical factors, each creating the opportunity and the excitement of possible resolution fraught with the concerns of failure.

Each confrontation with change poses a shift in the independent/dependent patterns each person has integrated over a lifetime.

Elderly persons are not immune to change and the necessity, at different points in older years maturational cycle, to shift temporarily from dependent/independent or independent/dependent modes.

A social problem presents the need to adapt. The style of interaction in an elderly person's relationship with significant others (i.e. family, professional caretaker) utilized in the past will predominate.

For most interdependence as described by Drago (1991) allows for the temporary disruption of the dominant (independent or dependent) resolution style.

The impact of constant loss over one's environment precipitates fear of the return to discarded dependency patterns or loss of dependency that marked the earlier adult development years.

For the older, frail adult for whom nursing home placement is necessary, the life change is perceived as permanent.

Interdependence is not recognized as an option. Dependency on others for life essentials takes precedence. Interaction patterns with the professional caregiver minimize individual effort for independence (Leibman-Tobias 1983).

ETIOLOGIES

EXTERNAL

SITUATIONAL CRISIS: Independent/Dependent: Retirement of spouse; loss of financial stability; loss of auto license due to health; loss of independent home environment. Dependent/Independent: Loss of spouse to divorce/death; alteration in family/social support network.

MATURATIONAL CRISIS: Altered health position; economic change due to age or health.

KNOWLEDGE DEFICIT: Aware of impact of external events impacting on individual life status.

PERCEIVED LOSS OF CONTROL: Life control ability dependent on external events/change.

INTERNAL

SITUATIONAL CRISIS: Potential alteration in familiar dominant interaction role (independent or dependent).

MATURATIONAL CRISIS: Resurrection of unresolved dependency or independency patterns of childhood/young adult development years; potential alteration of self concept, self-ideal.

KNOWLEDGE DEFICIT: Later adult years intelligence ability maintained unless presence of organicity—ability to judge/learn impact—need to change may temporarily be diminished.

PERCEIVED LOSS OF CONTROL: Inability to control placement because of ill health/helplessness—reinforces fear of earlier dependent/independent patterns that were discarded.

DEFINING CHARACTERISTICS

◆ Repeated verbal expressions of desire for independence (i.e. in situations that require some dependence: therapeutic, maturation, or social); repeated verbal expressions of desire for dependence; verbalized eliminate need for expression of anger; anxiety.

GOALS

◆ Reduction of independent/dependency conflict anxiety
◆ Determine recent life event that triggered conflict, its impact on present behavior
◆ Create realistic boundaries for new life mode (i.e. dependent or independent)
◆ Develop constructive outlet for expression of anger/anxiety
◆ Initiate social support system in present environment.

INTERVENTIONS

◆ Coordinate observations/source of potential behavioral problems with ancillary personnel/staff and nursing notes. (RN)
◆ Define increase or decrease in usual dependent or independent interaction patterns of client. (RN)
◆ Initiate (continue) daily interview (discussion) time to review with client occasions of change in behavior. (RN/LPN/NA)
◆ Discuss with client potential reasons for change: use of active listening skills, eye contact, body language, verbal empathy, affirmation; use of

observation skills, client language format, tone, body language congruency. (RN/LPN/NA)

◆ Define with client possible means of resolution to present crisis: use of past adapting; potential of full or partial use of these methods; client's power to change certain aspects of interaction. (RN/LPN/NA)

◆ Explore areas of unit activity that would enhance client ability to lessen dependency or independency (as indicated): assist in own health care (within limits); assist in planning unit activities; explore client perceived ability to care for certain areas of body care (i.e. signals for boundary exceeded). (RN/LPN)

◆ Utilize services of unit personnel to assist in gradual resolution of conflict status. (RN/LPN/NA)

12

Sexuality-Reproductive Patterns

Sheree Loftus
Richard S. Ferri

◆

SEXUALITY-REPRODUCTIVE PATTERNS

Sexuality and sexual expression are an essential part of human beings throughout their lifespan. From birth to death, sexuality is part of our identity, our masculinity, and feminity. Growing old does not cancel our sexual needs. The process of aging may change our bodies external features, but it does not change our internal desires. Society has stereotyped the aged as sexless beings. Those who continue to participate in sex into late life are often condemned as perverse, yet they may be our healthiest aged. Sexual dysfunction in the aged is the experience, or the risk of experiencing, a change in sexual health or sexual function that is viewed as unrewarding or inadequate.

The following information is focused on men over age fifty-five, and post-menopausal women. At this age, sex is not for procreation, but for recreation, communication, and love. The nurse plays an essential role in teaching the aged factual information about sexual function, encouraging the aged to participate in sexual expression if they so choose and providing options for them to do so.

SAFER SEX AND THE OLDER PERSON

No one is exempt from becoming infected with the human immunodeficiency virus (HIV) that causes Acquired Immunodeficiency Syndrome or AIDS—including the elderly. In fact, 10% of all AIDS cases reported involve persons over the age of fifty.

HIV is the virus that causes AIDS and is transmitted from person to person contact through the exchange of body fluids, such as blood and semen. The two safest methods to avoid HIV infection from sexual activity are abstinence, and mutually monogamous sex with a noninfected partner.

However, the elder may be sexually active with several partners or

294

may be experimenting with new sexual roles and options. It is critical that the nurse never assume an individual's sexual practices or orientation based on age.

Older people may be especially vulnerable for HIV infection as there is a normal decline in immune system function with aging. In fact, according to the Center for Disease Control HIV symptoms develop more rapidly than in younger patients.

An additional risk is the fact that the elderly are prime clinical candidates for blood and blood product infusions. Although the blood supply has been screened for the presence of HIV since 1985, and is considered very safe it still represents on additional risk exposure.

The nurse should perform a sexual assessment that includes knowledge level assessment on safer sex practices. Table 12-1 details Safer Sex Guidelines for all sexually active persons. These guidelines should be reviewed with the elder.

It is critical that safer sex education be incorporated into mainstream nursing knowledge in order to prevent the spread of HIV.

SEXUAL DYSFUNCTION

> ***Definition:*** An individual with a perceived problem in achieving desired satisfaction of preferred sexuality. The individual experiences changes in their sexual performance and/or expression that are self-identified as unfulfilling.

For many older individuals sexual dysfunction presents a significant problem which often goes untreated because of societal taboos regarding active sexuality of older people.

Sexual dysfunction may occur due to an overwhelming number of factors, such as drugs, lack of a suitable partner, monotony in sexual relations, preoccupation with career loss, physical infirmities, depression and mental illness, overindulgence in food or alcohol, fear of performance failure, and disuse atrophy.

ASSESSMENT

Assessment of sexual dysfunction may be difficult due to the hesitancy of the older adult and the nurse to discuss this issue. Discussion of sex and sexual problems may be taboo for religious reasons and/or conservative personal attitudes. The nurse must be open and willing to listen to any type of sexual diversity the older adult may choose to discuss. A matter of fact, nonjudgmental acceptance of the wide variety of human sexual expression, such as auto-stimulation, homosexuality, bisexuality, oral-genital sex, oral anal, and fantasy, will help the nurse to build a trusting, therapeutic relationship with the geriatric patient.

Assessment of possible reasons for sexual dysfunction must be accurate and comprehensive. Sexual preference, performance, and experience, all medications being taken—both prescribed and over the counter—religiosity, relationships with significant others, depression, and other psy-

TABLE 12–1 ◆ Safer Sex Guidelines

1. Risk-free behaviors:
   - ◆ Massage (without genital stimulation): As you discuss this behavior, you may also want to discuss with the client how massage can be a method of relaxation as well as shared intimacy. It may be helpful to discuss how both client and partner can use oils and lotions as well as create the environment to promote sensuality and erocticism.
   - ◆ Mutual masturbation/pleasuring techniques: These behaviors are relatively safe as long as the skin is healthy and free of lesions/open areas. Many people have not learned to masturbate, or may view these behaviors as "dirty" or "sinful," depending on their cultural/religious upbring. If this is the case they may need to be referrred to a counselor or sex therapist.
   - ◆ Social kissing and hugging.
   - ◆ Frottage (body-to-body rubbing): The behavior utilizes the erotic sensations of touch and can be combined with massage.
   - ◆ The use of sex toys (dildos) that are not shared with partners
   - ◆ Casual contact: hand holding, arm holding, shaking hands, etc.
   - ◆ Voyeurism and fantasy

2. Low-risk behaviors:
   - ◆ Intimate kissing (also known as deep kissing and/or French kissing): Penetration of tongue into partner's mouth. It is important that the mouth not have any open sores or lesions or any evidence of bleeding gums.
   - ◆ Fellatio (oral sex) without ingestion of seminal fluid or semen. Risk is further reduced with use of condom.
   - ◆ Cunnilingus (oral stimulation of the female genitals): Protective covering of the female genitalia will further reduce risk (dental dams, latex barrier).
   - ◆ Vaginal intercourse with the use of a properly applied condom
   - ◆ Rectal intercourse with the use of properly applied condom
   - ◆ Use of shared sex toys that are cleaned in between uses and covered with a condom for penetration

3. High-risk behaviors:
   - ◆ Ingestion of semen or vaginal/cervical secretions
   - ◆ Vaginal and/or anal intercourse without the use of a condom
   - ◆ Sharing sex toys
   - ◆ Analingus (oral-anal contact, also known as "rimming")
   - ◆ Piercing or drawing blood during sexual behaviors
   - ◆ Fisting: penetration of the anus with one's fist

SOURCE: Adapted from Bay Area Physicians for Human Rights, 1985; Bjorklund, 1987.

chological concerns, monitoring of nocturnal penile tumescence, evaluation of blood hormone levels, neurologic illnesses, arthritis, history of diabetes, cardiac, pulmonary, kidney, HIV illness and any other diseases, which may interfere with or impede performance, all must be evaluated to determine a cause or causes of sexual dysfunction.

Medications can cause significant problems in healthy sexual expression.

Changes such as Alzheimer's disease or Parkinson's dementia as well as any other problems that may impair cognitive function can contribute to sexual difficulties.

Physical insults, injuries, and other changes may cause irreversible impotence. Disruptions in health such as diabetes, spinal cord injury, some CVA's, radical prostatectomy, cancer, cardiac disease, endocrine dysfunctions, severe arthritis, and other maladies contribute to sexual dysfunction. These diseases need medical evaluation. Options for referral for the aged to continue sexual performance are available if the aged client chooses to do so. These options are dependent upon the health of the resident, but all may help to restore sexual function. The nurse must be sensitive to the needs of the resident and knowledgeable of the benefits and side-effects of each intervention.

The psychological and emotional factors that can cause sexual dysfunction may be difficult to decipher. Changes in body image, self-esteem, and multiple losses may all contribute. Psychological and emotional distress may be a result of physical changes and or may contribute to them.

Another key factor in obtaining a complete assessment of the elderly is the sexual history. To obtain a sexual history, the nurse should clarify her own values regarding sexual expression and avoid transferring them to the resident. There are several standardized sexual history forms, which can provide guidance. (See Diekelmann Sexual History form)

It is critical that all avenues of sexual expression be explored with the resident for assessment. In addition to heterosexual, homosexual, and bisexual behavior, the nurse should also consider past or current expression through prostitution, multiple sex partners, sado-machismism, and illicit drug use.

AGE-RELATED PHENOMENON

The research on age-related changes with sexual expression is sparse and inconclusive. Sexual activity, such as intercourse, masturbation, and fantasy, has a tendency to decrease in frequency with age, and past experience.

VISION

◆ Impaired color vision—Decreased ability to discern colors
◆ Decreased visual acuity—Reduced ability to see clearly/sharply.

These changes may directly affect the choice of colors in the environment and for dressing. Contrasting colors allow a sharper, more pleasurable view of the world. Red, orange, and yellow are more easily visualized, and should be considered for enhancement of sexuality. It is difficult to obtain enjoyment when the world appears gray. Glasses may be necessary to visualize other human beings. Contact lenses are suggested for those who may find glasses unattractive. It is usually more enjoyable and stimulating to be able to see the world clearly rather than as a blur.

TABLE 12–2 ◆ **Drugs That May Affect Sexual Function**

DRUG	POSSIBLE EFFECTS
Alcohol	Erectile problems, decreased libido with chronic intake, reduced potency in men, delayed orgasm in women
Antidepressants	Reduced libido and potency, delayed ejaculation
Aventyl-Nortriptyline	
Elavil-Amitriptyline	
Norpramine-Desipramine-Pertofrane	Peripheral blockage of nervous innervation of glands
Phenlzine sulfate-Nardil	
Sinequon	
Tranylcypromine sulfate-Parnate	
Tofranil-Impramine	
Vivactil-Protriptyline	
Doxepin	Decreased libido, erectile problems
MAO inhibitors	Impotence
Antihistamines	Block parasympathtic nervous innervation of sex glands
Diphenhydramine-Benadryl	
Promethazine-Phenergan	
Clorpheniramine-Chlor-Trimeton	
Antispasmodics/Anticholinergics	Inhibit parasympathetic innervation of sex glands
Methantheline-Banthine	
Glycoyrrolate-Robinul	
Hexocyclium-Tral	
Poldine-Nacton	
Diphenoxylate hydrochloride with atropine-Lomotil	
Belladonna alkakoids	Decreased libido, impotence
Amphetamine-Benzedrine	Reduced libido and potency
Benzodiazepines	Decreased libido
Bethanidine-Esbatal, Esbaloid	Impaired ejaculation
Benztropine	Decreased libido, impotence
Chlorthalidone	Impotence, loss of libido, and decreased vaginal secretion

TABLE 12–2 ◆ Drugs That May Affect Sexual Function *Continued*

DRUG	POSSIBLE EFFECTS
Cimetidine	Decreased libido, impotence
Clonidine-Catapres	Reduced libido, impotence, retrograde ejaculation
Defrisoquine-Declinax	Reduced potency, impaired ejaculation
Dextroamphetamin-Dexedrinee	Reduced potency, impaired ejaculation
Dextroamphetamin-Dexedrine	Reduced libido and potency
Diphenhydramine	Erectile, decreased libido
Disulfiram-Antabuse	Reduced potency, impotence
Disopyramide	Impotence
Diuretics	Chronic use may cause impotence
Ethacrynic acid-Edecrin	
Furosemide-Lasix	
Guanethidine-Ismelin-Esimil	Reduced potency, impaired ejaculation
Haloperidol-Haldol	Reduced potency
Levodopa-L-dopa	Increased libido (in some men and women)
Lithium	Reduced potency
Mecamylamine-Inversine	Cause of impotence in men and decreased vaginal lubrication in women
Methyldopa-Aldomet	Decreased libido, and potency, inability to maintain erection, and difficulty in ejaculation
Phenothiazides	
Chlorpromazine-Thorazine	Reduced libido, potency, erectile problems
Pramazine-Sparine	Impaired ejaculation (occasionally)
Triflupromazine-Vesprin	
Prochlorperazine-Compazine	
Phenoxybenzamine-Dibenayline	Impotence and impaired ejaculation
Primidone-Mysoline	Reduced libido and potency
Propantheline	Decreased libido and impotence
Reserpine-Serpasil	Reduced libido, potency and impotence
Sedatives/Hypnotics	When used regularly causes reduced libido and potency
Nembutal	
Seconal	
Barbiturates	

Table continued on following page

TABLE 12–2 ◆ Drugs That May Affect Sexual Function *Continued*

DRUG	POSSIBLE EFFECTS
Spironolactone-Aldactone	Gunecomastia and impotence
Thiazide diuretics	Reduced libido (occasionally in some men)
Diuril	
Enduron	
Esidrix	
Hydrodiuril	
Nagua	
Renese	
Tranquilizers	
Thioridazine-Mellaril	Ejaculation difficulties, decreased libido, reduced libido and potency
Equanil, Miltown-Meprobamate	Block autonomic innervation of sex glands
Prochlorperazine-Compazine	
Mesoridazine-Serentil	
Chlordiazepoxide-Librium	
Diazepam-Valium	
Phenoxybenzamine-Dibenzyline	
Chlorprothizene-Taractan	
Trimethaphan-Arfonad	Cause impotence in men and decreased vaginal lubrication in women

HEARING

◆ Conductive hearing loss—Reduced ability to hear low-pitched sounds

◆ Sensorineural hearing loss—Reduced ability to hear high-pitched sounds.

These changes may directly effect sexual interactions/attraction between aging humans. Speech discrimination may be impaired. Speech heard may sound garbled or muffled. This may inhibit approach between older adults or turn an interested partner off. Hearing aids are often helpful, but carry a social stigma. Enhancement of communication through the other senses—touch, vision, and using gestures—may be necessary. Modify the environment to maximize residual hearing function, decrease background noise, and maintain face-to-face communication.

SMELL

◆ Loss of olfactory receptors—diminished ability to smell and taste.

Loss of smell impairs the ability of the older person to detect body odors, when present. Daily hygiene, using deodorants, and bathing will decrease offensive odors and may improve interactions with other humans. Using colognes, aftershave lotions, and sachets strengthen the olfactory stimulus, as well as sniffing flowers and food. Memories of olfactory experiences may also provide enhancement.

The aging female experiences changes in sexual function, which are due to the normal aged-related changes of the reproductive system. Drugs, illness, or injuries, changes in self-image, social stereotypes, loss of a spouse, lack of privacy, poverty, sensory losses, and family pressures all may contribute to anorgasm. Women experience the climacteric. The climateric represents the cessation of reproduction for woman. This may occur in the fourth or fifth decade. This event does not represent the end of sexual function. Women remain sexually active into their seventh, eighth, and ninth decades and need not fear pregnancy at this time of life. Good health and regular sexual activity contribute to sustained sexual function in late life. Some women may experience a feeling of loss due to the inability to continue to produce children. These feelings may also contribute to anorgasm.

The same diseases, accidents, and injuries that may contribute to impotence in men may also contribute to anorgasm in women. The following are other common physical (organic) causes of anorgasm:

1. Cystocele, prolapsed uterus, rectocele.
2. Mastectomy.
3. Pruritus vulvae and painful uterine contractions
4. Obesity.
5. Atrophic vaginitis and vaginal irritation.
6. Removal of the adrenal glands.
7. Incontinence.

The aging male also experiences changes in sexual function, which are due to the normal age-related changes of the reproductive system. The same factors that affect female sexuality impact on the male. Older men can maintain sexual function into their seventh and eighth decade; some even have been known to father children at that age. Good health and regular sexual activity contribute to sustained sexual function in late life.

The following are examples of the most common physical (organic) causes of impotence:

1. Diabetes mellitus.
2. Arteriosclerosis and other diseases of the blood vessels.
3. Surgery involving the pelvic area, such as radical removal of the prostate, bladder, or rectum.
4. Diseases of the erectile tissue of the penis, including Peyronie's disease and priapism.

5. Hormonal abnormalities.
6. Alcoholism and drug abuse.
7. Medications, especially those prescribed for high blood pressure.
8. Neurologic diseases, such as Parkinson's disease and epilepsy.
9. Chronic diseases, for example kidney or liver failure.
10. Pelvic fractures, spinal cord injuries, and perineal trauma.

ETIOLOGIES FOR ORGANIC CAUSES OF SEXUAL DYSFUNCTION (FEMALE AND MALE)

◆ Ineffectual or absent role models
◆ Physical abuse
◆ Psychosocial abuse (e.g. harmful relationships)
◆ Vulnerability
◆ Misinformation or lack of knowledge
◆ Values conflict
◆ Lack of privacy
◆ Lack of significant other
◆ Altered body structure or function.

◆ Nursing Diagnosis

Sexual dysfunction due to normal physical and social age-related changes.

DEFINING CHARACTERISTICS

◆ Verbalization of problem in sexuality
◆ Alterations in achieving perceived sex role
◆ Actual or perceived limitation imposed by disease and/or therapy
◆ Conflicts involving values (cultural, religious)
◆ Alteration in achieving sexual satisfaction
◆ Inability to achieve desired sexual satisfaction
◆ Frequent seeking of confirmation of desirability
◆ Alteration in relationship with significant other
◆ Change of interest in self and others.

GOALS/OUTCOME CRITERIA

◆ Verbalizes rewarding or adequate sexual function
◆ Identifies alternative methods of sexual satisfaction
◆ Lessening of frustration, anxiety, depression
◆ Positive change in sexual health or sexual function.

INTERVENTIONS

1. Encourage the resident to discuss sexual concerns and needs with nurse or other appropriate counselor and/or sex partner. (RN, SW)

2. Provide resident with information regarding age-related changes that affect sexual expression. (RN, SW)

3. Explore the individual's belief about resuming sexual activity after the death of a sex partner/lover/spouse. (RN, SW)

4. Discuss attitudes regarding, and techniques of, masturbation. (RN, SW)

5. Assess any pain experienced during sexual relations. (Additional lubrication may be necessary either vaginally or rectally. Individuals with coronary artery disease may require nitrates prior to sex. Position adjustments may be necessary). (RN, MD)

6. Provide privacy for the resident to express sexual needs without interruption or fear of "being caught." (RN)

7. Form group sessions regarding sexuality available to all residents. In addition to the formal group leader, are there any social service and community agencies that can provide speakers, information, and referral? (RN, SW)

8. Kegel exercises—These exercises are designed to strengthen the pubococcygeus muscle and surrounding musculature. The muscle and its adjuncts help to control the urinary outlet; however, they also appear associated with the capacity for receiving sensory pleasure in the vaginal and clitoral areas. Women who have practiced Kegel exercises for a period of time report increased muscle tonus in the vagina, ability to constrict the vagina voluntarily, and increased capacity for achieving orgasm. In order for a woman to learn what muscles are involved and how to contract them, she should first stand facing the toilet as though she were a man about to urinate. Then she should pretend to release a stream of urine and abruptly inhibit it before the first drops are released. The contraction involved in inhibiting the stream is the basic maneuver of Kegel exercises. Once having experienced the method of contracting, the woman can perform the contractions while driving an automobile, sitting, lying, or doing anything else that does not involve a great deal of moving about. She should contract the muscles, hold the contractions for a 1-2-3 (subvocal) count, release, and repeat the process. She may do as many a day as she likes—about 90 is fine. In a few weeks she will be able to constrict her vagina voluntarily with considerable strength. Another set of exercises involves bearing down as one does during labor or defecation. Again, a 1-2-3 count, release, and repetition is the procedure. Do a set of Kegels and a set of these exercises. They can be continued indefinitely.

9. Manual stimulation—The use of a finger, hand, or any part of the body on the genitals or another part of the body of a sexual partner.

10. Mental orgasm—Remembering or imaging (fantasizing) the sensations of physical orgasm.

11. Oils and lubricants—Each oil and lotion has its own characteristics and should be selected or tried for a special effect. One should experiment to find out what is pleasing. Each couple will develop their own preference for the type of oil or lotion that they like to use. Most oils and lotions can be purchased at drug or department stores or in specialized bath or body shops. Oils may be mixed with a favorite scent or flavor. However, it should be noted that there are two types of oil, mineral and organic (vegetable), and that they do not mix together. Water soluble lubricants are best for internal use, and should be used with latex condoms.

12. Stuffing technique—A method by which the woman can experience the sensation of the penis in her vagina even though the male does not have an erection. It is done by using the fingers to stuff or tuck the flaccid, soft penis into the vagina. By thrusting her hips and using the muscles of her vagina, the woman can draw the soft penis into her vagina with a sort of pulling or sucking movement.

13. Vibrators—There are many types of vibrators, which offer a variety of sensations and can add a new dimension of enjoyment and pleasure. Many department stores or small appliance stores sell the type that fits on the hand and can be used for body or facial massage. Others, with special attachments, can be purchased without too much difficulty. Vibrators or dildos that you may wish to try may be available at adult book stores or through mail order sources. (RN, SW)

14. Animals—Pet therapy may prove to be a healthy alternative for sexual tension as animals provide warmth, unconditional love, and companionship. (RN, SW)

SEXUAL HISTORY

A. Family information
1. Were your questions about sex answered freely, with embarrassment, evaded, or ignored?
2. Who was most likely to speak about sex with you?
3. How old were you when you learned about menstruation? Wet dreams? Sexual intercourse?
4. From whom did you learn? How was the information explained?
5. How demonstrative were your parents with each other?
6. How demonstrative were your parents with you?
7. What family member was most demonstrative with you?
B. Personal Information
1. What has been the greatest influence on your feelings about sex of any kind?

2. How did you feel about sex play as a child?
3. How old were you when you first engaged in sex play?
4. What kinds of things did you do?
5. How do you feel about masturbation?
6. How often did you masturbate as a child?
7. How old were you when you first masturbated?
8. Were you ever punished for masturbation or sex play?
9. Did you pet as an adolescent?
10. What did petting include?
11. When you petted did you feel worried about being caught?
12. How old were you when you had sexual relations for the first time?
13. Who was your first sex partner, and how did you feel about him (her)?
14. What is your preference in terms of a sex partner or sexual activities?
15. If you had premarital intercourse, how did you feel about it?
16. How many sex partners have you had?

C. Current Data

1. Are you now having a sexual relationship with anyone?
2. How would you describe it?
3. How long have you been involved with your current major sex partner?
4. How many sex partners have you had during the past year?
5. How important is sex to you (not to your partner or to the relationship)?
6. What do you like best about sex?
7. What do you like least about sex?
8. How often do you feel satisfied with sex?
9. How often do you have sexual relations?
10. How often does one of you want sex and the other does not?
11. How often do you have sex when you don't want to, to please your partner?
12. How often does your partner have sex just to please you?
13. What causes you to become aroused?
14. What causes your partner to become aroused?
15. How often do you have a climax (orgasm) in sex relations?
16. How often does your partner have orgasm?
17. Are you satisfied with your climax?

18. What kinds of things other than vaginal intercourse can excite you enough to reach a climax?

19. What is your opinion about who should initiate sex?

20. Is it all right for you to initiate sex?

21. How comfortable are you and your partner about dressing and undressing in front of each other? Touching genitals? Rectal stimulation? Rectal intercourse?

22. Do you and your partner talk about sex?

23. How does your sexual experience differ from what you thought it would be like before you had sex for the first time (or before you became sexually active)?

24. What would you like to change about your sex life?

25. Are there particular problems you would like to discuss?

D. Genital Health

1. How do you protect yourself from being exposed to a sexually transmitted disease, including HIV infection?

2. Have you ever experienced symptoms such as itching, pain, or burning on urination, or slight discharge or unpleasant odor, which cleared up on their own? (If the answer is yes, obtain details of symptoms, self-treatment, etc.).

3. What symptoms would cause you to suspect that you might have a sexually transmitted disease?

4. Have you ever been treated for a sexually transmitted disease? (If the answer is yes, obtain details of symptoms, diagnosis, treatment, and follow-up).

5. When was the last time you had a breast/vaginal/rectal and/or scrotal exam? What were the results?

In addition to the four parts of the sexual history—family information, personal information, current data, and genital health—the following parts can be included for the adult having sexual problems.

E. Specific Problems

1. Do you have trouble becoming sexually aroused?

   Frequently   Occasionally, but not a problem   Never

2. If you frequently have trouble being aroused:

   a. How often does this happen?

   b. When you are having difficulty, how long does it take you to eventually become aroused?

   c. Have you been aroused when interacting with another person?

   d. Have you been aroused from books, music, or daydreams (fantasy)?

   e. Do you fear pain? If yes, why?

3. Can you get an erection:

   Always   Sometimes   Never
   Often   Rarely   Not applicable

4. If you rarely or never get an erection:

   a. Have you ever been able to get an erection?

   b. Do you ever wake up with an erection?

   c. Can you get an erection by yourself? If yes, how?

5. If you have trouble keeping an erection, under what circumstances do you lose it?

6. Do you have pain with intercourse?

   Yes   No   Occasionally, but not a problem

7. If yes, you do have pain:

   a. How often?

   b. When do you get it?

   c. Where is it located?

   d. How long have you had it?

   e. Does anything make it better?

   f. How long does it last?

8. Do you climax (achieve orgasm):

   Too soon   Later than you wish
   Never   Too seldom

9. If you climax too soon:

   a. How long have you been aware of the problem?

   b. How long can you have intercourse before climaxing?

   c. How long do you expect to be able to have intercourse before climaxing?

   d. What have you tried to delay it?

   e. Is it getting worse?

   f. What is your partner's reaction?

10. If your climax takes too long:

    a. How long have you been aware of the problem?

    b. How long does it take you to climax?

    c. What have you tried to speed it up?

    d. Is it getting worse?

    e. How long can your partner have intercourse before climax?

    f. Does your partner know about your problem? What is his or her reaction?

11. Do you climax:

    a. From masturbation

       Yes   No   Sometimes

    b. From partner's mouth or hand stimulation

       Yes No Sometimes

    c. From vaginal intercourse

       Yes No Sometimes

    d. From rectal intercourse

       Yes No Sometimes

12. If no to any of the above questions:

    a. Have you tried to climax that way?

       Yes No

    b. Have you ever climaxed that way?

       Yes No

    c. Did you formerly climax that way but no longer can?

       Yes No

13. If you have never experienced climax (orgasm), what do you think is the reason for that?

14. Do you have diabetes, heart trouble, or high blood pressure? Does anyone in your family?

15. Do you take any drugs, including uppers, downers, marijuana, or prescribed medications? (List them).

16. On the average, what volume of alcoholic beverages do you drink in a week?

17. Have you had any major surgery?

For postmenopausal women only:

How old were you when menstruation completely stopped?

Are you currently on hormone replacement therapy?

    _____ Yes _____ No

    If yes, what are you taking?

Are you currently experiencing any symptoms that you attribute to having reached menopause?

    _____ Yes _____ No

In retrospect, how would you describe your feelings about menopause?

What impact has menopause had upon your life?

Although the signs of male menopause are more generalized, the nurse should include assessment in this area and encourage the client to discuss his feelings and perceptions.

    1. What symptoms have you experienced and how severe are they? (Use a scale of 0 = none; 1 = slight; 2 = moderate; and 3 = marked).

Symptoms	*Severity*
Hot flashes	_____
Sweating	_____
Anxiety	_____
Depression	_____
Forgetfulness	_____
Nightmares	_____
Worry	_____
Impatience	_____
Moodiness	_____
Touchiness	_____

2. How old were you when symptoms began?
3. Are you on any medication specifically for symptoms?

     _____ Yes   _____ No

   If yes, what are you taking?

4. Are you concerned or inconvenienced by any menopausal symptoms which you have not discussed with your doctor?

     _____ Yes   _____ No

5. How do you cope with the changes your body is currently undergoing?
6. How would you describe your feelings as you are experiencing menopause?
7. Compared with men you know, how would you rate yourself?

     _____ Having an easier time with menopause than most.

     _____ About the same as other men.

     _____ Having a harder time with menopause than most.

     _____ Do you have an explanation for this?

NORMAL AGE-RELATED CHANGES OF THE SEXUAL-REPRODUCTIVE PATTERN

◆ Aging Female

- ◆ Changes expected post-menopause due to steroid starvation
- ◆ Older women continue to have nipple erections
- ◆ Increase in size, areolar engorgement, flush prior to orgasm is diminished in intensity
- ◆ The sex flush caused by vasoscongestive skin response to tension is diminished

◆ Decrease in general muscular tension with arousal, diminished myotonia

◆ Decreased rectal sphincter contractions with orgasm

◆ Shrinkage of clitoris, but high degree of responsivity remains

◆ Minor labia vasocongestive thickening diminishes and color changes before orgasm diminish

◆ Bartholin's glands mucoid secretion during plateau diminishes

◆ Vaginal wall tissues become paper thin, noncorrugated, pinkish in color, vagina shortens, and expansive ability decreases. Less vaginal elasticity due to connective tissue changes

◆ Lubrication 1–5 minutes or more after stimulation. Reduced vaginal lubrication—estrogen responsive

◆ Orgasmic platform (swelling of outer vagina develops during plateau, constricting vagina). Engorgement is reduced, but constriction response continues. Reduction in duration of orgasm-resolution occurs more quickly, number of contractions of platform decrease during orgasm. Number of expulsive contractions with orgasm decrease

◆ During resolution rapid collapse of expanded portion of vagina

◆ Uterine elevation during excitement and plateau reactions are delayed and elevation is not as marked.

◆ Aging Male

◆ Nipple erection diminishes

◆ Reduction in size, firmness of testicles. Testosterone diminishes gradually

◆ Myotonia, diminished muscular tension, and involuntary muscular contractions

◆ Decrease frequency in rectal sphincter contractions during orgasm

◆ Erection of the penis may take 2–3 times longer over the age of 50, and a full erection may not be attained until just before an orgasm is about to occur

◆ Erection may be maintained longer without ejaculation

◆ When erection is partially lost, there may be difficulty in returning to full erection, which may be due to arteriosclerosis and reduced tissue elasticity

◆ Color changes of the glans penis may be diminished or absent

◆ Ejaculation: the expulsive contractions force during orgasm may be diminished and sensual experience may be reduced. Reduction in warning of inevitability

◆ Lengthening of refractory period, there may be a prolonged phase after orgasm before the next erection; rapid penile detumescence

◆ Ejaculation changes from a two-stage, well-differentiated process to a single stage expulsion of seminal fluid. There is a reduction in seminal fluid

◆ Prostatic contractions may become absent

◆ Older men may experience seepage rather than expulsion; fewer and less viable sperm than younger men

◆ Diminished response of scrotal folding patterns obliterated with sexual tension

◆ Testicular elevation in late excitement or early plateau; response is diminished, (increase in size) rapid descent of testicles.

RAPE-TRAUMA SYNDROME

Definition: Rape is an act of violence committed upon the resident without her or his consent. Rape is never an act of sexual passion. Vaginal and/or rectal penetration may be the form of sexual aggression committed upon the individual. Forced, nonconsensual sexual activity with or without penetration is considered rape. (The act of penetration is a factor of legal definition in many states. The Rape Trauma diagnosis does not limit itself to penetration and views any nonconsensual, forced act as traumatic.)

The sexual assault is usually followed by a syndrome that disorganizes the victim's life style with somatic, cognitive, psychological, and behavioral symptomology. The older individual is not immune or protected from rape or any act of violence. The institutionalized elder may be more fearful of reporting any incident for fear of staff/family disbelief or reoccurrence of trauma from the rapist. The nursing home resident is in a vulnerable position and may need to depend on her or his aggressor for basic care.

ASSESSMENT

Assessment of the resident that has been raped has two distinct, but overlapping, components—physical and emotional assessments.

The physical assessment of an elderly rape victim should be comprehensive and done with calm, understanding approach. It is vital that the nurse examine the body for any lacerations, abrasions, or any other marks indicating physical violence. The elderly victim should be carefully assessed for any hematomas, joint pain, or inability to move extremities. Assess the hips bilaterally for any pain, trauma, or misalignment. Examine for vaginal and rectal trauma. All victims should have a culture for sexually transmitted diseases sent to the lab.

Blood work for syphilis and the presence of the HIV antibody should be done with the expressed informed consent of the victim. Many states require signed informed consent for HIV antibody testing, and the nurse should be very well versed in her practice state(s) laws.

It is also critical to counsel the victim on the significance of HIV antibody testing post rape trauma. The client should be informed about the current information regarding HIV infection, transmission, and incubation period. Since antibodies to HIV can take anywhere from 3 to 6 months to be detectable after infection the client needs to be informed of serial HIV antibody tests. The series is usually done in three phases: the first is at the time of the rape; the second is three months post rape; and the last is six months past the rape. If the client is HIV negative six months after the rape then she or he is generally considered free of the virus from the assault.

The nurse should access any local support from area AIDS Service Organizations (ASO's) to help the client cope with any related anxiety or concerns.

It is important to remember that rape is a crime, and crimes require evidence to prosecute attackers. Care must be taken not to destroy any physical evidence by bathing or douching the resident after the incident prior to physical exam and the collection of specimens. Very few nursing homes have a rape trauma protocol for nurses to follow if a resident is attacked. Nursing home residents should be taken to the nearest hospital emergency room for examination. It is critical that a nursing home staff member go with the victim, and stay with her or him throughout.

It has been said that rape is the ultimate violation of a person. A rapist more than penetrates an orifice—the very essence of the individual is violated. In order to assess and treat the rape victim's emotional needs the nurse should be supporting, non-judgmental, and accepting. The nurse should respond to and treat the rape victim as a healthy individual who has suffered significant emotional (and possibly physical) trauma. The victim should not be labeled and recorded as a "raped woman or man." They are a woman or man who has been raped. The nurse should also help the victim clarify and understand their options regarding being victimized, treated, and the law. Finally, the nurse should assist the individual to explore how their significant others are going to respond, and discuss personal safety.

Rape trauma syndrome has two phases. The acute phase displays emotional reactons such as fear, humiliation, embarrassment, and self-blame. Numerous physical manifestations may also occur, such as genitourinary pain, gastrointestinal distress, and disruption in sleep disturbance.

The long-term phase displays changes in life style (i.e. relocation) and occurrence of repetitive nightmares. Individuals usually seek out family and social supports.

Rape victims that do not disclose information about the rape to anyone are prone to develop "silent rape trauma." The individual cannot resolve feeling about the trauma and develop increased levels of anxiety. They may also develop a sudden phobic reaction. Changes in behavior may occur including depression, suicidal actions, acting out, and somatization.

AGE-RELATED PHENOMENON

It is sad reality that rape is committed upon the institutionalized elderly. Nursing home residents may be violated by family, friends, visitors, staff, or intruders. The resident is at special risk because of his or her physical status. Even the healthiest of elders will probably have great difficulty in physically defending themselves from a rapist. The frail elderly virtually stand no chance in self-defense.

The assailant may indeed be a "trusted" individual who provides basic needs for the individual. The older person may fear withdrawal of these needs (i.e. bathing, feeding, etc.) if they tell someone they have been raped. The rapist may threaten the older individual with bodily harm, destruction of personal property, or worse.

Confusion, dementia, or psychiatric disorders of some nursing home residents further complicate rape-trauma.

Victims of rape frequently fear their home environment that they once considered safe but which was violated. The nursing home resident may become angry and distrustful of the staff and the environment.

The older adult has specific fears and concerns following rape. These are concern over physical safety, fear of death, reputation, and respectability.

ETIOLOGIES

Etiologies of rape do not apply to the victim. No individual ever asked to be raped. Rape is an act of violence forced upon a person.

Etiologies may be appropriate for a discussion on why a rapist attacks. The rape trauma diagnosis focus on the victim, not the attacker.

Nearly 80 percent of all rapes are violent, planned attacks not based on physical attractiveness. Rapists will typically attack a smaller and physically weaker person and threaten them with weapons. Rape statistics show that victims range from age 3 months to over 90 years.

◆ Nursing Diagnosis

Rape-trauma syndrome related to forced, non-consensual sexual activity upon the resident.

DEFINING CHARACTERISTICS

ACUTE PHASE

◆ Resident reports forced, non-consensual act
◆ Anger and hostility
◆ Embarrassment and humiliation
◆ Fear of being left alone
◆ Fear of attacker's return
◆ Guilt
◆ Panic
◆ Denial.

LONG TERM PHASE

◆ Fear and phobias
◆ Sleep disturbances

◆ Anxiety
◆ Change in life style (i.e. relocation).

GOALS/OUTCOME CRITERIA

◆ Decrease the immediate negative responses to rape and increase disclosure.
◆ Resident will experience a decrease in any physical symptomology.
◆ Resident will develop trust of criminal justice system.
◆ Resident will identify support persons and systems.
◆ Return to pre-rape event level of functioning.
◆ Experience optimal psychosocial adjustment past event.

INTERVENTION AND ACCOUNTABILITY

◆ Calm and effective physical assessment with injury repair (RN, MD)
◆ Establish "safe person" to stay with resident throughout exam.
◆ Do not leave resident alone. (RN, SW)
◆ Brief individual on expected police and hospital procedures that are going to occur. (RN, SW)
◆ Maintain non-judgmental attitude and approach. (RN, Staff, Family)
◆ Counsel immediate family and/or support persons. (RN, SW)
◆ Preserve evidence. Assist with personal hygiene requests *after* examination. (RN, LPN, NA, STAFF)
◆ Obtain permission to contact rape crisis counselor (and do so, if permission granted). (RN, SW)
◆ Explain the examination process.

References

Barnhart, Edward R. *Physician's Desk Reference.* 41st edition. Oradell, NJ: Medical Economics Co.; 1987.

Bay Area Physicians for Human Rights. (1985, June). *AIDS safe-sex guidelines.* Available from San Francisco AIDS Foundation, 333 Valencia Street, Fourth Floor, San Francisco, CA 94103.

Bjorklund, E. (1987). Prevention: Reducing the risk of AIDS. In J.D. Durham and F.L. Cohen (Eds.), *The person with AIDS: Nursing prospectives,* (pp. 178–191). New York: Springer.

Botwinick, J. *Aging and Behavior,* 2nd edition. New York: Springer Publishing Co.; 1978.

Brecher, EM. *Love, Sex and Aging.* Boston: Little, Brown & Co.; 1984.

Burnside, IM. *Nursing and the Aged.* New York: McGraw-Hill, Inc.; 1981.

Carpenito, Lynda Juall. *Nursing Diagnosis: Application to Clinical Practice.* 3rd edition. Philadelphia, PA; J.B. Lippincott Co.; 1988.

Fletcher, David J. *Counseling Elderly Patients About Sex.* In *Geriatric Consultant*; September/October 1982.

Jarvis, L. *Community Health Nursing: Keeping the Public Healthy.* Philadelphia: F.A. Davis; 1981.

Kenney, RA. *Physiology of Aging a Synopsis.* Chicago: Year Book Medical Publishing, Inc.; 1982.

Kimmel, DC. *Adulthood and Aging.* 2nd edition. New York: John Wiley & Sons; 1980.

Kjervik, D and Marrtinson, I. *Women in Health and Illness.* Philadelphia: W.B. Saunders; 1986.

Murry, R, Huelskoetter, MM and O'Driscoll, D. *The Nursing Process in Later Maturity.* Englewood Cliffs, NJ: Prentice-Hall, Inc.; 1980.

National Institutes of Health. *Age Page: AIDS and the Older Adult.* Public Health Service; 1989.

Rehabilitation Nursing Institute. *Rehabilitation Nursing: Concepts and Practice, A Core Curriculum.* Evanston, IL: Rehabilitation Nursing Institute; 1981.

Rockstein, M and Sussman, M. *Biology of Aging.* Belmont, CA: Wadsworth Publishing Co.; 1979.

Shives, L. *Basic Concepts of Psychiatric Mental Health Nursing.* Philadelphia: J.B. Lippincott; 1986.

Slonick, RL. *Sexuality and Aging.* The University of Southern California Press, the Ethel Percy Andrus Gerontology Center, publisher; 1978.

Thompson, J et al. *Clinical Nursing.* 2nd edition. St. Louis: C.V. Mosby; 1989.

Walz, TH and Blum, NS. *Sexual Health in Later Life.* Lexington, MA: D.C. Heath & Co.; 1987.

Coping Stress Tolerance Patterns

James J. Kane

◆

COPING PATTERNS

Coping is an ongoing process employed by all persons in the face of stress. Physical and mental make-up, personality, support systems, and learned behaviors all contribute to individual and family coping styles.

Numerous developmental tasks have been mastered by elders: careers, coupling, child-rearing, educating, health changes to list a few. These tasks have provided arenas for finely tuning coping skills. Elders, then, are faced with many major physical and social changes, which tax their learned coping styles. The nurse can play a vital role in fostering the use of the elder's learned coping skills and promoting flexibility and mastery to obtain new techniques.

The following section describes coping patterns common to elder populations and interventions useful to facilitiate adaptation.

INEFFECTIVE COPING: INDIVIDUAL

Definition: Impairment of adaptive behaviors and problem-solving abilities for meeting life's demands and roles. Methods of handling stressful life situations are insufficient to control anxiety, fear, or anger.

Individuals may lack the resources to deal with the rapid and numerous changes of aging. Depression, loneliness, isolation, feelings of helplessness and uselessness inhibit continued growth and wellness.

ASSESSMENT

Assessment of coping can be challenging and complex due to the interrelatedness of physical symptoms and coping behaviors. Initially, a comprehensive physical assessment provides a screening tool to indicate the pres-

The author wishes to acknowledge Jill Bormann MSN, RN, CS for her help in reviewing the manuscript.

ence of biological causes for stress-related symptoms. The relationship the nurse establishes with the older person is key to establishing the trust needed to understand the individual, his or her prior history of coping with crises, and current bio-psycho-social-cultural well-being. The goal of the assessment is to look at the person's cognitive and physical resources since these are the basis from which the person perceives a threat and copes.

Accurate mental status assessment is an essential component of cognitive assessment. Hays and Borger (1985) suggest using the Glasgow Coma Scale (GCS) (see Table 13–1) to help quantify state of consciousness in older individuals. Another simple tool, the SET Test, is used to assess cognitive status. This is composed of four categories, Fruits, Animals, Color, and Towns (FACT), of which the older person is asked to name ten of each. One point is given for each accurate reply. A score of below 15 indicates severe dementia (see Table 13–2).

Altered communication patterns, social isolation, behavioral disturbances—fear, anger, agitation, self-destructive activities, anxiety, inability to care for oneself, increase in accidents, poor problem-solving—all are manifestations of ineffective coping. Abusive behaviors towards self or others indicates ineffective coping and can require prompt emergency treatment. A sudden change in normal functioning warrants examination. The source of this information can expand from the resident to all those involved. Changes in the ability to meet role expectations and inappropriate use of defense mechanisms, including verbal manipulation, can indicate ineffective coping. Combined with all of the symptoms, physical complaints of pain and gastrointestinal changes (nausea, anorexia, weight loss, diarrhea, constipation), including changes in weight and sleep patterns, are considered to indicate inadequate coping.

TABLE 13–1 ◆ The Glasgow Coma Scale

Eyes Open	Spontaneously	4
	To speech	3
	To pain	2
	None	1
Best Verbal Response	Oriented	5
	Confused	4
	Inappropriate words	3
	Incomprehensible words	2
	None	1
Best Motor Response	Obeys commands	6
	Localized pain	5
	Flexion withdrawal	4
	Abnormal flexion	3
	Abnormal extension	2
	Flaccid	1
	TOTAL:	

TABLE 13-2 ◆ The SET TEST

SET TEST	
(10 each)	Fruits
	Animals
	Colors
	Towns
Total Score:	

The SET TEST is a useful test to assess overall mental function of the elderly client. By naming ten items in each category (score 1 point for each), it is thought that motivation, alertness, concentration, short-term memory, and problem-solving are demonstrated. Scores below 15 indicate severe dementia. Scores between 16 and 24 indicate the need for further evaluation.

AGE-RELATED PHENOMENON

Developmentally, aging presents numerous challenges to an individual's ability to cope and adapt, and thus place the elder population at risk for ineffective coping. Physically, changes in sensory systems (visual and hearing loss, mobility, sexuality, and cognitive abilities) are adapted to with age. Simultaneously, many major life events occur between 65 and 75 years of age. Retirement (self or spouse), oldest child leaving home, widowhood, illness requiring hospitalization, and relocation are some common stressors confronted by this age group.

Examination of older populations' response and adaptation to the stress of age provides useful insights into potential areas for nursing intervention. Studies have consistently suggested that older people experience little personality change. For example, when rigidity is seen, it is a defense against a perceived threat or actual crisis, not a characteristic of aging.

Older populations cope and adapt to stress differently from younger populations, and older populations have a wide range of adaptive styles. Yet their ability to cope can be severely hampered due to the number of stresses and losses encountered with aging. The adaptive processes of the older person that are utilized to cope with loss differ from those utilized to deal with stress. Therefore, a crisis for an elder must be defined in terms of the amount of change required versus the perception of the crisis in terms of the meaning of the event or the loss entailed.

Cognitive and physical resources are the factors that determine the adaptation and coping abilities of the elderly. Yet the presence of these resources does not necessarily assure effective coping. Utilization and promotion of available resources is key to the adaptation of the elderly.

Emphasis on dealing with age is counterproductive. The focus of treatment must be on the identification of the type of problem elder individuals encounter, the changes required, and the resources available to cope with these changes. Fostering coping is an essential role of the nurse, who has contact with the aged individual, either in the community or extended-care facility.

ETIOLOGIES

ENVIRONMENTAL

◆ Situational crises: institutionalization, widowhood, loss of colleagues and friends, relocation, closing the family home, economic changes, isolation

◆ Maturational crises: retirement, oldest child leaves home, role changes, response of others to aging

◆ Personal vulnerability: decreased social contacts

◆ Knowledge deficit

◆ Perceived loss of control

◆ Belief in self: cultural conditions may enforce sense of uselessness, ineffective use of coping styles, decisions about them made without their being included.

INTERNAL

◆ Situational crises: illness requiring hospitalization

◆ Maturational crises: self-concept/ideal as effected by aged, physical and cognitive changes of aging—sensory decrease, mobility decrease, etc.—declined level of wellness, less resistance to illness, decreased ability to utilize resources, personality factors preventing acceptance of resources, i.e. pride

◆ Problem-solving skill deficit: inability to utilize public transport due to physical changes, cognitive/physical changes limit self care ability

◆ Perceived loss of control; belief in self: self-ideal affected by rapid changes—"life isn't as expected"—self-image—affected by changes due to age—independence prevented by physical changes—leads to questions of self worth—no sense of worth/satisfaction.

◆ Nursing Diagnosis

Ineffective coping due to situational crisis or problem solving deficit (i.e., forced relocation, retirement, or institutionalization). (See also Social Isolation) Given as examples, some of these may present greater maturational crises and vice versa.

DEFINING CHARACTERISTICS

◆ Verbalizes inability to cope

◆ Inability to ask for help

◆ Anxiety, fear, anger.

◆ Change in societal participation
◆ Gastrointestinal changes (bowel, appetite disturbance)
◆ Inability to meet role expectations (including self-care)
◆ Inappropriate use of defense mechanisms.

GOALS/OUTCOME CRITERIA

◆ Verbalizes ability to cope
◆ Identifies alternate methods of dealing with anger
◆ Initiates new social activity
◆ Subjectively GI symptoms are resolved
◆ Performs ADL and role expectations (i.e., house cleaning, gardening)
◆ Denial will be used appropriately
◆ Asks for help.

INTERVENTIONS

1. Encourage talking about the recent change in nondirective manner on a frequent basis a few minutes daily. (RN, LPN, NA)
2. Assess coping strategies used in past when confronted with major environmental changes. (RN, LPN)
3. Facilitate problem description by the resident.
   a. Explore possible options, reinforce prior coping experiences.
   b. Discuss advantages and disadvantages.
   c. Discuss factors preventing acceptance of viable alternatives. (Do not badger or coerce client into acceptance of alternatives; let them make choice.)
   d. Assure exploration of viable alternatives. (RN, LPN, NA)
4. Promote utilization of social supports. (RN, LPN, NA)
   a. Is family aware of the impact the crisis has had? (See Family Coping: Compromised).
   b. Encourage family to provide emotional support.
   c. Explore interests in social activities in the past. Encourage continued activity in new settings (make sure resident knows viable choices).
   d. Foster networking. Mobilize peers as indicated. (RN)
   e. If possible and appropriate, allow visits to old friends at old location to ease the transition. (This provides the opportunity for closure or termination, ending and saying goodbye to something that can be no longer.) (RN)
   f. Encourage talking about the new changes in relationships with old friends.

g. Allow verbalization about the loss due to the change (see Grieving Dysfunctional).

5. At all times employ principles of therapeutic communication. (RN, LPN, NA)

a. Acknowledge and accept feelings.

b. Encourage hopeful perspective without negating the client's reality.

6. Encourage experiences that promote feelings of self-worth in the new environment. Support steps towards acceptance of the change.

7. Help resident discuss and choose factors and people that will allow acceptance of the change.

8. Severe maladaptive coping requires referrals to appropriate specialists.

9. Be aware of the potential for violence (see appropriate diagnosis category) and refer to nurse therapist as indicated.

10. Use a sense of humor.

◆ Nursing Diagnosis

Ineffective coping (individual) due to perceived loss of control; belief in self (see Powerlessness).

DEFINING CHARACTERISTICS

◆ Cannot ask for help

◆ Inability to problem solve

◆ High rate of accidents.

◆ Excessive food, alcohol intake

◆ Anxiety

◆ Digestive, bowel, appetite disturbance; chronic fatigue or sleep pattern disturbance

◆ Cannot meet role expectations

◆ Cannot care for self (not necessarily due to physical cause)

◆ Change in socialization, communication

◆ Destructive behavior (to self or others)

◆ Manipulation.

GOALS/OUTCOME CRITERIA

◆ Within 2 weeks of treatment will be able to identify when help is needed to cope

◆ Decreased frequency of accidents

◆ Able to list alternatives to problems objectively

◆ Subjective and objective decrease in anxiety

◆ Return of digestive/sleep pattern to pre-crisis levels

◆ Role resolution—performing as expected

◆ Initiates self-care activities

◆ Initiates social contact once alternatives are explored

◆ Absence of self/other destructive behaviors (emergency measures taken as needed).

INTERVENTIONS

◆ Assessment of prior and present coping pattern completed within three days of contact. (RN)

◆ Initiate emergency measures as indicated for suicidality. (See Potential for Violence.)

◆ Reinforce attempts to cope, even when resident only acknowledges the need to cope better, i.e. reflect or observe: "I can see you're trying to cope with a great deal." (RN, LPN, NA)

◆ Allow opportunities for ventilation on daily basis. Sit with client every day. Listening has been described as crucial to fostering self-esteem of the elderly.

◆ Acknowledge feelings.

◆ Foster sense of mastery whenever possible by summarizing attempts at coping the client makes.

◆ Facilitate the problem-solving process by helping client explore alternatives. Whenever possible allow client to suggest options. This fosters a sense of competency and control. Simplifying complex abstract concepts into simple, concrete tasks may facilitate problem-solving.

◆ Allow residents as much control as possible over their environment and praise positive attempts to master tasks. Foster independence. Allow opportunity for privacy and to be alone. Allow time for transition. (RN, LPN)

◆ Encourage exploration of new interests, hobbies, or social events. Support rebirth of old hobbies.

◆ Encourage physical activity, walking, shopping, gardening.

◆ Encourage family support. Teach and allow client to ask friends/family for help when needed.

◆ Allow expression of concern regarding bowel/sleep changes. Don't focus on these symptoms while still acknowledging and treating their presence. Help the individual to recognize the stressors and feelings of worth that may be related to physical symptoms. Reinforce mastery of physical signs/symptoms. (RN, LPN, NA)

◆ Note and identify for the resident the impact they have on others, since negative sense of self-worth may prevent this, i.e. "Your roommate really appreciates you listening to his problems, it helps him."

◆ Encourage positive discussions about the client's prior experiences, skills, and achievements. This fosters the sense of accomplishment, potentially identifies areas for continued pursuit, and allows the client to feel as though someone listens and is interested.

◆ Allow time for privacy and to be alone.

◆ Pets are useful to promote feelings of being needed, and provide companionship and affection. When appropriate, encourage and support this.

◆ Nursing Diagnosis

Ineffective individual coping as related to maturational crises (marital problems, death of spouse (see Grief), physical deterioration, loss of self-ideal, role changes, empty nest).

DEFINING CHARACTERISTICS

◆ Anxiety, fear, irritability (withdrawal)

◆ Tension

◆ Presence of life stressor

◆ Unable to meet basic needs

◆ Role conflict or not meeting role expectation

◆ Destructive behavior to self or others

◆ Inappropriate use of defense mechanisms

◆ Change in communication (argumentative with spouse, family, staff)

◆ Refusal of assistance

◆ Ineffective use of defense mechanisms (regression, somatization, introjection, dependency, repression)

◆ Subjective inability to cope

◆ Depression.

GOALS/OUTCOME CRITERIA

◆ Resident will identify numerous stressors

◆ Subjective decrease in fear, anxiety, tension

◆ Assumption of alternate role expectations. Role resolution

◆ Able to more actively assume part of self-care

◆ Make reasonable effort to accept and deal with sensory loss (i.e. uses hearing aid or glasses)

◆ Marital couples and family given opportunity to talk about recent changes

◆ Absence of destructive behaviors

◆ Defenses will be used appropriately.

INTERVENTIONS

◆ Resident routinely given opportunity to talk about recent changes on a daily basis. Sit with client daily. Identify the stressor. (RN, LPN, NA)

◆ Fears and anxieties related to maturational changes are identified through gently probing and encouraging client to talk about concerns. (RN, SW)

◆ Problem-solving skills need examination and alternatives need to be explored (see Intervention in Ineffective Coping, Situational Crises, Problem-Solving.) (RN, LPN)

◆ Pay attention to and acknowledge physical problems and treat acceptingly, without focusing on negative aspects of a disability. (RN, LPN, NA)

◆ Appropriate use of defense mechanisms is supported. When denial is used, acknowledge its presence and give client permission to take charge. (RN, LPN)

◆ Allow talking about fears. Introduce resident (as appropriate) to other persons with the same change (stressor). In order to share coping ideas and learn they are not alone. (ALL)

◆ Environmental changes may help cope with maturational stressors (or others). A move may be indicated once grieving over the loss of a spouse is completed. A smaller home may be suggested in cases of large empty nests. (ALL)

◆ When possible, reduce the impact of stressor so defenses can be relaxed. Support defenses when appropriate. (ALL)

◆ Maintain hope in future events. (ALL)

◆ Allow appropriate expression of anger. (ALL)

◆ Have psychiatric experts evaluate and treat when symptoms continue or are life-threatening. (RN, MD)

◆ Keep the resident involved in the treatment, to foster a sense of competency. (RN, LPN, NA)

◆ Remain supportive, helpful, interested, and intervening. (RN, LPN)

◆ Encourage pursuit of old and new social contacts. Present alternatives that encourage physical activity within limits of abilities (i.e. walking, outdoor activities). (ALL)

◆ Nursing Diagnosis

Ineffective individual coping related to personal vulnerability (decreased resistance to illness, decreased social supports, decreased physical resources, personality variables).

DEFINING CHARACTERISTICS

◆ Subjective inability to cope

◆ Ineffective problem-solving

◆ Physical risk
◆ Not meeting ADL
◆ Changes in socialization
◆ Changes in physical symptoms
◆ Ineffective use of defense mechanisms.

GOALS/OUTCOME CRITERIA

◆ Vulnerability identified
◆ Alternate problem-solving described
◆ Self-care increased, decline in (somatic) physical signs/symptoms
◆ Defenses supported appropriately.

INTERVENTIONS

◆ Assessment of coping resources completed. (RN)
◆ Problem-solving skills explored. Alternatives examined (see Situational Crises. Teach Problem-Solving). (RN, LPN)
◆ Positive steps to independence encouraged in area of self-care.
◆ Promote and encourage interests in outside activities (social events, friends, family, recreational events). (RN, LPN, NA)
◆ Risk factors identified and addressed directly.
◆ Experiences and feelings are talked about and catharsis encouraged.
◆ Attempt to modify stressor when possible to fall within range of coping abilities.
◆ Support appropriate use of defenses. Provide alternate defenses or support when inappropriate use of defenses impairs coping (teach new coping). (RN, LPN)

AVOIDANCE COPING

Definition: Prolonged minimization or denial of information when a situation requires active coping. Ambiguity with respect to the problem or resources leads to continued absence of an appropriate response. [See also Individual Coping: Ineffective.]

ASSESSMENT

Full assessment of the individual's personal resources (including physical and cognitive) is indicated. Examination of social supports (family, friends, and group supports), personality characteristics (defenses, flexibility) and coping skills (including prior coping strategies) lays the foundation to begin to understand the etiology of avoidance of a stimulus. This comprehensive assessment includes a goal to understand why a particular stressor elicits fear, misperception, or intimidation.

Several key areas require assessment: (1) the resident's ability to contain the stress within tolerable limits; (2) the impact of the stressor or ability to maintain self-esteem; (3) the interpersonal relationships involved and their continued presence in the face of the stress; and (4) resources and adaptability to a new environment. In addition to assessment of these four categories, establish a pattern of avoidance with regard to a certain problem. The clues of avoidance being present include passivity or the "ideal patient syndrome," depression, anger, hostility, and anxiety. Cognitive deterioration may accelerate in elders where prior deterioration has occurred. [NOTE: Denial and numbness is an adaptive response to the loss of a significant other and a normal part of a grief reaction. (See Grief: Dysfunctional.)]

AGE-RELATED PHENOMENON:

Elders have had years to develop and refine coping patterns. In some cases these patterns may be less useful than in others. Psychological and social denial, and an adaptive response in which the elderly withdraw, have been identified as three of the common coping mechanisms of elders. Additionally, passive coping and denial or avoidance strategies are useful in cases of some institutionalizations and types of specific diseases. Changes in cognitive and physical resources can determine the mechanisms chosen by the elder to cope. Overall, individuals who accurately perceive a stress are able to begin the changes in the thought process that bring about an adaptation to the environment.

Key factors in coping and the use of avoidance are the level of perceived stress and preoccupation with the stress. These concepts form the basis for understanding the elder avoiding a particular stressor. The use of avoidance is contingent on perceived availability of support to deal with a stressor.

Rather than attack avoidance directly, treatments are devoted to fostering an improved sense of mastery and better use of resources.

ETIOLOGIES

INTERNAL

◆ Perceived competency

◆ Perceived powerlessness

◆ Support system deficit (cognitive, physical).

EXTERNAL

◆ Support system deficit (social support).

◆ Nursing Diagnosis

Avoidance coping, as related to perceived competency/powerlessness (see also Powerlessness).

DEFINING CHARACTERISTICS

◆ Presence of perceived threat to health, self-image, values, life style, or relationships

◆ Minimizes, ignores, or forgets information following clear communication or observation

◆ Mislabels events

◆ Absence of problem-solving, information-seeking, incorporation of new information into future planning

◆ Repressive dependency

◆ Anxiety, depression, passivity, or anger.

GOALS/OUTCOME CRITERIA

◆ Emergency treatment as indicated is taken in cases of potential health danger due to passivity or depression

◆ Individuals will be able to list available strengths.

◆ Problem-solving alternatives are explored

◆ New coping mechanisms are discussed

◆ Support systems are mobilized

◆ Self-help group information is given

◆ The individual will eventually describe perceived stress in a manner showing greater objectivity (not immediate goal)

◆ Autonomy, mastery and control are fostered

◆ Individual is encouraged to pursue accurate information regarding stressor.

INTERVENTIONS

◆ Assess current strengths, coping strategies, and perceived problem. (RN)

◆ Validate nature of crisis through ancillary sources as necessary (i.e. family members, physicians). (RN)

◆ Treat emergency symptomatology: call a consult with appropriate expert if clinically depressed, withdrawn, or physical health is in peril. (RN)

◆ Have client list as objectively as possible all assets (include prior coping strategies, social supports, physical strengths, positive attitudes). Support attempts to do this. (RN, LPN)

◆ Explore problem-solving skills. Discuss alternatives. (See Individual Coping: Ineffective). (RN, LPN)

◆ Discuss concerns in terms of outcomes, not necessarily by directly confronting individual with stressor at this time.

◆ Attempt to deal with altered perception of reality by exploring etiologies of this altered reality.

◆ Provide information regarding self-help groups (see Intervention: Family Coping: Potential for Growth). (RN, LPN, NA)

◆ Allow the client time, when possible, to assimilate resources and information that conflicts with reality. (RN, LPN, NA)

◆ Promote the exercising of autonomy by encouraging the making of choices and listing alternatives.

◆ Encourage use of family resources to support client (see Family Coping: Potential for Growth and Compromise). (RN)

◆ Allow client to identify knowledge deficits in open-ended fashion. (RN, LPN, NA)

GERIATRIC FAMILY COPING

FAMILY COMPOSITION

The family is a vital source of satisfaction, nurturance, and growth throughout an individual's life cycle. Four-fifths of all older people in the United States have living children. The composition of a family is unique individually and can vary from multi-generational large groups to small sets of siblings. An elder's comments that a certain family member is no longer contacted usually indicates this relationship has great emotional content as well as those with whom the elder relates more directly.

Family composition is in a state of flux. Improved health care and birth control bodes a change from multi-sibling groups to families of small numbers over several generations. This means more people will be relating to other family members as adults.

Filial responsibility for aging parents both physically and financially is a societal expectation. Some welfare laws require depletion of family resources prior to an elder receiving benefits. Adults with more than one aged parent and grandparents would be unfairly burdened. Stress of this type could adversely affect the positive aspects of the family relationships with the older persons. Institutionalization is described as a serious stressor for adult children of aged parents, due to unresolved guilt that affects continued support of the elder.

COMMON VARIABLES

Several common variables help clarify how family members relate together as a system to cope with stress. Structure, process, and communication are core components of analysis in family work.

Structure refers to the boundaries and relationships between members in addition to the goals and purposes that affect these. Process refers to the covert and overt movement of the family through the phases or stages of development. Communication refers to the verbal and nonverbal interactions of members. Communication patterns can indicate problems in structure or process and are useful sites for treatment. These components form the foundation of all family interaction, and also provide useful places for assessment and intervention.

FAMILIES AS SYSTEMS

It has been stated that older people remain involved with their families. The crises that affect these individuals affect the whole family. Even the youngest members of a family react emotionally to the problems of the grandparent. Adult children sense the impact of an elder on a family and react based on their resources. These adults understand that their children's attitude toward aging will be developed during this time and reflected later in their life.

Numerous stressors are unique to geriatric families. The units or subsystems of these families must be flexible, exchange resources through their boundaries, and allow for individual growth to promote coping and homeostasis.

STRESS ON THE FAMILY

Four sources of stress on the family have been identified and are significant in understanding the coping of families.

1. Stressful contact of one (unit) member with an outside force requires family interaction to cope. All the problems faced by an individual affect the whole. Forced retirement, relocation, changed finances, and physical changes of the elder affect the whole system.

2. A second source of stress occurs when the entire family faces an outside stress. Relocation of the whole group is an example of this stress. The assimilation of a new environment or culture tests all family members. The inclusion of an elder to an established family household results in changes in roles, responsibility, and coping by the entire family.

3. A major problem facing families with geriatric members occurs with family development at transition points. The transition of the mature parent to the role of older adult is a major stressor for families.

The elder member may be forced to assume a role as grandparent. Not all elders may appreciate the positive aspects of this role. Myths associated with this role include the over-intrusive, domineering elder. Reality is that grandparents potentially can experience biological continuity, vicarious accomplishment, and emotional self-fulfillment in the role of grandparenting. Problems can occur when old, unresolved conflicts with adult children are acted out through grandchildren. Other grandparents may feel exploited.

A major developmental stressor involves filial maturity. The growth of children to adulthood and the assumption of responsibilities and roles left by aging parents is a normal part of family development. In addition to accepting their own aging, adult children are responsible for children, professional careers, and now aging parents. Prior perception of all powerful and nurturing parents are challenged. The societal pressures, as discussed, can place financial and physical burdens on the relationship adults have with elder parents. The adults must recognize their parents as individuals, with rights, needs, limits, and history. Adult children must complete their emancipation from the parent to be free to help the parent.

Post-parenting couples are at risk for problems in coping. Older couples are faced with accepting the physical changes in their spouse. Several expectations of these couples are care during illness, household management, and emotional gratification. Marriages are sites for individual and mutual growth. Yet not all marriages grow together in the later years of the couples' lives. Conflicted expectations, loss of parental roles (empty nest), physical changes in one person draining the physical and emotional resources of the caretaker, retirement leading to increased contact and more free time, altered patterns of dominance, all occur with the transition to aging for mature couples. Couples have years to develop dysfunctional patterns and these are now faced with age.

   4. The fourth major problem families face is idiosyncratic stresses. Long-term illness can be categorized in this area. Death of an elder is a great stress requiring restructuring and multiple changes in a family. The need for institutionalization has been described as the second major cause of geriatric family dysfunction (the first being filial maturity). Families have been shown to go to inordinate lengths to prevent institutionalization of elder parents. Anxiety about one's own aging, denial of older parent's disabilities, projection of guilt onto the institution, and profound grief, leading to avoidance of the parent after separation, occur when families are inadequately supported during an elder's institutionalization.

FAMILY ASSESSMENT

The goal of a family assessment of coping is to examine the way in which the family as a whole supports one another in the face of changes caused by the aging of one member. The concepts of structure, process, and communication form useful areas to assess the potentially overwhelming dynamics of family interaction.

   Structure is examined at by observing the boundaries between the individuals and subsystems (i.e. spousal, sibling, parent-child) within the family. Simply, boundaries refer to the distance or closeness of members. Do the spouses maintain mutual support or does a child interfere? Does a parent interfere with the marriage of a child? Are all parties afforded mutual respect for freedom of choices and privacy? Does one subsystem (i.e. sibling) continually advise another how to relate (i.e. spousal-elder couple)? These areas require observation in light of the changes aging causes to the elder member.

   Process is the manner in which the family moves through the phases or stages of development towards explicit or implicit goals. An overview of the process in which an elder was accepted into a household is observed. The process of deciding that institutionalization is indicated (or is not indicated) is another example of family dynamics. Process is the way things are done in a family. The way change is dealt with, the mutual acceptance of responsibility, or use of available resources are all examples of process.

   Communication patterns are useful to assess to understand family function. These spell out how a family works. What feelings are permitted? Can everyone speak freely? What might be inhibiting expression of feelings? How has the aging of one family member affected communication? Is the elder member allowed individual expression? Do family members listen to one another? Where are conflicts? Is conflict allowed? Is communication clear?

   The role of the nurse in the extended care facility can easily include family meetings for discussion and support. Symptoms evidenced in a resident only reflect the problems of the whole. In addition to clarification of problems, support is fostered in meetings of this type and useful observations can be made.

FAMILY COPING: POTENTIAL FOR GROWTH

Definition: Family member has effectively managed adaptive tasks involved with the client's health challenge and is exhibiting desire and readiness for enhanced health and growth in regard to self and in relation to the client. Family gathers information, makes and implements decisions, resolves conflict, and provides for individual growth and development, creates an emotional context fostering self-disclosure, trust, cooperation, and acceptance.

ASSESSMENT

Boundaries between family members and subsystems are clear. Decisions are made by appropriate members (subgroups). Individuals are allowed privacy and receive support, when asked or as needed. Rules of the family are conducive to individual growth toward self-actualization. Stressors can be clearly described and the impact that these have on family goals is recognized. Limitations are recognized and outside help is sought. Wellness is optimized by choosing activities that promote this for all members. (See Assessment of Families.)

AGE-RELATED PHENOMENON

Potential for growth is promoted when individual family members and subsystems have clear boundaries, which have been established throughout the history and culture of the group. Stressors of aging members have been anticipated and are dealt with through the mutually supportive relationships that have been established. Self-actualized families support goals of the individual, aging is viewed as a challenge, free time is looked at as opportunity, interests and values have been maintained over the life cycle of the elder members.

ETIOLOGIES

INTERNAL AND EXTERNAL

Self-actualization (sense of satisfaction, completion, mutual support is present).

◆ Nursing Diagnosis

Family coping: potential for growth as related to self-actualization.

DEFINING CHARACTERISTICS

- ◆ Little or no mutual decision making
- ◆ Limited access to related resources

◆ Individual members not included in communication or process of growth.

GOALS/OUTCOME CRITERIA

◆ Members decribe crisis in terms of values, goals, or relationships
◆ Members promote health and enriching life styles that support maturational processes, monitor treatment, choose treatment wisely
◆ Seek assistance from individuals having similar experiences.
◆ Family talks about current changes in useful terms
◆ Members participate in the treatment of the elder.
◆ Members are knowledgeable regarding self-help groups.

INTERVENTIONS

◆ Family is assessed. Meetings of all significant family members are conducted initially on contact with the resident when changes necessitate, and more frequently as needed. (RN, LPN)
◆ Communication is encouraged between members.
◆ The nurse models clear communication.
◆ Encourage continued family participation in the elder's treatment.
◆ Allow open discussion regarding concerns specific to current crisis or change.
◆ Support the family's healthy use of available resources.
◆ Promote and support the family's need for feelings of "universality" or of not being alone in their problems. Introduce the family to others with recent similar changes, as appropriate.
◆ Provide available resources regarding self-help groups (i.e. National Institutes of Health (1979) *A guide to medical self-care and self-help groups for the elderly* (Publication No. NIH 80-1687). Washington, DC. Provide information regarding SAGE (Senior Actualization and Growth Exploration) groups in the area.
◆ Support elder participation in peer assistance groups.

FAMILY COPING: COMPROMISED

Definition: Usually supportive primary person (family member of close friend) providing insufficient, ineffective, or compromised support, comfort, assistance, or encouragement needed by the resident to manage or master adaptive tasks related to health challenge. Individual use of resources is inhibited. Interpersonal conflict among family members inhibits usual manner that stress is dealt with.

ASSESSMENT

The following signs and symptoms may be present upon assessment. The structure of family is not flexible in response to stress. Modification in roles required by an elder's physical, cognitive, and developmental changes does not occur smoothly. During interactions, family members fail to assume necessary responsibility. In the case of illness or death, the old structural alliances are inadequate (i.e. daughter-father alliances are inadequate to help mother when father is unable to deal with his own illness). The process that fosters mutual growth, although present, is inhibited. Communication is inadequate. Frustration may ensue. Individuals focus on personal problems. The group may acknowledge "not knowing what to do." Decisions may be made for the individual without usual concern for independence and capability. Autonomy is ignored. Members may speak, answer, and decide for each other rather than mutually. The family is "stuck." (See Universal Family Assessment.)

AGE-RELATED PHENOMENON

In families with histories of decreased coping or less than optimal maturity, the stress of an aging individual may be unanticipated. The longstanding, unresolved emotional conflicts, which occurred due to overly diffuse or rigid boundaries, become explosive causes of conflict. Numerous stresses, as described, can contribute to a continued drain on available supportive resources. Adult children may be unable to accept the aging of parents and therefore withdraw support. The threats of aging lead to personal anxiety of the family so that mutual coping is incomplete. The individual in greater need of support is abandoned. Necessary role changes fail to occur in a family suffering compromised coping. A sense of loss due to changes necessitated by the crisis of developmental change permeates the group. Elders may fear relinquishing control, or young adults are afraid to assume control, and available resources are compromised.

ETIOLOGIES

INTERNAL

◆ Knowledge deficit (i.e. illness or available support services)

◆ Emotional conflicts (between subsystems)

◆ Exhaustion of supportive capacity (i.e. caretaker spouse is drained)

◆ Role changes (i.e. no one assumes role of absent roles or has lack of knowledge of how to assume role)

◆ Family disorganization (chaos among members, restructuring hampered)

◆ Developmental and Situational Crises (as described, see prior section).

EXTERNAL

◆ Emotional conflicts (with outside forces, i.e. institution)

◆ Exhaustion of supportive capacity (financial supports from government organization unknown or absent).

◆ Nursing Diagnosis

Ineffective family coping: compromised, related to knowledge deficit.

DEFINING CHARACTERISTICS

◆ Family members acknowledge inadequate knowledge regarding how to continue to be supportive
◆ Family member attempts to be supportive ineffectively (old supportive methods repeated unsuccessfully).

GOALS/OUTCOME CRITERIA

◆ Family is made aware of available resources
◆ Family is able to repeat demonstrated necessary procedures to help member in need
◆ Family continues to seek help when needed
◆ Members able to more clearly identify areas of knowledge deficit.

INTERVENTIONS

◆ Assess family, provide safe environment for disclosure. (RN)
◆ Encourage communication between members.
◆ Allow the family to discuss conflicts.
◆ Explore areas of knowledge deficits to clarify these more specifically.
◆ Allow the family to explore available resources to solve problem prior to advising or providing the answer. This fosters a sense of mastery. (RN, LPN)
◆ Provide information regarding available self-help groups (see Interventions: Family Coping: Potential for Growth).
◆ Identify for the family perceived areas of necessary education and provide this (use resources as needed). Expect a repeat demonstration as an evaluation of having mastered the material.
◆ Be prepared to refer, if needed, to appropriate family experts.

◆ Nursing Diagnosis

Ineffective family coping: compromised, related to emotional conflicts.

DEFINING CHARACTERISTICS

◆ Significant person is preoccupied with personal reactions to an elder's health, disability or change with age
◆ Significant person displays overly protective behavior disproportion-

ate (too much or too little) to the resident's needs and autonomy (diffuse boundaries)

◆ Significant person is absorbed in limited communication with client at time of need

◆ Old patterns of coping and interaction ineffective to cope with crisis or change.

◆ Established structure of subsystems is adequate to allow proper use of available resources.

GOALS/OUTCOME CRITERIA

◆ Family members will identify available resources to deal with the crisis

◆ Individuals will recognize the impact the change/crisis is having on other family members

◆ Individual members will recognize the importance of self-sufficiency among other family members

◆ The resources of all available family will be involved in dealing with the crisis

◆ New structural relationships will be identified by the family.

◆ New coping modalities will be described by family members.

INTERVENTIONS

◆ Family assessment. Provide a safe environment for self-disclosure. (RN, LPN)

◆ Family members are encouraged to discuss their perception of the problem. This is clarified and validated by family.

◆ Available strengths of individual members are elicited and discussed (including physical and emotional resources).

◆ Prior problems requiring a family response are explored, to foster a sense of mastery and recall coping mechanisms.

◆ Communication from each person is promoted and expected to help re-establish individual autonomy.

◆ The feelings individuals have regarding the change/crisis are explored to foster an awareness among the family of the impact of the crisis. (RN, LPN)

◆ Suggestions of how to use available resources are offered.

◆ In cases of over-involvement of one family member with another, the intruded upon one is given opportunity to speak for himself or herself. His or her own ideas on how to deal with the problem are considered by the group.

◆ Old subsystems will be identified by the nurse.

◆ Refer to experts when emotional conflicts, old coping continues or the crisis remains unresolved.

◆ Nursing Diagnosis

Ineffective family coping: compromised, related to developmental or situational crises, or exhaustion of supportive capacities (i.e. physical deterioration of elder, institutionalization, long-term illness requiring physical care, financial depletion, forced retirement).

DEFINING CHARACTERISTICS

- ◆ Significant person withdraws into limited interaction with client at time of need
- ◆ Client expresses concern about family member's response to his/her problem
- ◆ Significant person is preoccupied with personal feelings of fear, guilt, grief, anxiety) to the client's change/crisis or situational disability
- ◆ Significant person's attempt to support are ineffective
- ◆ Significant person displays protective behavior disproportionate (too little or too much) to the client's ability or autonomy
- ◆ Significant person may state inability to "go on" or physical exhaustion
- ◆ Usual coping alternatives are exhausted in view of new crisis
- ◆ Structure of family is unable to make necessary changes to support the elder.

GOALS/OUTCOME CRITERIA

- ◆ Dysfunctional patterns will be identified
- ◆ Resources will be made available for use
- ◆ Problem will be clearly described by the family
- ◆ The impact of the crisis on each person will be described and understood by all family members
- ◆ The autonomy of individual members will be supported
- ◆ Limitations will be recognized
- ◆ Individual personal feelings will be described as related to current crisis.
- ◆ Self-help resources will be made available to the family
- ◆ Alternate coping mechanisms will be suggested
- ◆ New structure of subsystems will be fostered to promote coping and use of group strengths
- ◆ Appropriate referrals will be made.

INTERVENTIONS

- ◆ Family assessment completed in a safe environment for self-disclosure. Time limits and frequency of meetings is announced. (RN)
- ◆ The problem is identified and discussed as seen from individual family members' perspectives.

◆ The impact of the crisis on individuals is explored.

◆ Feelings about the problem are elicited from individual members.

◆ The nurse asks for clarification regarding the current crisis from individual members.

◆ Available strengths, alternatives to deal with the crisis are elicited and tallied. (RN, LPN)

◆ Using the knowledge regarding the stress of institutionalization:

   a. the nurse explores directly feelings of guilt, abandonment, and exploitation individual members may experience.

   b. continued involvement in the elder's life is modeled as an expectation.

   c. families are taught ways they continue to be needed and useful. The elder is asked to identify these.

   d. The limitations of the family are discussed freely by exploring these directly. Acceptance and acknowledgement of these is fostered (i.e. everyone is asked: "Do you agree grandma can't continue to care for grandpa considering . . . (list difficulties)."

◆ All family members are treated openly at all times and opinions encouraged (autonomy fostered).

◆ Prior experiences requiring mutual support are reminisced to foster mastery and remind the group of coping skills. (RN, LPN)

◆ Nonverbal clues of old conflicts will be addressed and explored.

◆ When crisis, anxiety, continued dysfunction persists, referral to appropriate family expert is made.

◆ Dysfunctional patterns are noted and addressed openly.

◆ Self-help groups are made available as appropriate (see Family Coping: Potential for Growth).

◆ Family members are introduced as appropriate to persons and families with similar experiences.

◆ Provision to support physically and emotionally those persons exhausted by the crisis are explored and a time table for implementation is developed.

◆ Nursing Diagnosis

Ineffective family coping: compromised, as related to role changes or temporary family disorganization (due to stress on individual members of idiosyncratic stress, i.e. the death of a family member).

DEFINING CHARACTERISTICS

◆ Client expresses concern about significant other's response to crisis.

◆ Significant person dwells on the personal impact (guilt, anxiety, grief, fear) the crisis has.

◆ Client or significant person asks for help.

◆ Significant person's attempts to be supportive are ineffective

◆ Significant person withdraws into limited personal communication with client at time of need

◆ Significant person displays protective behaviors disproportionate to the client's abilities

◆ Family members do not allow time for assimilation of the impact of the change

◆ Previously filled responsibilities are not performed by anyone in the family

◆ Old structural subsystems are ineffective to deal with the crisis

◆ Family members acknowledge a lack of a certain role being filled due to the change.

GOALS/OUTCOME CRITERIA

◆ The problem will be clarified

◆ The impact on individual members will be discussed

◆ Resources will be identified

◆ Family will recognize blocks to using resources

◆ Feelings related to the crisis will be talked about by the family

◆ Alternate coping/problem-solving will be discussed

◆ Individual autonomy is fostered

◆ The behaviors of the absent "role" are identified

◆ Responsibilities will be redistributed

◆ Family members will support those needing time to accept the change

◆ More effective subsystems will be developed

◆ Plans for continued meetings confirmed

◆ Appropriate referrals, as necessary.

INTERVENTIONS

◆ Assess the family in a safe environment that promotes self-disclosure. Structure the time length and frequency of meetings. (RN, LPN)

◆ Have individual family members discuss their perceptions of the problem.

◆ Have members describe the feelings and personal impact the crisis has had on them.

◆ Available strengths and resources are elicited.

◆ Descriptions of problems that prevented coping are discussed only to identify blocks to coping. This is not dwelled upon.

◆ Alternate methods to deal with the crisis are explored.

◆ All members are given opportunity to speak and be recognized for their contributions.

◆ The role changes necessitated by the change are explored. Alternate means to fulfill the responsibilities caused by the change should be listed and suggestions to implement these encouraged.

◆ The nurse identifies patterns of subsystems and questions the group regarding their continued efficacy.

◆ Alternate supports, and subsystems to promote the use of resources are explored.

◆ Continued blocks to coping, obsession with personal problems, and rigidly developed dysfunctions, all indicate need for referral to family experts.

◆ Self-help groups are made available (see Interventions: Family Coping: Potential for Growth).

INEFFECTIVE FAMILY COPING: DISABLING

Definition: Behavior of significant person disables own capacities and the resident's capacities to effectively address tasks essential to either person's adaptation to the crisis. The coping mechanisms used are harmful to the individuals. Continued deterioration could be expected. Boundaries are diffuse, and serious physical signs and symptoms may be present.

ASSESSMENT

Patterns of coping are detrimental in the face of the new challenges faced by aging. Subsystems undermine any potential useful coping. The actual problem may be unclear or denied. More than one family member may be discounted as a valuable contribution to solving the problems. Individuals may be abandoned. Violence may be present. Numerous physical symptoms are presented by more than one person. Individuals may resort to substance abuse to cope. Coalitions of subsystems may threaten or already have seceded from the family. The elder may serve as the scapegoat in the family, "It's all their fault." Communication is poor. Individuals may monopolize conversation. Some persons may be absent or quiet. (The absent persons may be greatly significant). The environment is one of chaos with high energy or none.

AGE-RELATED PHENOMENON

A family's years of established patterns of structure, communication, and interaction are confronted with the multiple developmental and situational stresses of aging. Unresolved conflicts between elder parent and adult child are inflamed in the face of physical and cognitive changes the elder experiences. The immature adults are forced to face their parent's limitations and the realities of their own aging. Unfulfilled or never established goals hang like shadows around feelings of dissatisfaction with accomplishments. Overly dependent children are confronted with helplessness.

The adult children must begin to accept their own inadequacies due to overly involved parents. A sense of loss or anger can permeate. The parents have their individual losses to accept in unrealized expectations of children or their lives. The culture and rules of these families rarely foster open communication. Guilt, anger, anxiety, hostility, resentment are all feelings that have been lying dormant and can explode freely upon the now failing elder. The absence of individual growth and actualization is evidenced by the inability to deal with the developmental tasks of an individual's aging. Longstanding mixed feelings towards parents or towards children come to light in nonverbal and verbal ways. The problem of potential institutionalization causes feelings of guilt, anger, abandonment on the part of the adult child. Cycles of criticism, hostility recur. These pains will reverberate through the generations of the family. Young children will be drawn into the patterns.

When the elder is institutionalized, the adult child is confronted with the loss of the idealized parent as though dead. This loss, combined with their own death anxiety, can lead to a grief reaction too profound to confront. The adult child is forced to withdraw and indeed abandon the elder. The elder too then deteriorates without the nurturance and support needed to deal with changing physical and cognitive resources.

These two things, filial maturity and institutionalization, can present the greatest strain on the ambivalent relationships in marginally functioning families.

ETIOLOGIES

INTERNAL

◆ Ambivalent relationships (filial immaturity)
◆ Unexpressed guilt, anger, hostility.

EXTERNAL

◆ Institutionalization.

◆ Nursing Diagnosis

Ineffective family coping: disabling, as related to ambivalent family relationships (filial immaturity, absence of individuation).

DEFINING CHARACTERISTICS

◆ Neglect of the elder with regard to basic human needs
◆ Reality distortion, including denial, regarding the client's health problem
◆ Intolerance, rejection, taking on physical signs/symptoms of the client
◆ Family decisions negatively affect economic and social health of the family
◆ Psychosomaticism

◆ Usual routines continue without regard for the client's needs
◆ Agitation, depression, hostility, anxiety, despair, guilt (suicidality).
◆ Neglect of other family members
◆ Elder develops helpless dependence.

GOALS/OUTCOME CRITERIA

◆ Basic human needs will be met for the client
◆ Appropriate local social service agencies are notified in cases of neglect or abuse
◆ Emergency measures implemented to treat profound major depression
◆ Family members receive care, as necessary
◆ The family is allowed to clarify and recognize the impact of the problem
◆ Family communication is enhanced
◆ Appropriate family experts are involved
◆ Appropriate expression of feelings caused by the changes is encouraged
◆ Pathological patterns of interaction are noted and described to the family
◆ Physical health needs are met for all family members.

INTERVENTIONS

◆ Potential emergency situations are identified promptly and appropriate treatment initiated. (RN, LPN)
  a. Suicidality is assessed, appropriate referral is made to mental health agencies.
  b. In cases of neglect or abuse of the elder, the Department of Protective Social Services is notified. The safety of the elder is assured by any means (use of law enforcement may be necessary).
  c. Family members being neglected are referred for treatment to appropriate local agencies.
  d. Referral to appropriate family treatment expert is initiated promptly.
◆ Family assessment is completed.
◆ Patterns of coalition among subsystems are identified by the nurse.
◆ Family members are provided autonomy by eliciting individual perceptions of the crisis.
◆ The impact on individual family members is discussed.
◆ Communication in clear terms, acceptance of all members is encouraged and modeled.

◆ Ambivalent feelings are elicited when present. Common feelings among family members are looked for and expected.

◆ Safety for self-disclosure is paramount for a severely disabled family. An environment of nurturance and support is fostered.

◆ Long-standing symptoms of depression in the elder or other family members indicate the need for expert intervention. (RN, LPN)

◆ Competency of the family to deal with the changes necessitated by the aged members is fostered by instilling hope and expressing unconditional acceptance of fears and concerns.

◆ Social service agencies will be mobilized as needed to deal with potentially deleterious financial decisions the impaired family has made.

◆ Families with diffuse boundaries, or rigid subsystems, evidencing strong psychosomatic symptoms, require expert intervention.

◆ Nursing Diagnosis

Ineffective family coping: disabling, related to unexpressed guilt, hostility, despair (potential in institutionalization).

DEFINING CHARACTERISTICS

◆ Abandonment or desertion of the elder

◆ Intolerance of the elder

◆ Rejection of the elder

◆ Neglect of the resident's basic needs

◆ Agitation, depression, aggression, hostility, despair, guilt (projection of anger)

◆ Impaired restructuring of life, lack of individuation, prolonged overconcern of resident

◆ Resident develops helpless dependence

◆ Reality is distorted regarding nature and severity of health crisis

◆ Other family members may be neglected.

GOALS/OUTCOME CRITERIA

◆ Basic human needs will be met

◆ Appropriate local social service agencies are notified in cases of neglect or abuse

◆ Emergency measures to treat depression (suicidality) are implemented

◆ Other family members receive needed care

◆ Feelings regarding guilt are expressed

◆ Family participation is encouraged to continue

◆ The need for continued mutual support is identified

♦ Autonomy and competence of individuals is fostered
♦ Pathological patterns of reaction to stress are noted and presented to the family
♦ Necessary support from self-help groups is elicited
♦ Referrals for family treatment are completed.

INTERVENTIONS

♦ Appropriate emergency measures initiated (see Ineffective Family Coping: Disabling, related to ambivalent relationships). (RN)
♦ Family assessment is completed. Safety for self-disclosure is paramount for severely disabled families. An environment of nurturance and support is fostered. (RN)
♦ Patterns of communication and structure are identified and presented to the family for reflection, as appropriate. (RN)
♦ All family members are allowed time to identify their perception of the problem. (RN, LPN)
♦ Guilt is actively explored (especially regarding institutionalization) and resolved through mutual support of all members.
♦ Problem-solving is achieved by recognition of available individual strengths and coping mechanisms.
♦ Clear communication, acceptance of all persons is modeled by the nurse.
♦ Anger, hostility, aggression are recognized and appropriately directed. The process is identifed.
♦ Self-help group resources are mobilized (see Potential for Growth: Family Coping).
♦ Referral to family experts is indicated in cases of depression, persistent dysfunctional structures and communication or harm to an individual.

References

Benner, P. *The Privacy of Caring: Stress and Coping in Health and Illness.* Menlo Park: Addison Wesley; 1989.

Burggrof, V. *Nursing the Elderly: A Care Plan Approach.* Philadelphia: Lippincott; 1989.

Burnside, IM. *Nursing and the Aged.* New York: McGraw Hill; 1976.

Butler, R and Lewis, M. *Aging and Mental Health: Positive Psychosocial and Biomedical Approaches.* 3rd Edition. St. Louis: Mosby; 1982.

Carpenito, LJ. *Nursing Diagnosis: Application to Clinical Practice.* Philadelphia: Lippincott; 1992.

Dreher, B. *Communication Skills for Working with Elders.* New York: Springer Publishing; 1987.

Gorman, L, Sultan, D, and Luna-Raines, M. *Psychosocial Nursing: Handbook for the Nonpsychiatric Nurse.* Baltimore: Williams & Wilkins; 1989.

Hallal, JC. Nursing diagnosis: An essential step to quality care. In *Journal of Gerontological Nursing.* 1985; 11:35–40.

Hays, A and Borger, F. A test in time. In *American Journal of Nursing.* 1985; 85:1107–1111.

Hogarth, CR. Families and family therapy. In BS Johnson (ed.) *Psychiatric Mental Health Nursing.* 2nd ed. 1989; 222–248.

Lieberman, MA. Adaptive processes in late life. In N Datan and L Ginsberg (Eds.) *Life Span Developmental Psychology: Normative Life Crisis.* New York: Academic Press; 1975; 132–139.

Love, C. Applying the nursing process with the elderly. In H. Wilson and C. Kneisl (eds.) *Psychiatric Nursing.* 3rd ed. Menlo Park: Addison Wesley; 1989.

Maas, HS and Kuypers, JS. *From Thirty to Seventy.* San Francisco: Jossey-Bass; 1974.

Minuchin, S. *Families and Family Therapy.* Cambridge: Harvard University Press; 1974.

National Institutes of Health. *A guide to medical self-care and self-help groups for the elderly.* (Pub. No. NIH 80-1687) Washington, DC; 1979.

Osgood, N. *Suicide in the Elderly.* Rockville, MD: Aspen Systems; 1985.

Pelletier, L. *Psychiatric Nursing: Case studies, diagnoses and care plans.* Springhouse, Pa: Springhouse; 1987.

Rogers-Seidl, F. *Geriatric Nursing Care Plans.* St.Louis: Mosby-Year Book; 1991.

Sedgwick, R. *Family Mental Health: Theory and Practice.* St. Louis: Mosby; 1980.

Shanas, E. Older people and their families: The new pioneers. In *Journal of Marriage and the Family.* 1980; 42.

Siegler, I. The psychology of adult development and aging. In E Buose and D Blazer (Eds.) *Handbook of Geriatric Psychiatry.* New York: Von Nostrand Reinhold; 1980.

Sussman, MB. Relationships of adult children with their parents in the U.S. In E Shanas and GF Strieb (Eds.) *Social Structure and the Family: Generational Relationships.* Englewood Cliffs, NJ: Prentice-Hall; 1965.

Teasdale, G and Jennett, B. Assessment of coma and impaired consciousness: A practical scale. In *Lancet.* 1974; 7:81–84.

Van Servellen, G. *Group and Family Therapy: A Model for Psychotherapeutic Nursing Practice.* St. Louis: Mosby; 1984.

Value-Belief Pattern

Verna Carson

◆

VALUE-BELIEF PATTERN

The choices and decisions made throughout a lifetime are guided by the values, goals, and beliefs of an individual. These choices reflect what the individual perceives as important in life. Conflict with established values and beliefs can impact on health.

The older individual reviews values, beliefs, and the decisions and choices that were made in a major psychological and spiritual developmental task. Successful completion of this task results in wisdom and a sense of wholeness. Failure to complete this task results in a sense of despair regarding the value of one's life. This process may involve reminiscing about the past in an effort to accept it, forgive it, and relive it, so as to create a new order in the present.

Another interpretation regarding the importance of spiritual beliefs to the elder is the identification of spiritual behaviors, such as prayer and looking for the "silver lining," as a major source of coping. The nurse can be instrumental both in helping the elder to complete the task of reviewing values and beliefs and also to identify and use spiritual beliefs and activities to cope with stress.

The following section describes the importance of spirituality; situations that result in spiritual distress; and interventions to eliminate or alleviate this distress in elder populations.

SPIRITUAL DISTRESS (DISTRESS OF THE HUMAN SPIRIT)

> *Definition:* The individual questions the meaning of life and the values and beliefs that have guided decisions and choices. Inability to recognize the transcendent values attached to living and relationships leaves the individual feeling empty.

Because spirituality is at the core of an individual's being, the sense of meaninglessness may be manifested in both physical and emotional behaviors and could easily be misinterpreted. The individual feels cut off from God (however God is perceived), from other individuals, and from meaningful activity. There is a sense of futility and detachment that emanates from the person. Expressions of despair, related to present circumstances, but more importantly to a life which seems without value, are common.

The elder experiencing spiritual distress contradicts the meaning in Robert Browning's poem which states:

"Grow old along with me, the best is yet to be,
The last of life, for which the first was made.
Our times are in His hands."

The elder does not believe that the last of life is the best time of all. The elder may only focus on the physical and social losses that accompany aging.

This perspective, so unlike Browning's, fails to recognize that there are gains that come from aging. These gains are primarily spiritual ones that deepen the enjoyment of the later years. Old age is the most satisfactory period for religious activity. There is a strong correlation between conventional religious beliefs and activities and life satisfaction, morale, happiness, and wholesome adaptations to the total sociocultural milieu.

As the demands of life slip away, individuals are left with time to enjoy the fruits of life's labors and to reflect on the beauty of small things so often overlooked in the frantic activity of youth. The spiritually healthy person is able to substitute alternative activities if former ones are no longer possible. The jogger may learn to stroll; the traveler may learn to enjoy reading. The individual learns to slow the pace of life to derive from doing and accomplishing to enjoying and being. There is time to pursue relationships just because they are a source of joy, pleasure, and appreciation of life. Although disengagement may occur from nearly everything else in the late years of life, those who reach them with spiritual health find that spiritual well-being is not dependent upon physical and material circumstances. The inability of the elder to shift to a spiritual focus may leave the individual clinging to an idealized youth and feeling bitter, negative, and overdependent.

Even though formally organized religious participation decreases, the religious beliefs, feelings, and personalized ritualistic practices, like prayer and spiritual readings, become more intense for the religious elder.

The spiritual focus that characterizes the endeavors of aging is present in whatever setting elders find themselves—their own homes, the homes of family members, senior apartments, or institutional settings. The accomplishment of the spiritual task of aging can be helped or hindered by the environment. The environment must allow for enough solitude to encourage reflection, but not so much that the individual feels isolated. There should be enough opportunity for activity and interaction that the individual still feels there is purpose in living, but not so much activity that the individual is tired and overstimulated.

A poem written by Father Joseph Breighner (1988) and appearing in *The Catholic Review* aptly reflects the spiritual focus of the elderly.

I wish you could have known me then
Full of life and strong.

I wish you could have known me when
I wasn't sick so long.

I've turned a few heads in my day,
I've dazzled them with charm.
I've helped some people on my way
And protected them from harm.

I have been someone's relative
I've tasted family life.
I didn't want a sedative
Or need a surgeon's knife.

I've lived out life's familiar rhymes
I've watched as new life grew.
I didn't need these pills those times
Nor have viruses and flu.

I've built ideas in people's minds,
And I've repaired the old.
I missed diseases of all kinds,
And rarely caught a cold.

Yes, I lived a life of hope,
Of laughter and of tears.
But sickness makes it hard to cope
With a past that no one hears.

Oh, I wish you could know all I was
Those things that fill my dreams.
So please treat me with respect because
My life's more than what it seems.

ASSESSMENT

Assessment of spirituality is a challenge because many of the behaviors that indicate spiritual distress could also indicate an emotional or physical problem. First, the nurse must observe the individual's nonverbal behavior and affect. The person may be displaying signs of sadness, anger, agitation, or anxiety. These behaviors might reflect a spiritual concern that was being expressed through emotional channels. Does the individual pray or read religious material? Does the individual have the physical capability to pray and read religious material, if he or she so desired?

The content of the elder's statements also provides insights about feelings and needs. For instance, does the elder complain excessively in relation to the severity of present disabilities? Does the elder state that sleeping is difficult? Are repeated requests made for pain medication or sedation? These behaviors may indicate a physical need, but they may also provide clues that the individual is experiencing spiritual distress. It is important to note whether the elder talks about a God and in what manner. Sometimes the presence of a deep spiritual need is revealed through joking or lighthearted reference to the "man upstairs." Does the elder mention specific religious issues such as faith, hope, forgiveness, or prayer? Does the topic of church-related functions enter the conversation?

A third area for the nurse to observe is the quantity, and more importantly, the quality of interpersonal relationships in which the elder is involved. Does the individual have visitors or are visiting hours spent alone? What effect do the visitors have on the elder? Do the visits leave the individual feeling happy and relaxed or agitated and emotionally upset? Do visitors come from the elder's place of worship? Does the individual interact with the staff and other residents? Does the individual receive telephone calls? If these observations lead the nurse to conclude that the elder does not have a supportive system with which to interact, and people with whom love and concern is communicated, then the elder may also be experiencing a similar estrangement from faith or God. After all, much of one's knowledge of God's love is from the quality of love that is exchanged with significant others.

The fourth area that the nurse is concerned with is the environment of the elder. The presence of a Bible, Book of Mormon, Torah, or other religious reading material might indicate that religious matters are important. Other things for the nurse to observe would be whether the individual wears religious medals, pins, or articles of clothing or possesses religious statues, pictures, or other such items.

An adequate assessment also involves interviewing the individual. At present, most nursing histories merely identify the elder's religious affiliation and do not elicit specific spiritual needs. These needs can be ascertained through the use of specific questions geared to five areas of spiritual concern:

◆ the individual's source of strength and hope
◆ the importance of specific religious practices to the individual
◆ the individual's personal concept of God
◆ the individual's perception of a relationship between personal spiritual beliefs and health
◆ the individual's thoughts about what gives life meaning.

The nurse needs to be aware that spiritual matters are often a difficult area for individuals to discuss. The best approach avoids asking numerous questions, one after another, but rather questions are used to respond to verbal and nonverbal clues that indicate the presence of a spiritual need. In addition, it is important for the nurse who is undertaking a spiritual assessment to approach the elder with acceptance, a gentle manner, and a sensitivity to timing and to the elder's feelings. Generally, questions related to psychosocial and spiritual issues are left until the end of the interview when the elder and the nurse are feeling more at ease with each other. It is also helpful for the nurse to share with the elder the rationale for seeking information about spirituality. The elder should know that this information increases the nurse's knowledge about the elder's sources of strength and allows the nurse to plan care more effectively.

AGE-RELATED PHENOMENON

Although the review of life events and the reflection of life's meaning are the spiritual and psychological tasks of the elderly, many of the life events that occur between 65 and 75 years of age have the potential for causing spiritual distress as well as spiritual well-being. For instance, retirement can cause a spiritual crisis if the elder is unable to find meaning in life outside of an occupation. Other events that have this same dual potential include the last child leaving home, widowhood, relocation, and illnesses requiring hospitalization. Each of these events must be evaluated and a meaning attributed to them. The ability to successfully do so depends on the elder's perception of the event and past ability to deal with stress.

Catastrophic illness of self or a loved one may challenge the fiber of deeply held beliefs and values. A woman who watches her spouse slowly deteriorate from Alzheimer's may question her own beliefs about the sanctity of marriage as she considers the possibility of divorce to preserve some jointly held assets. An individual may question the character of a God who permits intense suffering without relief. An elderly daughter may wonder about the value of the life of her mother, who is comatose in a nursing home. These situations cause a person to reflect intensely about beliefs that perhaps at an earlier point in life seemed unquestionable.

Another source of spiritual distress arises from the inability to practice religious rites and rituals that once provided solace and meaning. This separation from what was once so familiar and comfortable produces feelings of anxiety, guilt, sadness, grief, and a sense of loss. Separation can result from a decrease in mobility that interferes with the elder's ability to go to a place of worship, or it can result from confinement to an institution for continuous care. A feeling of separation can be related to lack of privacy in the setting in which the elder resides. This lack of privacy prohibits spontaneous personal expressions of religious feeling.

Coping with events that threaten the spiritual integrity of the elder depends greatly on how they responded spiritually to crises that have gone before. If they have consistently been able to find meaning in stress, then those skills will be helpful in present life circumstances. If they have struggled to integrate past crises into a meaningful view of life, then new crises will only intensify that struggle. Successful coping has been demonstrated with the changes of aging and strong religious faith. Nurses can assist the elderly in this process by recognizing the need to discuss life events in terms of the deeper meaning that an elder ascribes to them, by recognizing the importance of a life review to the elder in coming to terms with the life that is past, in recognizing the importance of maintaining religious rites and rituals regardless of the setting in which the elder resides, and in facilitating this religious participation.

ETIOLOGIES

ENVIRONMENTAL (EXTRINSIC)

◆ Situational crises: Institutionalization, loss of colleagues, relocation, closing the family home, economic changes, isolation.

◆ Maturational crises: Retirement, last child leaving home, role changes, response of others to aging

◆ Personal vulnerability: Decreased social contacts

◆ Perceived loss of control/belief in self: Cultural conditions may enforce sense of uselessness, meaninglessness; decisions made about them without their being included; may feel left out of church-related programs that focus on youth.

INTERNAL (INTRINSIC)

◆ Situational crises: Illness requiring widowhood, hospitalization

◆ Maturational crises: Self-concept/ideal as affected by aging; physical and cognitive changes of aging, i.e., sensory decrease, mobility decrease; declined level of wellness; less resistance to illness

◆ Personal vulnerability: Unable to get to a place of worship

◆ Perceived loss of control/belief in self: Self-ideal affected rapid changes—"life isn't as expected"; self-image affected by changes due to age; independence prevented by physical changes; leads to questions of self-worth; or life satisfaction

◆ Knowledge Deficit: Hospitalization may provide certain religious dispensations regarding dietary laws and other rituals.

◆ Nursing Diagnosis

Spiritual distress due to situational crisis: institutionalization, widowhood, loss of colleagues, loss of friends, relocation of home, economic changes, isolation.

DEFINING CHARACTERISTICS

1. Verbalizes that life has no meaning without spouse, friend, etc.
2. Anxiety, anger, sadness, depression.
3. Shows little energy to participate in any activity.
4. May verbalize anger at God for allowing loss to occur.
5. May express feelings of abandonment by God.
6. Unable to participate in usual religious activities.
7. Change in societal participation.
8. Inability to meet role expectations.
9. Gastrointestinal changes (bowel, appetite disturbance).
10. Altered sleep patterns (difficulty falling asleep, staying asleep, and having nightmares).

GOALS/OUTCOME CRITERIA

1. Verbalizes that situational crisis had meaning within the broader context of life.

2. Able to express and work through feelings of anger, sadness, and loss.
3. Energy levels increase so that participation in daily activities is possible.
4. Expresses feelings toward God and is able to resolve these feelings.
5. Able to resume religious practices.
6. Individual seems less preoccupied with loss and begins to enjoy life.
7. Able to perform expectations (i.e. homemaker, gardening)
8. Subjectively GI symptoms are resolved
9. Reports that sleep is more restful and refreshing.

INTERVENTIONS

1. Encourage talking about the recent change in a nondirective manner. This can be done individually or in a group setting (RN, LPN, NA).
2. While sitting with the individual, ask what this event has meant. Ask the person how they will cope with this situation; how they have coped in the past? What do they see as their future? Their hope? Ask what you can do to help. Communicate that you believe the elder is a person of value. (RN, LPN)
3. Encourage ventilation of feelings of anger, sadness, depression. Let the individual know that these feelings are a normal response to loss and can result in a sense of spiritual malaise. (RN, LPN)
4. Assess spiritual issues using the suggestions given in the assessment section. (RN, LPN)
5. Encourage the individual to use past coping responses to deal with present situation. Suggest other strategies. These could include prayer, religious reading, viewing religious programs on television, listening to religious broadcasts on radio, talking to clergy, talking with the nurse, participating in religious services, journaling (writing about the individual's perception of the situation), and reminiscing in a group setting with other elders. (RN, LPN)

◆ Nursing Diagnosis

Spiritual distress due to maturational crisis (retirement, oldest child leaving home, role changes, response of others to aging).

DEFINING CHARACTERISTICS

1. Verbalized doubt about ability to cope with new role.
2. Speaks disparagingly about personal aging process.
3. Verbalizes a sense of uselessness.
4. States concerns that others will find individual a burden.
5. See Defining Characteristics #2–10 for Spiritual Distress: Situational Crisis.

GOALS/OUTCOME CRITERIA

1. Verbalizes ways to cope with role changes.
2. Verbalizes positive remarks about present life stage.
3. Able to verbalize that usefulness is not a by-product of what the individual produces but rather a reflection of the individual's being.
4. See goals #2–9 for Spiritual Distress: Situational Crisis

INTERVENTIONS

1. Identifies alternative activities to replace those that are no longer appropriate due to role change. These could include volunteer work, taking up a new hobby, resuming a once discarded hobby, joining a senior center, etc. See nursing interventions #1–8, Spiritual Distress: Situational Crisis. (RN, LPN)
2. Offer to contact a clergy person. (RN, LPN, NA)
3. Suggest the use of music and/or literature to assist the individual to experience spiritual peace. (RN, LPN, NA)
4. Encourage individual to eat a balanced diet and to get adequate exercise. (All Staff)

◆ Nursing Diagnosis

Spiritual distress due to personal vulnerability (decreased social contacts, unable to get to place of worship).

DEFINING CHARACTERISTICS

1. Verbalizes that isolation is a problem.
2. Verbalizes guilt regarding inability to get to place of worship.
3. Expresses fear related to feeling alone and unloved.
4. See defining characteristics #3–10 for Spiritual Distress: Situational Crisis.

GOALS/OUTCOME CRITERIA

1. Identify ways to decrease time spent alone.
2. Identify alternative ways to worship God.
3. Devise a system that will promote a feeling of security.
4. See goals #2–9 for Spiritual Distress: Situational Crisis.

INTERVENTIONS

1. Provide information on activities for the elderly such as eat togethers, bus trips, senior centers that provide social activities and other services designed to increase social interaction. (RN, LPN, SW, Activity Director)

2. Obtain information on services for the elderly that provide transportation to the activities mentioned in goal #1. (RN, LPN, NA, SW, Activity Director)

3. Explore the use of private prayer, religious reading, viewing televised religious services, and listening to religious radio broadcasts and music, and journaling. (RN, LPN)

4. Explore the possibility of having a person visit from the elder's church. (RN, LPN, SW, Family)

5. Identify a support system and a mechanism to provide a sense of security to the elder. It could consist of a family member, neighbor, or church member, as well as a home health-care provider who agrees to visit or call the elder on a regular basis. (RN, LPN, SW)

6. See interventions #1–8 for Spiritual Distress: Situational Crisis.

◆ Nursing Diagnosis

Spiritual distress due to perceived loss of control/belief in self (cultural conditions may enforce sense of uselessness, meaninglessness, self-image affected by changes due to age, etc.)

DEFINING CHARACTERISTICS

See first two sections of Spiritual Distress.

GOALS

See goals for first two sections of Spiritual Distress.

INTERVENTIONS

See interventions for first two sections of Spiritual Distress. (RN, LPN)

◆ Nursing Diagnosis

Spiritual distress due to knowledge deficit (some religions provide dispensations for the elderly from participation in religious activities and rituals).

DEFINING CHARACTERISTICS

1. Verbalizes guilt regarding inability to participate in prescribed religious activities, such as fasting and worship services.

2. Expresses fear of Divine retribution.

GOALS/OUTCOME CRITERIA

1. States realistic expectations for own participation in religious activities.

2. Able to accept own limitations regarding participation in religious activities.

3. Able to identify alternative religious activities that are appropriate for present health status.
4. Verbalizes value in personal expressions of religiosity.

INTERVENTIONS

1. Encourage discussion of feelings and concerns regarding change in participation in formal religious activities. (RN, LPN, SW)
2. Encourage discussion with church representative regarding the church's position about participation of the elderly in religious activities. (RN, LPN, SW)
3. Explore the use of private prayer, religious reading, viewing televised religious services, and listening to religious radio broadcasts, and journaling. (RN, LPN)

References

Beard, BB. Religion at 100. In *Modern Maturity.* 1969; 12:1–4.

Breighner, J. Can you name the patron saint for the elderly? In *The Catholic Review.* 1988; 53:7.

Bromley, DB. *The Psychology of Human Aging.* Baltimore: Penguin Books; 1966.

Brooke, V. The spiritual well-being of the elderly. In *Geriatric Nursing.* 1987; 8:194–195.

Carson, VB. Spirituality and the nursing process. In VB Carson (Ed.). *Spiritual Dimensions of Nursing Practice.* Philadelphia: W.B. Saunders & Co. (in press).

Goleman, D. Now in their 80's, Eriksons develop fresh insights into the psychology of aging. In *The Baltimore Sun.* June 19, 1988; 5.

Groeschel, BJ. *Spiritual Passages: The Psychology of Spiritual Development.* New York: Crossroad; 1987.

Jourard, S. *The Transparent Self.* Princeton: Van Nostrand; 1964.

Manfredi, C and Pickett, M. Perceived stressful situations and coping strategies utilized by the elderly. In *Journal of Community Healthy Nursing.* 1987; 4:99–110.

Moberg, DO. Religiosity in old age. In *Gerontologist,* 1965; 5:78–87.

Moberg, DO. Spiritual well-being in later life. In JA Thorson & Cook, TC (Eds.), *Spiritual Well-Being of the Elderly.* Springfield, Illinois: Charles C. Thomas Publisher; 1980.

Moberg, DO and Taves, MJ. Church participation and adjustment in old age. In AM Rose and WA Peterson (Eds.), *Older People and Their Social World.* Philadelphia: F.A. Davis Co. 1965; 113–124.

Stallwood, J and Stoll, R. Spiritual dimension of nursing practice. In IL Beland and JY Passos (Eds.), *Clinical Nursing.* 3rd edition. New York: Macmillan Publishing Company; 1975; 1088.

Stoll, R. Guidelines for spiritual assessment. In *American Journal of Nursing.* 1979; 79:1574–1577.

Index

Note : Page numbers followed by t refer to tables.